The recognition and management

The treatment of early psychosis has been bedevilled by an entrenched pessimism, stemming from the asylum era and the Kraepelinian model of schizophrenia. More recently, however, there has been a surge of interest in preventively oriented treatment of patients showing the first signs of psychotic illness, with the realization that these illnesses are frequently highly responsive to early treatment, as well as a corresponding recognition of the suffering and lost opportunities resulting from untreated or partially treated psychosis in young people.

This is the first text to focus on the potential of early detection of psychosis, and the practicalities of treatment during the intensive critical phase, drawing on advances in biological and psychosocial treatment, and reforms in service delivery. Based on the pioneering experience and research of a now well-established prevention and intervention centre, and with contributions from international authorities, the book outlines a framework for intervention, reviews the evidence available to guide clinical practice, and describes models of treatment and intervention.

Providing a solid foundation for future developments, this is an up-to-date handbook for clinicians of optimal practice in this burgeoning area of psychiatry. Incorporating many personal narratives and case histories, it is strong on theory, sensitive on practical issues, and will challenge, inform and guide clinicians seeking to provide optimal care for younger patients with early psychosis.

Patrick D. McGorry is Professor of Psychiatry at the University of Melbourne and Director of the Youth Program of a new service for children and young people covering a catchment area of one million people.

Henry J. Jackson is Associate Professor of Psychology and Convenor of the Postgraduate Clinical Psychology Program at the University of Melbourne.

The recognition and management of early psychosis

A preventive approach

Edited by
PATRICK D. MCGORRY
and
HENRY J. JACKSON
University of Melbourne

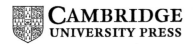
CAMBRIDGE
UNIVERSITY PRESS

PUBLISHED BY THE PRESS SYNDICATE OF THE UNIVERSITY OF CAMBRIDGE
The Pitt Building, Trumpington Street, Cambridge, United Kingdom

CAMBRIDGE UNIVERSITY PRESS
The Edinburgh Building, Cambridge CB2 2RU, UK http://www.cup.cam.ac.uk
40 West 20th Street, New York, NY 10011-4211, USA http://www.cup.org
10 Stamford Road, Oakleigh, Melbourne 3166, Australia

© Cambridge University Press 1999

This book is in copyright. Subject to statutory exception
and to the provisions of relevant collective licensing agreements,
no reproduction of any part may take place without
the written permission of Cambridge University Press.

First published 1999

Typeset in Palatino and Frutiger [VN]

A catalogue record for this book is available from the British Library

ISBN 0 521 55383 0 hardback

Transferred to digital printing 2004

Every effort has been made in preparing this book to provide accurate and up-to-date information which is in accord with accepted standards and practice at the time of publication. Nevertheless, the authors, editors and publisher can make no warranties that the information contained herein is totally free from error, not least because clinical standards are constantly changing through research and regulation. The authors, editors and publisher therefore disclaim all liability for direct or consequential damages resulting from the use of material contained in this book. Readers are strongly advised to pay careful attention to information provided by the manufacturer of any drugs or equipment that they plan to use.

This book is dedicated to our parents
Desmond and Margaret McGorry and
Henry George and Elizabeth Jackson

Contents

List of contributors	ix
Foreword by CARLO PERRIS	xiii
Preface	xvii
Acknowledgments	xxvii

Part I. Introduction

1. 'A stitch in time'... The scope for preventive strategies in early psychosis. PATRICK D. MCGORRY — 3

Part II. Onset and detection of psychosis

2. The onset of psychotic disorder: clinical and research aspects. ALISON R. YUNG AND HENRY J. JACKSON — 27
3. Pathways to care in early psychosis: clinical and consumer perspectives. CLARE LINCOLN AND PATRICK D. MCGORRY — 51
4. Promoting access to care in early psychosis. ALISON R. YUNG, LISA J. PHILLIPS AND LORELLE T. DREW — 81
5. Studies of biological variables in first-episode schizophrenia: a comprehensive review. ANJAN CHATTERJEE AND JEFFREY A. LIEBERMAN — 115

Part III. Assessment and clinical management of early psychosis

6. Initial assessment of first-episode psychosis. PADDY POWER AND PATRICK D. MCGORRY — 155
7. Initial treatment of first-episode psychosis. JAYASHRI KULKARNI AND PADDY POWER — 184
8. Home-based treatment of first-episode psychosis. JAYASHRI KULKARNI — 206
9. Early intervention in psychosis: the critical period. MAX BIRCHWOOD — 226

10. Recovery from psychosis: psychological interventions.
HENRY J. JACKSON, JANE EDWARDS, CAROL HULBERT
AND PATRICK D. MCGORRY 265
11. Preventive case management in first-episode psychosis.
JANE EDWARDS, JOHN COCKS AND JAMES BOTT 308
12. Suicide and early psychosis. PADDY POWER 338
13. Early psychosis and substance abuse. DONALD H. LINSZEN
AND MARIE E. LENIOR 363
14. Family intervention in early psychosis. JOHN GLEESON,
HENRY J. JACKSON, HEATHER STAVELY AND
PETER BURNETT 376
15. The role of day programmes in recovery in early
psychosis. SHONA M. FRANCEY 407

Part IV. Conclusion
16. Sharpening the focus: early intervention in the real
world. PATRICK D. MCGORRY, JANE EDWARDS AND
KERRYN PENNELL 441

Appendix 1. A consensus statement on strategies for
prevention in early psychosis 471

Appendix 2. International Early Psychosis Association 475

Index 477

Contributors

MAX BIRCHWOOD
Northern Birmingham Mental Health NHS Trust
Archer Centre
All Saints Hospital
Lodge Road
Winson Green
Birmingham B18 5SD
UK

JAMES BOTT
Early Psychosis Prevention and Intervention Centre
Parkville Centre
35 Poplar Road
Parkville, 3052 Victoria
Australia

PETER BURNETT
Early Psychosis Prevention and Intervention Centre
Parkville Centre
35 Poplar Road
Parkville, 3052 Victoria
Australia

ANJAN CHATTERJEE
Department of Psychiatry
Medical School, Wing B, CB 7160
University of North Carolina
School of Medicine
Chapel Hill, NC 27599–7160
USA

JOHN COCKS
Early Psychosis Prevention and Intervention Centre
Parkville Centre
35 Poplar Road
Parkville, 3052 Victoria
Australia

LORELLE T. DREW
Early Psychosis Prevention and Intervention Centre
Parkville Centre
35 Poplar Road
Parkville, 3052 Victoria
Australia

JANE EDWARDS
Early Psychosis Prevention and Intervention Centre
Parkville Centre
35 Poplar Road
Parkville, 3052 Victoria
Australia

CONTRIBUTORS

SHONA M. FRANCEY
Early Psychosis Prevention and
Intervention Centre
Parkville Centre
35 Poplar Road
Parkville, 3052 Victoria
Australia

JOHN GLEESON
Early Psychosis Prevention and
Intervention Centre
Parkville Centre
35 Poplar Road
Parkville, 3052 Victoria
Australia

CAROL HULBERT
NEMPS (Larundel)
Plenty Road
Bundoora, 3083 Victoria
Australia

HENRY J. JACKSON
Department of Psychology
University of Melbourne
Parkville, 3052 Victoria
Australia

JAYASHRI KULKARNI
Department of Psychiatry
Dandenong Psychiatric Hospital
134 Cleeland Street
Dandenong, 3175 Victoria
Australia

MARIE E. LENIOR
Department of Psychiatry
University of Amsterdam
PO Box 22700
1100 DE Amsterdam
The Netherlands

JEFFREY A. LIEBERMAN
Department of Psychiatry
Medical School, Wing B, CB 7160
University of North Carolina
School of Medicine
Chapel Hill, NC 27599–7160
USA

CLARE LINCOLN
Early Psychosis Prevention and
Intervention Centre
Parkville Centre
35 Poplar Road
Parkville, 3052 Victoria
Australia

DONALD H. LINSZEN
Department of Psychiatry
University of Amsterdam
PO Box 22700
1100 DE Amsterdam
The Netherlands

PATRICK D. MCGORRY
Early Psychosis Prevention and
Intervention Centre
Parkville Centre
Locked Bag 10
Parkville, 3052 Victoria
Australia

KERRYN PENNELL
Early Psychosis Prevention and
Intervention Centre
Parkville Centre
35 Poplar Road
Parkville, 3052 Victoria
Australia

CONTRIBUTORS

LISA J. PHILLIPS
Early Psychosis Prevention and
Intervention Centre
Parkville Centre
35 Poplar Road
Parkville, 3052 Victoria
Australia

PADDY POWER
Early Psychosis Prevention and
Intervention Centre
Parkville Centre
35 Poplar Road
Parkville, 3052 Victoria
Australia

HEATHER STAVELY
Early Psychosis Prevention and
Intervention Centre
Parkville Centre
35 Poplar Road
Parkville, 3052 Victoria
Australia

ALISON R. YUNG
Early Psychosis Prevention and
Intervention Centre
Parkville Centre
35 Poplar Road
Parkville, 3052 Victoria
Australia

Foreword

This book gives a thorough presentation of the work that Professors McGorry and Jackson and their colleagues, notably Dr. Jane Edwards, have been carrying out for several years in Melbourne and represents the first really comprehensive treatise of targeted interventions for young individuals at risk of developing a long-term psychotic condition. Nearly five years ago I was fortunate enough to be able to pay a visit to the unit led by Professor McGorry and was impressed by the pioneer work that he and his group were implementing. Now, a few years later, I feel privileged to have the opportunity of introducing the present volume that brings a valuable and so far neglected perspective to understanding and helping in a phase of their life that could be the beginning of a long, painful and disruptive career as a psychiatric patient.

For a long time, looking back at the practice of psychiatry, I have been struck by the tenacious adherence to traditional conceptions of the mental illnesses and their treatment that still dominate in our specialty. Not even the dramatic changes which have occurred in the administration of psychiatric care during the last few decades seem to have exerted any radical impact on the way in which the *major* disorders are approached. Treatment has been split into distinct psychosocial or somatic therapy approaches, and these have not taken account of the uniqueness of each patient with their special needs. Furthermore, there are relatively few centres of excellence where patients can be seen with high levels of competence and sufficient frequency.

Even though a large body of evidence has been available for a long time concerning the possible negative long-term effects of a delay in appropriate intervention, thoroughly reviewed in Chapter 3, and despite an awareness for several decades of the paramount importance of preventive action, everyday practice seems to have consistently been to wait until a manifest psychotic condition has become established before implementing a suitable treatment. For no other condition has such an unduly passive attitude been so dominant until quite recently as for those mental disorders characterized by a psychotic breakdown, among which those of the schizophrenic type represent the most important group. Several factors have contributed to fostering such an attitude, one of the most important being that psychiatrists, by and large, have felt reluctant to move from the familiar settings of hospitals, mental health centres or clinics and, instead, orient their work toward the community. In addition, while the introduction of neuroleptic drugs, as discussed in Chapter 5, has been both good and bad from the perspective of the study and treatment of psychotic illness, it has also helped to create, at least in an earlier era, a naïve optimism about the possiblity of radically changing the subsequent course of already established psychotic syndromes. The neo-Kraepelinian trend that apparently inspires current classification systems and, in particular, their shortcomings in taking into account prodromal manifestations, has also tended to divert attention from the need for early interventions aimed at influencing the course of schizophrenic disorders. Not least, there has been a relative reluctance of politicians and administrators alike toward a radical change of the organization of care. This derives from concern about a possible increase of costs in the short term, paradoxically restraining any enthusiasm for activities which could prove to be less expensive in the long run.

On the other hand, early interventions also have important ethical implications of which the authors of the various chapters are well aware. Undoubtedly, a balance has to be achieved between the appropriateness of an even earlier intervention and the risk of encroaching upon the personal integrity of a young person. The components of the comprehensive programme described in Chapter 4, and later on in Chapter 8, purposefully contribute in suggesting strategies which minimize this risk, and greatly contribute in reducing the risk of stigmatization.

While I cannot comment on all the important material reported in this book, I would like to underscore the deeply humanistic stance that consistently inspires the work of the Melbourne group. Respect for the patient's integrity and uniqueness, flexibility in the choice of the most appropriate strategies of intervention, attention to the necessity of an integrated approach in which family members are involved from the very beginning and due consideration is paid to their grief and trauma, are manifest throughout the volume. What cannot be sensed from a written text is the warm empathic concern for the patients which characterizes all the members of McGorry's group and of which I have personally had an experience at close quarters.

FOREWORD

Finally, the broad scope of the text – which encompasses many models of intervention, all described in a manual-like fashion and richly illustrated clinically, and summarizes most of the available knowledge on preventive strategies and early intervention in psychosis, complemented by its focus on empirical work – makes this volume a landmark contribution. The approaches described and carefully documented in it suggest that psychiatry is entering one of the most exciting phases in its history, and indicates that a paradigm shift may be under way. For such a shift to become a reality, it will be necessary that several centres like that in Melbourne will have to be developed. Fortunately, it seems that this process is now under way in many quarters.

Carlo Perris
November 1998
University of Ureâ, Sweden

Preface

Prevention in psychotic disorders has been a cherished ideal since the early years of this century. However, the seeds of a preventive endeavour were sown in very stony ground, comprising the intrinsic pessimism of the Kraepelinian framework, the serious nature of the disorders involved, and the ineffective and iatrogenic approaches to their treatment, which continue to the present day. The prevailing climate for the germination and growth of these seeds has remained hostile until very recently for a variety of additional reasons, yet there are increasing signs that this may be changing. Partly as a result of the entrenched pessimism associated with schizophrenia in particular, hopes for prevention have rested to an excessive degree on the emergence of effective forms of primary prevention. This, in turn, is dependent upon the clarification of a range of significant causal risk factors for these syndromes – a process which has been frustratingly slow. A key shift in thinking has been the recognition that variants of secondary prevention, notably early intervention and indicated prevention, are not only the 'best bet' at present in schizophrenia and psychosis, but are very likely to prove cost-effective as well as more humane. This, combined with recent advances in psychopharmacology, psychosocial treatment and service delivery, has liberated thinking among clinicians, researchers and health planners, so that a more realistic form of prevention now has the chance to flower. While the ecosystem for this growth is highly variable across the world, we should see increasing elaboration of models and understanding over the next few years. It is an exciting time because there is a real chance of enhanced well-being and quality of life for many people who will develop these distressing, dangerous and potentially disabling disorders. We have a clear responsibility to nurture this process in a careful and scientific manner, so that growth is not only steady but sustainable. We need to tread a middle path between maintaining momentum and progress on the one hand, and over-reaching or over-selling the prospects on the other. The latter is a risk in any area which has been held back or constrained, but the issues are too important to allow any further false dawns. Yet we also need to strive and persevere, because, in our opinion at least, we are finally on firm foundations. Contained within this book is an attempt to lay some of these foundations. Readers will be able to make up their own minds about the solidity or otherwise of this base of knowledge and experience.

Following the introductory Chapter 1 (Part I), the subsequent 15 chapters in the book are contained within Parts II, III and IV. Part II contains four chapters, and is concerned with 'Onset and detection of psychosis'. Part III contains 10 chapters and is concerned with 'Assessment and clinical management of early psychosis', beginning with initial assessment of the first episode and concluding with the role of day programmes in early psychosis. The final stand-alone chapter (Part IV) is concerned with service delivery models and a range of strategies for implementing change.

In the first chapter, entitled '"A stitch in time"... The scope for preventive strategies in early psychosis', Patrick McGorry makes the case for realistic preventive strategies in early psychosis, utilizing a modern, elaborated framework for prevention devised by Mrazek and Haggerty. The concept of early psychosis is described as part of a phase-oriented approach to classifying psychosis. A preventive framework for research and clinical care in the psychotic disorders linked to this classification is proposed. The rationale and evidence supporting a specialized clinical focus upon the early stages of psychotic disorders is established.

Chapter 2 is the first chapter in Part II and is entitled 'The onset of psychotic disorder: clinical and research aspects'. Written by Alison Yung and Henry Jackson, it examines conceptual issues and terminology, defining onset and the concept of prodrome, together with issues involving retrospective description. The authors then examine the phenomenology and duration of the onset phase in psychotic disorders covering early pre-DSM-III and DSM-III descriptions, and 'other alternative' descriptions they have incorporated into their own work. Selected research findings conducted within their own unit are included. These have focused upon the reliability and specificity of the DSM-III-R group of prodromal features in community and clinical samples. The authors then make the case for 'indicated prevention', describing their attempt to prospectively identify the 'prodrome' or 'at-risk state' of a first-ever psychotic episode. They suggest that this potentially could help to prevent, modify or attenuate the onset of 'full-blown' psychosis.

PREFACE

Conceptual issues surrounding other markers and risk factors are discussed, since these will almost certainly be required for more accurate prediction and specific interventions.

In the third chapter of the book, 'Pathways to care in early psychosis: clinical and consumer perspectives', Clare Lincoln and Patrick McGorry tackle the notion of 'delay', focusing first on the pathways to care involved in first-episode psychosis, arguing that there may be scope for reductions in delay for those with schizophrenia. They cite data which suggest that more than one month of untreated psychosis, but less than six months of psychosis, may constitute boundaries of a 'critical period' for detection and initiation of treatment, since beyond this period it seems more difficult to enhance recovery. The consequences of delay are discussed, with cost-reductions, better prognosis, and outcome, all being linked to the reduction of delay. The 'topography of the initial pathway' based on data obtained within their unit is presented, along with four illustrative cases. Under the heading of 'Delay as a paradox', there is discussion of factors affecting delay including illness recognition, help-seeking (emphasizing symptoms and coping), and referral pathways (focusing on diagnosis by mental health professionals and the pathways experience). Specific risk factors for delay are also considered, including stigma, clinical features, gender and inaccessible services. In the discussion, emphasis is given to the twin aims of promoting access to early care and rendering pathways accessible and 'user-friendly'.

Chapter 4, contributed by Alison Yung, Lisa Phillips and Lorelle Drew, is entitled 'Promoting access to care in early psychosis' and focuses on case detection and how it is affected by help-seeking, recognition and referral factors. Engagement of patients in treatment and strategies aimed at facilitating patients' access to care are discussed. This chapter then describes two service models which address some of the barriers to care in early psychosis. The first is an extended hours, mobile assessment team set up purely to seek and attract referrals of young people with a first episode of psychosis. This involves the capacity for rapid response assessments and a significant community and professional education role. A description of the modus operandi of the mobile assessment team is provided, including the intake system, the actual clinical service it provides and its role in community education. Data are provided on the total number of referrals, response time, police involvement, and the effects on duration of untreated psychosis. Illustrative case examples are provided. The second service model is a special clinic for older adolescents and young adults who have developed significant role and relationship difficulties and are believed to be at risk of incipient psychosis (i.e. they may be 'prodromal'). This clinic, known as the Personal Assistance and Crisis Evaluation Clinic, is based at a non-stigmatizing centre for adolescent health adjacent to the campuses of two teaching general hospitals. A description of the clinic is provided along with some preliminary data including total referrals, referral sources, reasons for referral, psychopathology levels, and transition rates to psychosis. A case example of a young person 'at risk' is given.

Part II of the book concludes with Chapter 5 by Anjan Chatterjee and Jeffrey Lieberman entitled: 'Studies of biological variables in first-episode schizophrenia: a comprehensive review'. In recent years, research activity in first-episode psychosis has increased dramatically and has led to an emerging body of knowledge regarding the biology of first-episode psychosis. This chapter provides an overview of the current status of this rapidly expanding field of research, which will be of interest to clinicians and researchers working with this group of patients. The chapter covers neuroimaging (MRI, PET, SPECT, and magnetic resonance spectroscopy) and neurophysiology (EEG and sleep, event-related potential studies, electrodermal) studies in first-episode psychosis. Progress in neuropsychology, neuroendocrinology and neurochemistry is also carefully reviewed. Findings from studies of movement disorder and neurological abnormalities are described, including extrapyramidal signs, circling behaviours and spontaneous dyskinesias. Coverage of immunological and treatment studies completes the chapter. Summaries are provided within each major biological domain, permitting the reader to gain an overview of progress within each.

Part III, which is concerned with 'Assessment and clinical management of early psychosis' begins with Chapter 6 by Paddy Power and Patrick McGorry. In this chapter the authors delineate the 'Initial assessment of first-episode psychosis'. The entry phase is characterized as an avoidable crisis and the clinical landscape of onset is described from the perspective of biopsychosocial assessment. Key issues highlighted are the difficulties in determining the onset of disorder and the lack of clarity and stability in psychotic syndromes. Guidelines are then provided for engaging with the client and family. Emphasis is given to understanding the person and their context, their supports, and the parameters of their illness. Also stressed is the need for a comprehensive clinical assessment, including the taking of a clinical history, mental state examination, and assessments for risk (suicide, neglect and death, violence and victimization by others), and comorbidity. A rationale is provided for a neuroleptic-free assessment period of at least 48 hours. Factors influencing the decision concerning when and how to hospitalize are discussed. A section on biomedical evaluation of first-episode psychosis contains discussion of the physical examination, laboratory investigations, neuropsychological evaluation and social and vocational assessment. The chapter concludes with a discussion of the issues relevant to diagnosis and formulation.

Chapter 7, by Jayashri Kulkarni and Paddy Power, covers misconceptions about 'Initial treatment of first-episode psychosis', and the principles of early treatment are delineated. These include the need for: comprehensive biopsychosocial assessment, identification of the phases of illness, consideration of the location of treatment (hospital or community), the addressing of precipitating events, the use of integrated or multi-modal treatment interventions, and the avoidance or minimization of the potential harmful effects of treatments. Specific biological and psychological treatments for first-episode psychosis are then outlined. The use of very low doses of neuroleptics with slow and careful titration is stressed, and novel antipsychotics are preferred as first-line treatment. The use of adjunctive benzodiazepines, mood stabilizers and antidepressants, is discussed, and the *process* of drug therapy at this phase of illness is also considered. A decision tree for initial drug therapies is provided. Under the rubric of psychosocial interventions, cognitive, nursing, and family interventions are each described in turn. The chapter concludes with a description of some subgroups of patients requiring special consideration, including treatment-resistant first-episode patients, patients with complicating substance abuse disorder and, finally, patients with mental retardation.

Chapter 8, written by Jayashri Kulkarni, is concerned with 'Home-based treatment of first-episode psychosis'. The key difference in the approach described is that, while later phases of illness are treated in the community in many settings, here even the most acute initial phase is treated in the home, rather than having recourse to hospitalization. Following an introductory section, in which the rationale for this style of treatment is outlined, the chapter focuses on the key factors in successful home-based management of first-episode psychosis. These are discussed under headings labelled 'the individual', 'the family', and 'the treating team'. Then specific management strategies for home-based treatment of these patients are delineated, strategies which are delivered according to phases: the immediate or 'crisis' phase, the acute phase, the recovery phase, and the follow-up phase. The tasks and foci of each phase are carefully outlined. The following aspects are described: medication management, physical investigations, psychoeducation, psychosocial issues, and hospital back-up for the treatment of first-episode patients treated predominantly at home. The chapter concludes with results from a pilot study of home-based treatment of patients with first-episode psychosis.

Chapter 9, by Max Birchwood, addresses 'Early intervention in psychosis: the critical period'. The chapter reviews a range of evidence and suggests that, in the early course of psychotic disorders, interventions may have a greater influence on current and eventual outcome. Following a review of relevant literature including that from the pre-neuroleptic era, Birchwood mounts the argument that there is a plateau effect between 2 and 5 years following the onset of illness, in which the course of psychotic disorder will stabilize and may even relent among those who initially deteriorate the most. Topics such as early relapse, long-term outcome and suicide, are briefly reviewed and this is followed by a section on a broad range of predictors of outcome. Birchwood concludes by summarizing and evaluating the concept of the 'critical period'. Potentially helpful interventions are then suggested, such as reducing delay in treatment, relapse prevention, cognitive therapy, promoting early social recovery, and managing early treatment resistance.

Chapter 10, by Henry Jackson, Jane Edwards, Carol Hulbert and Patrick McGorry, is concerned with 'Recovery from psychosis: psychological interventions'. A historical perspective outlines three distinct eras in psychological approaches to therapy in the psychoses, illustrating a belated shift recently to a more cognitive framework. The chapter covers two distinct types of cognitive approach, with the first focusing on the adaptation of the person in the wake of the initial psychotic episode, and the second dealing with more specific strategies for the treatment of delusions and hallucinations derived from experience with patients with treatment-resistant symptoms. The material in the first area covered establishes the need for a new paradigm, emphasizes the self and normal psychosocial development, and highlights the impact of psychosis on both. The need for a new therapy is established, and then the four phases of cognitively oriented psychotherapy for early psychosis, or COPE, are described under the headings of: assessment, the therapeutic alliance, adaptation and, finally, secondary morbidity. Research progress is documented. The second major theme of the chapter deals with the treatment of delusions and hallucinations. Initially, work with people with persistent treatment-refractory symptoms is described. This is followed by a description of how this work has been modified for use in early psychosis, particularly those patients with prolonged recovery. The chapter concludes by emphasizing that the two lines of therapeutic development are synergistic, and both appear very promising in terms of their potential benefits for patients.

Chapter 11, by Jane Edwards, John Cocks and James Bott, focuses on 'Preventive case management in first-episode psychosis', delineating the principles of preventive case management within this population.

PREFACE

After describing the EPPIC case management context, guidelines and issues are discussed under five headings: the clinician–patient relationship; case management tasks in each phase of the disorder – acute, early recovery, and late recovery; prolonged recovery; use of an integrated biopsychosocial model; and management of the case management team. The authors consider the evidence for the role of maintenance and targeted drug therapy in the wake of an initial psychotic episode and emphasize the importance of flexibility and process issues in relapse prevention. The early identification of treatment resistance is stressed and an integrated biopsychosocial strategy to tackle the phenomenon is outlined. Throughout the chapter vignette fragments are used to illustrate points and issues.

Chapter 12, by Paddy Power, deals with 'Suicide and early psychosis'. Suicide is an unfortunately salient issue in the course of early psychosis. After providing initial facts and figures about suicide in general, the chapter focuses on suicide in serious mental illness, specifically on suicide in affective disorder, schizophrenia, and in those with complicating alcohol- and substance-abuse disorders. A model of suicidality and suicide behaviours in psychosis is proposed, within which risk factors and protective factors are discussed, and the clinical application of the model to early psychosis is outlined. Possible preventive strategies to tackle suicide risk in early psychosis are considered. Primary prevention is briefly considered; however, secondary and tertiary prevention is seen as more immediate and relevant for service providers and clinicians. Factors helpful in the detection and assessment of suicide risk in early psychosis are described, along with some specific suicide prevention interventions for this population. The latter include psychological and psychosocial, as well as pharmacological and physical treatments.

Chapter 13, written by Donald Linszen and Marie Lenior, is concerned with 'Early psychosis and substance abuse'. After establishing the extent of the comorbidity, via prevalence rates, two main hypotheses are advanced. The first is the vulnerability hypothesis that drug and alcohol abuse may contribute to the development of psychosis, or may precipitate signs and symptoms of the illness. The second is the self-medication hypothesis, which proposes that psychotic patients may attempt to alleviate the symptoms of the illness or the side effects of medication via the use of alcohol and drugs. The authors acknowledge the difficulty of answering the question as to whether substance abuse precipitates, or is a consequence of psychosis. The authors proceed to examine the onset of substance abuse and psychosis, initially independently, then conjointly. The effect of substance abuse on the early course of psychotic illness is described, the chapter concluding with some practical treatment guidelines for the patient with this type of comorbidity.

Chapter 14, by John Gleeson, Henry Jackson, Heather Stavely and Peter Burnett, concerns 'Family intervention in early psychosis'. The chapter highlights the critical importance of family support, education, and involvement in the early stages and subsequently in psychotic illness. Most people experiencing an initial psychotic episode are in close contact with relatives and, particularly in the era of community psychiatry, relatives have the opportunity to play an essential caring and support role in the recovery process. In the setting of prolonged illness, the patient and the clinicians involved need to form a healthy partnership with the carers, who have significant needs of their own. This chapter deals with family interventions in early psychosis, commencing with a rationale for a preventive model in family work and then focusing on empirical work with 'first-episode families'; examining, first, the expressed emotion literature regarding relapse and its ability to predict the same and, secondly, the family burden literature. Studies examining the efficacy of family interventions with the first-episode psychosis population are reviewed, and it is concluded that there is a need to develop a tailored approach to meet the needs of first-episode families. A four-stage model is proposed to cover family needs around these stages in early psychosis: 'before detection'; 'after detection'; 'towards recovery'; and 'first relapse and prolonged recovery'. A description of the EPPIC family services model of staged support and intervention is provided, with emphasis being given to: the engagement and assessment process, psychoeducational work, and multiple-family group work. Particular emphasis is given to the need for family support, but with a view to empowering the family members. Suggestions are made for future directions in this line of work.

Chapter 15, written by Shona Francey, is concerned with 'The role of day programmes in recovery in early psychosis'. The chapter begins by examining both the definitions and the efficacy of day programmes and briefly reviews the needs of recovering patients in general. The function of day programmes is described and presented as a new element in facilitating recovery. The EPPIC day programme is then described in some detail, beginning by looking at the way in which referrals and assessments are organized; this is followed by an account of the structure and content of the streams within the overall programme. The latter includes social, recreational, vocational, creative expressional, health promotion, personal skills development and focus group streams. The consensual monitoring of the progress of participants and the evaluation of elements of the programme and of the overall

PREFACE

programme is undertaken. Data are reported for day participants from the broader EPPIC follow-up sample.

Chapter 16, which concludes the book, is entitled 'Sharpening the focus: early intervention in the real world', and addresses future challenges and service models in early psychosis. Written by Patrick McGorry, Jane Edwards and Kerryn Pennell, it focuses on the range of emerging issues in the field of early psychosis and how services in different geographical settings can focus preventively on vulnerable young people in this key phase of illness. A deliberately practical stance is taken with the hope of stimulating 'bottom up' initiatives in a wide variety of clinical settings. For optimal implementation and wide-ranging reform, however, a synergy between 'bottom up' and 'top down' processes is clearly required. To mobilize systemic and global support is a complex endeavour which depends on a number of essential elements. These are discussed, and the importance of the evidence-based paradigm is highlighted. In addition to emerging evidence, other powerful forces are identified which will ultimately determine the fate of this reform agenda. These fall generally under the heading of ideology. The key questions of effectiveness and cost-effectiveness of an early intervention approach are central to matters of both evidence and ideology. The chapter also contains summary information about some of the pioneering efforts in the early psychosis field, and gives a sense of the momentum which has built up around the world in this area in recent years.

In conclusion, this book aims to capture the conceptual basis and the range of current clinical practice in this emerging area of early psychosis. In addition to the clinical emphasis, interwoven through the book is a comprehensive review of the core research data in early and first-episode psychosis. It is our hope that it will prove a helpful guide to clinicians and researchers working with people at this phase of illness. We look forward to further expansion of knowledge and expertise in the years to come.

The editors would like to acknowledge the efforts of all of the contributing authors to the book, and all of the clinical and research staff within EPPIC and other clinical or research settings who have contributed in a myriad of ways to the knowledge and experience distilled in this book. We have drawn inspiration in our efforts from pioneers in the field of psychosis, notably John Strauss, Tom McGlashan, Silvano Arieti and Paul Meehl. The growing international cohort of colleagues and friends working in this frontier is a tremendous source of encouragement and support, and here we acknowledge particularly Jan Olav Johannessen, Marco Merlo, Don Linszen, Richard Wyatt and Johan Cullberg. We would also like to acknowledge the enduring support of

PREFACE

Professor Bruce Singh to this enterprise and to Rhonda Galbally and Professor Gustav Nossal of the Victorian Health Promotion Foundation, who took a calculated risk in supporting our Melbourne-based explorations in early psychosis. Similarly, the Victorian Department of Human Services provided essential support for the development of a clinical model which was essentially an experiment, yet one which has allowed a range of benefits, including this book, to flow. Jennifer Williams and Andrew Stripp deserve our gratitude in this respect, as does their predecessor, Dr Peter Eisen. More recently, George Shaw, as Chief of Clinical Programs at our parent North-Western Health Care Network has been highly encouraging and supportive of our clincial and research endeavours. We thank Samantha Albert for diligently cleaning up final drafts of each chapter and securing the files, and Dominic Miller for his creative input into the various figures. Thanks also to our editor Dr Richard Barling for standing by us and waiting patiently for us to supply the 'end-product'. Most importantly, we would like to thank our patients and their families, from whom we have learned so much and who are the intended beneficiaries of this global effort.

Finally, we sincerely acknowledge our families, our partners Merilyn and Anne, respectively, and our children, Liam, Niall and Fionn McGorry and Carl Jackson, for the sacrifices imposed upon them through the writing of this book and all that went into its creation.

Patrick D. McGorry
Henry J. Jackson

Acknowledgments

An earlier draft of the text of Chapter 1 appeared as McGorry, P. (1998). A stitch in time . . . the scope for preventive strategies in early psychosis. *European Archives of Psychiatry and Clinical Neuroscience*, **248**, 22–31.

Figure 1.1 is reprinted with permission, from Mrazek, P. J. & Haggerty, R. J. (eds.) (1994). *Reducing Risks for Mental Disorders*. Copyright 1994 by the National Academy of Sciences. Courtesy of the National Academy Press, Washington, D.C.

Table 2.1 is reprinted with permission from *Schizophrenia Bulletin*, from Yung, A. R. & McGorry, P. D. (1996). The prodromal phase of first-episode psychosis: past and current conceptualizations. *Schizophrenia Bulletin*, **22**, 353–70.

For Figure 4.1 permission is given by the Royal College of Psychiatrists, from Yung, A. R., Phillips, L. J., McGorry, P. D., McFarlane, C. A., Francey, S., Harrigan, S., Patton, G. C. & Jackson, H. J. (1998). Prediction of psychosis: a step towards indicated prevention of schizophrenia. *British Journal of Psychiatry*, **172** (Supplement 33), 14–20.

Figure 6.1 is reprinted with permission from Blackwell Science Pty. Ltd., from McGorry, P. D. (1995). A treatment-relevant classification of psychosis. *Australian and New Zealand Journal of Psychiatry*, **29**, 555–8.

Permission to publish Figure 9.1 has been given by Cambridge University Press. The Figure was published previously as Figure 3 in Shepherd, M., Watt, D., Falloon, I. & Smeeton, N. (1989). The natural history of schizophrenia: a five-year follow-up in a representative sample of schizophrenics. *Psychological Medicine*, Monograph Supplement 15.

Permission to publish Figures 9.2 and 9.3 has been given by *Behaviour Change*. The Figures have been adapted from Figures 3 and 4 in Birchwood, M. (1995). Early intervention in psychotic relapse: cognitive approaches to detection and management. *Behaviour Change*, **12**, 2–19.

ACKNOWLEDGMENTS

Permission to publish Figure 9.4 has been given by the *British Journal of Psychiatry*. The Figure was published previously as Figure 1 in Drury, V., Birchwood, M., Cochrane, R.,& Macmillan, R. (1996). Cognitive therapy and recovery from acute psychosis: a controlled trial. I. Impact on psychotic symptoms. *British Journal of Psychiatry*, **169,** 595–601.

For Figure 15.2 permission is given by the Royal College of Psychiatrists, from Albiston, D. J., Francey, S. M. & Harrigan, S. M. (1998). Group programmes for recovery from early psychosis. *British Journal of Psychiatry*, **172** (Supplement 33), 117–21.

Figure 16.1 is reproduced with permission from Gardiner-Caldwell Communications Ltd., from McGorry P. D. & Edwards, J. (1997). *Early Psychosis Training Pack*. Cheshire: Gardiner-Caldwell Communications.

Part I
Introduction

'A stitch in time'... The scope for preventive strategies in early psychosis

PATRICK D. MCGORRY

It is of the greatest practical importance to diagnose cases of dementia praecox with certainty and at an early stage (Kraepelin, 1896/1987, p. 23)

The sooner the patients can be restored to an earlier life and the less they are allowed to withdraw into the world of their own ideas, the sooner do they become socially functional (Bleuler, 1908/1987, p. 63)

Introduction

The notion of prevention in psychotic disorder has a long yet tenuous pedigree. In one sense, drawing on the ideas of the early pioneers of the schizophrenia field is like quoting from the Bible. One can usually find something to support one's perspective, even if it is essentially out of sympathy with the original author's main thesis. Kraepelin and Bleuler, observing the scene during the pre-neuroleptic era, were heavily and understandably influenced by the devastation wrought by the unchecked erosive force of the disorders they witnessed. Kraepelin in particular, at least initially, through his concepts and classification, became the architect of an entrenched pessimism which continues to exert its influence. Yet even he hints at some preventive implications of early diagnosis.

Sullivan also observed many years ago: 'The psychiatrist sees too many end states and deals professionally with too few of the pre-psychotic' (Sullivan, 1927, p. 106). This is undoubtedly true of a range of mental disorders not merely the psychoses; nevertheless, the surprisingly prolonged delays in treatment for first-episode psychosis patients

(Loebel et al., 1992) and the concentration of those patients with the most persistent and disabling forms of illness in services, mean that the sensitivity of the average clinician to the issues and preventive possibilities surrounding the onset phase of illness are severely blunted. Such a distortion of clinical experience is closely related to the clinician's illusion (Cohen & Cohen, 1984), a phenomenon of which Bleuler in particular was well aware:

> Only a very small proportion of all schizophrenics come under observation in our institutions, and when it comes to individual groups of the illness we see only a selective sample. For example, patients who recover after one attack are observed only during that initial attack. (Bleuler, 1908/1987, p. 71)

The corrosive influence of this illusion upon therapeutic optimism can be readily seen in everyday clinical practice. Thomas McGlashan has recently illustrated the common effect upon the morale of the treating clinician of such experience:

> I remain convinced that with them [refers to specific patients] I came upon the scene too late; most of the damage was already done. I remain convinced that with schizophrenia in its moderate to severe form, our current treatment efforts amount to palliation and damage control (McGlashan, 1996, p. 198)

He goes on to indicate how this experience can, paradoxically, help to provide momentum for a more preventive approach.

Indeed, as the concept of schizophrenia enters its second century, we are at an unusually favourable point in the understanding and clinical care of people with psychotic disorders. A building sense of optimism is heightened by the realization that these developments are long overdue. Throughout the last 100 years, dark clouds of pessimism have cast a shadow over the prospects for people developing these disorders, particularly schizophrenia. While these originated in the reality of the serious prognosis of these illnesses at that time, prior to the discovery of effective treatments, pessimism has been deeply entrenched by the flawed conceptual framework devised by Kraepelin (Boyle, 1990; McGorry, Copolov & Singh, 1990). The fundamental conceptual error which was exposed during Kraepelin's own lifetime and led him to alter his opinions, was the decision to allow course and outcome to substitute as an interim validating criterion in place of pathophysiological criteria. Unfortunately, the nosological model has survived essentially intact and has created a barrier to research progress, preventive efforts, and good clinical care (McGorry et al., 1990). The best efforts of generations of researchers and clinicians alike have been unable to disperse the clouds of pessimism, although some sunshine has occasionally pierced the gloom with significant, often serendipitous, advances such as the discovery of neuroleptic medications. Unfortunately, the clouds always re-gathered, since even our effective weapons, ranging from drug and psychological therapies to systems of health care, have generally been crudely or inexpertly deployed. At best, treatment has been less effective than could otherwise have been the case, and at worst it has created additional iatrogenic misery, morbidity and mortality. Examples of this include the past abuses of psychosurgery (Sachdev & Sachdev, 1997; Valenstein, 1986), the still widespread use of neuroleptic medications in excessively high doses (Lader, 1997), the use, beyond their use-by date, of forms of psychotherapy which were ineffective in psychotic disorders (Jackson et al., 1996), and which inhibited the development of more useful and humane approaches, and the warehousing of patients (Scull, 1979). The latter has been followed more recently by a well intentioned, but, in most countries, poorly planned, irresponsibly executed and inadequately funded process of deinstitutionalization (Bachrach, 1994). In many respects, the history of treatment and care of our most serious mental disorders has mirrored the natural history of the disorders themselves, and reinforced the pessimistic aura surrounding them.

Although the neuroscientific revolution has not yet truly delivered in terms of enhanced treatments, the adoption of a clinical epidemiological perspective highlighting the preventive opportunities which exist, combined with encouraging advances in psychopharmacology and psychosocial treatment, has begun to create a climate of optimism. The limitations of our societies, our concepts, and our cultures of care, and of the capacities of clinicians, have combined to retard and prejudice the recovery process for many decades for those (mainly) young people who developed these potentially serious illnesses. As the services designed for the pre-neuroleptic era gradually dissolve away, we have the chance to replace them, in optimal circumstances, by better-funded and more efficient models in tune with the twenty-first century and the needs of community-based patients and their families. There have been a number of false dawns and the preventive seeds sown by Sullivan (1927) and Cameron (1938) did not immediately germinate within a barren ecosystem of care. Even the optimism and reform of the 1960s bypassed and ultimately failed people with schizophrenia and other serious mental illnesses. The question immediately arises: is the current optimism more securely based? It will need to be to interrupt the familiar cycle of enthusiasm followed by dissipation and disappointment. Let us consider the logic, the evidence, and future directions.

Early intervention in psychotic disorders is increasingly seen as having the potential to produce better outcomes in these potentially disastrous conditions, which generally strike during the critical developmental phase of adolescence or early adulthood (Birchwood & Macmillan, 1993; Birchwood, McGorry & Jackson, 1997; McGlashan, 1996; Wyatt, 1991). This idea has logic and a substantial amount of circumstantial evidence to support it, but, to date, relatively little direct evidence. The logic translates directly from mainstream preventive medicine (Mrazek & Haggerty, 1994), from which this zone of psychiatry has been effectively insulated, and rests on several pillars. First, delays in initiating treatment are often prolonged, and the duration of untreated psychosis (DUP) is associated with substantial functional decline, treatment resistance and increased subsequent rates of relapse (Helgason, 1990; Jones et al., 1993; Johnstone et al., 1986; Loebel et al., 1992; Wyatt, 1991). Secondly, intensive and sophisticated intervention following detection during the early phase of the illness could minimize iatrogenic damage and more effectively promote recovery (McGorry et al., 1996), which frequently occurs anyway later on. This is potentially critical, since such late recoveries are often seriously incomplete and seem to occur despite treatment efforts. Much of the damage is to the patient's personal development, social environment and lifestyle, and is very difficult to repair after years of neglect. This is particularly poignant in people who have had a dramatic late remission in response to clozapine. Their experience is analogous to that depicted in *Awakenings* (Sacks, 1982) and highlights the distinction between the core illness and its consequences. Thirdly, targeting failure of initial remission or early treatment resistance with recently developed enhanced drug and psychosocial interventions, could result in a lower rate of prolonged treatment resistance, relapse and disability (Edwards et al., 1998). Fourthly, maintaining remission and preventing or limiting relapse, by reducing the total duration of active psychosis and its deleterious consequences, is a post-psychotic analogue of reducing DUP (Curson et al., 1986; Johnson et al., 1983). In addition to improving outcomes for first-episode patients and those moving through the critical period (Birchwood & Macmillan, 1993) of the first several years after onset, it may even be possible to conceive of, and offer interventions for, those people who are probably experiencing the pre-psychotic phase of illness. This form of preventive intervention, known as *indicated prevention*, could be closer than we think. I now propose to outline briefly a framework for preventive interventions in psychosis and build upon this to further examine the logic and the evidence relating to the preventive clinical foci listed above. Subsequent chapters will develop these foci in greater detail.

A practical framework for preventive intervention in psychosis

Since preventive intervention around the onset of frank psychosis has been regarded until recently as beyond our present capacities (McGlashan & Johannessen, 1996), it is important to be clear about the conceptual basis for approaching it. In particular, the notion of treatment even prior to the onset of fully-fledged schizophrenia attracted an earlier generation of clinicians (Cameron, 1938; Meares, 1959; Sullivan, 1927), but the conceptual and practical obstacles have not hitherto been adequately addressed (McGorry & Singh, 1995; Yung & McGorry, 1996). It is useful to consider more generally the spectrum of intervention in mental disorders prior to focusing specifically on pre-psychotic intervention and early intervention (Mrazek & Haggerty, 1994). Broadly, interventions can be classified into prevention, treatment and maintenance.

Within prevention, drawing on the ideas of Gordon (1983), Mrazek & Haggerty (1994) subclassify interventions as universal, selective, and indicated, as shown in Figure 1.1. *Universal* preventive interventions are targeted to the general public or a whole population group which has not been identified on the basis of individual risk, e.g. the use of seat belts, immunization, and prevention of smoking. *Selective* preventive measures are appropriate for subgroups of the population whose risk of becoming ill is above average. Examples include special immunizations for people travelling to areas where yellow fever is endemic, and annual mammograms for women with a positive family history of breast cancer. The subjects are clearly asymptomatic. *Indicated* preventive measures apply to those individuals who, on examination, are found to manifest a risk factor which identifies them, individually, as being at high risk for the future development of a disease, and as such could be the focus of screening. Gordon's (1983) view was that such individuals should be asymptomatic and 'not motivated by current suffering', yet have a clinically demonstrable abnormality. An example would be asymptomatic individuals with hypertension. Mrazek & Haggerty (1994) adapted Gordon's concept as follows: 'Indicated preventive interventions for mental disorders are targeted to high-risk individuals who are identified as having minimal but detectable signs or symptoms foreshadowing mental disorder, or biological markers indicating predisposition for mental disorder, but who do not meet DSM-111-R diagnostic levels at the current time' (p. 494).

This major definitional shift allows individuals with early and/or subthreshold features (and hence a degree of suffering and disability)

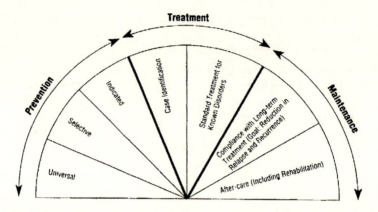

Figure 1.1. The spectrum of intervention in mental disorders (modified from Mrazek & Haggerty, 1994).

to be included within the focus of indicated prevention. Some clinicians would regard this as early intervention or an early form of treatment; however, the situation with these individuals is not so clear-cut. While some of these cases will clearly have an early form of the disorder in question, others will not. They might, however, have other less serious disorders, and many individuals, subthreshold for a potentially serious disorder like schizophrenia may have nevertheless crossed a clinical threshold where they either require or request treatment. Eaton, Badawi & Melton (1995) have warned that the absence of firm data on the validity of the classification system enjoins us to be careful about conceptualizing the process of disease onset. Parenthetically, many of the issues discussed here are relevant to defining 'caseness' and thresholds for initiating treatment in a range of mental disorders (Mrazek & Haggerty, 1994). In schizophrenia, the threshold has been set high and requires not only the presence of positive psychotic symptoms but also a six month duration of illness. This is due to a combination of historical factors, a degree of therapeutic nihilism and the social implications of the diagnosis. The height of the bar is set at a much lower level for other disorders, e.g. depression, where the above factors do not apply. The high threshold may have contributed to treatment delay (Loebel et al., 1992) and hence added to the risk of poor outcome. It may therefore be worthwhile to question the clinical threshold for treating 'psychosis spectrum disorders'. Ultimately, however, while we might not agree with the threshold set by DSM or ICD for receiving a diagnosis of a mental disorder such as schizophrenia, if this is the current criterion for 'caseness', then an intervention aimed at preventing the further evolution of symptoms such that the threshold is reached, does strictly meet

1 PREVENTIVE STRATEGIES IN EARLY PSYCHOSIS

the definition of indicated prevention, since it is aiming to reduce the occurrence of new cases. If we can argue successfully for interventions at this phase or level of symptoms and disability, then by current convention it should be regarded as indicated prevention and not (early) treatment *per se*, although this distinction may be of dubious relevance to the patient. All the same, Eaton et al. (1995) has emphasized that the implications of offering a preventive intervention are different from offering treatment for a fully-fledged disorder, since there is a finite chance that, in the first instance, the person may not go on to develop the disorder in question.

Even though it is currently only just within reach, Mrazek & Haggerty state very clearly that they view the cusp of the onset phase as the current frontier of preventive effort in schizophrenia: 'The best hope now for the prevention of schizophrenia lies with indicated preventive interventions targeted at individuals manifesting precursor signs and symptoms who have not yet met full criteria for diagnosis. The identification of individuals at this early stage, coupled with the introduction of pharmacological and psychosocial interventions, may prevent the development of the full-blown disorder' (Mrazek & Haggerty, 1994, p. 154).

Moving beyond purely preventive interventions, the framework focuses upon case detection, and this involves the potential for early intervention, a form of secondary prevention under the older conceptual framework. Early intervention can be further subdivided into a series of elements, each with the potential to contribute to a secondary preventive effort. Both indicated prevention and early intervention will now be considered in more detail, as dual foci for preventively oriented intervention in psychosis.

Focus 1: Indicated prevention in psychotic disorder

What are we waiting for?
Several authors have highlighted the potential for people who ultimately develop a schizophrenic disorder to have been identified as ill prior to the onset of frank psychotic symptoms (Cameron, 1938; Meares, 1959; Sullivan, 1927). Until recently, it was believed that, given the non-specificity of pre-psychotic features (Sullivan, 1927), a prospective approach to the study of onset in psychosis was impossible (Häfner et al., 1995). Bleuler alluded to this as follows: 'Thus when we speak of the initial symptoms of schizophrenia, we must limit ourselves to the first symptoms which come to notice. All too often we do not know the first real manifestations' (Bleuler 1911/1950, p. 252).

Häfner and colleagues (1995) have made a valiant effort to overcome this obstacle, yet residual problems clearly exist with a retrospective approach (Yung & McGorry, 1996). With the advent of the framework of Mrazek & Haggerty (1994), the notion of sequential screening (Derogatis, Della Pietra & Kilroy, 1992) or a 'close-in' research strategy (Bell, 1992), and the epidemiological work of Eaton et al. (1995), we are now able more clearly to formulate how to go about such an endeavour, and to appreciate the potential pitfalls. In retrospective studies of first-episode psychosis (e.g. Häfner et al., 1995; Yung & McGorry, 1996), only those cases who have developed a psychosis are included in reconstructions of the pre-psychotic phase. Hence, the predictive power of particular clinical features cannot be assessed. The pre-psychotic features are described as prodromal since in this sample they are always followed by psychotic symptoms. Such features are thus regarded as the earliest manifestations of the disorder itself (even though, at that point, they would be below threshold for diagnosis) and, hence, interventions would be seen as variants of secondary prevention. Many clinicians, extending as far back as Bleuler, have difficulty seeing what problems could arise in treating such patients as if they have schizophrenia. In fact, Bleuler himself eschewed the notion of prodrome because he believed that these early, yet highly variable, features which he meticulously described were merely the initial phases of a presumably inevitably progressive disorder (Bleuler, 1911/1950). This was also the original approach of Ian Falloon and colleagues in Buckinghamshire in the 1980s (Falloon, 1992; Falloon et al., 1996). However, looking at the issue from a prospective standpoint reveals the dilemma. The clinical features identified retrospectively in first-episode samples are mostly non-specific (McGorry et al., 1995; Yung & McGorry, 1996) and have only a limited predictive power in relation to subsequent psychosis (and thus the diagnosis of a fully-fledged disorder). We have suggested the term 'at risk mental state' (McGorry & Singh, 1995) to denote this state of affairs, while Eaton et al. (1995) have developed the notion of 'precursor' features for the same purpose. These terms indicate clinical features which can be assigned a finite estimate of both relative and attributable risk for the fully-fledged disorder. This means they have a looser link with the fully-fledged disorder than the notion of 'prodrome', and allow for a significant false positive rate. Drawing on the 'close-in' strategy referred to above and the conceptual tools of clinical epidemiology (Kraemer et al., 1997), we have sought to identify additional risk factors and markers to improve our predictive capacity. This strategy has great potential to overcome some of the weaknesses of traditional high-risk research while retaining genuine preventive credentials.

What do we know so far? Well, we now know that it is possible to identify and engage a sample of young people at greatly enhanced risk of early transition to psychosis. Our early findings indicate that 40–50% of such individuals identified via operational clinical criteria will develop a fully-fledged psychotic disorder within 12 months of detection (Yung et al., 1996, 1999). Admittedly, those who do make the transition are probably an unrepresentative subset of the universe of first-episode psychosis. It is also likely, parenthetically, that some of those who do not make an early transition are nevertheless still covertly vulnerable to psychotic disorder and constitute what we have termed 'false false positives' (Yung et al., 1996). This is the possibility with which the traditionalists have a problem, because they believe that schizophrenia is characterized by inevitability. Murray has characterized this loosely as 'doomed from the womb' (Murray, 1987). Such a model implies a 'sufficient' or even a 'necessary and sufficient' causal model as in Huntington's disease, a scenario we are already confident does not exist in most cases of schizophrenia. This is a fundamental logical flaw underpinning the thinking of many clinicians, and even the intervention strategy in the Falloon (1992) study, and sees the patient inevitably programmed to develop the disorder – an analogy would be with some form of computer virus. The alternative is a risk factor model where a mix of potential contributory causal factors will influence the expression of the disorder. Within such a model, it may ultimately be possible to identify and influence malleable causal risk factors to prevent the full expression of the disorder. In the meantime, with more accurate characterization of risk and high level prediction, we are approaching the stage where more intensive treatment, including time-limited, low-dose neuroleptics and psychosocial interventions, could be evaluated in a carefully controlled manner in potentially pre-psychotic individuals. The latter could involve a blend of stress reduction, lifestyle restructure and enhanced coping, using modern cognitive–behavioural interventions. With this phase, however, as argued elsewhere (McGorry et al., 1996; Vaglum, 1996), we simply do not yet know that interventions developed for one phase of illness are optimal or even appropriate for another.

Essentially, the answer to the question, 'why wait?', is that we have to take account of the risk:benefit ratio for patients, including issues of stigma, and carefully evaluate the optimal duration of treatments to be offered at this phase. Some people have expressed an appropriately cautious view that it could be potentially iatrogenic to treat at this phase, particularly when it comes to applying a diagnosis and using neuroleptic medication. Others have emphasized the imperative to 'do something' when it is clear that a young person is in trouble, with their lifestyle and prospects collapsing around them, as, in a substantial proportion of cases, they slide into a serious psychotic disorder. This is an exciting area with huge potential for patient care and cost-effectiveness, and hence for further exploration. It is likely to yield interesting new data from a number of centres. Such data will be an essential foundation for an evidence-based clinical approach.

Focus 2: Early intervention

What's the hurry?

A series of recent studies have highlighted the relationship between the DUP and clinical outcome in psychotic disorders (Helgason, 1990; Larsen, McGlashan & Moe, 1996; Loebel et al., 1992; McGorry et al., 1996; Wyatt, 1991). This is not a new idea but dates back to the 1920s (Cameron, 1938; Sullivan, 1927) and the delays in recognition were also described by Bleuler (Bleuler, 1911/1950). What has surprised and shocked many people however, is the extent of the delays in treatment, even in developed countries with more than adequate psychiatric services (Larsen et al., 1996). Even after the person has developed a fully-fledged psychosis, the duration of the delay in obtaining treatment averages a year or even more in such developed countries. There is strong face validity to the idea that such a prolonged delay in treatment during the critical developmental phases of adolescence and early adult life could profoundly negatively influence the capacity for psychosocial recovery, even if the biological disturbance could be successfully treated. There is an additive theory that the biological change may itself prove less responsive to treatment if it is present for a long period before the person is exposed to anti-psychotic medication, and this is supported by several lines of evidence (Wyatt, 1991, 1995).

Interestingly enough, despite this face validity argument, the lines of evidence which provide partial support for the strategy and the enthusiasm generated in many parts of the world for interventions aimed at shortening this period of untreated psychosis, there is a significant degree of scepticism. Why should this be so? First, it has its roots in the Kraepelinian pessimism referred to above and has been nurtured by more recent incarnations of this, such as the 'doomed from the womb' notion, an unnecessarily pessimistic interpretation of the neuro-developmental model of schizophrenia (Murray, 1987; Weinberger, 1987). Secondly, apart from the Camarillo study (May, Tuma & Dixon, 1976), which has its flaws, and others reviewed and re-analysed by Wyatt (1991, 1995) and by Wyatt, Green & Tuma (1997), there are no contemporary high grade randomized controlled trials (RCTs) comparing timely versus delayed intervention. Nevertheless, even those who are sceptical, or are attempting to remain so, of the early intervention paradigm, regard it as unethical to delay intervention for a first episode of psychosis (McGlashan & Johannessen, 1996). This is a revealing clue to the depth of conviction of such scepticism! Other sceptics argue that brief psychoses with a short DUP which have a good outcome are somehow 'a different beast' with a different psychopathological basis and an intrinsically good prognosis. This is a variant of the notion that if you recover you did not really have schizophrenia. It is difficult to argue with such circularity and fatalism which derives, as argued, from Kraepelin's legacy, and which would find little support in other medical disciplines, where aetiopathology and outcome have been separated, e.g. nephrology.

On the other hand, a genuine reason for scepticism derives from the possibility that the relationship between DUP and outcome is at least partially explained by a third factor which contributes both to an increased risk of treatment delay *and* poor outcome, at least in an important subgroup. This could most likely occur via certain clinical features, e.g. negative symptoms of insidious onset, or persecutory delusions, which might be not only markers of poorer outcome but also mediators of delayed treatment. In the light of this possible alternative explanation for the link, it therefore seems worthwhile to look as McGlashan has done, at alternative ways (other than the RCT of delayed versus timely treatment) of testing the hypothesis that reduction of the DUP results in an improvement in outcome (McGlashan, 1996). Successful experimental manipulation (reduction) of the DUP variable in an experimental sample while eschewing such early detection efforts in a control sample would enable conclusions to be drawn concerning the degree of influence of this factor on course and outcome. Such samples could need to be geographically separated, and randomization, at least at the level of the individual, would be impossible. There may be alternative possibilities, for example, cluster randomization, although even here there would be obstacles (Peter Jones and Shôn Lewis, personal communication).

What's so special about the first episode?
This question turns on the nature and intensity of interventions offered at this phase of illness, and raises the question of how different they need to be from treatment approaches derived and delivered in later phases and with more chronic subsamples of patients. Even with treatments essentially similar to those employed in patients with established illness, remission rates are excellent in first-episode psychosis, at least as far as positive symptoms are concerned (Lieberman et al., 1993). However, when one considers neurocognitive functioning,

psychological recovery, relapse rates and functional outcome, the short-term prospects are probably much more guarded. This is where a careful consideration of the needs of patients and their families is critical. We have argued elsewhere that the treatment of first-episode and early psychosis patients in general requires a highly modified approach in contrast to that offered in later phases of the disorder (Edwards et al., 1994; McGorry, 1992; McGorry et al., 1996). These modifications are required across the whole spectrum of treatment and challenge therapeutic errors derived from the clinician's illusion referred to above. Thus, the approaches relevant to the subgroup of cases with definite relapsing and disabling illnesses, including complex co-morbidities, may be unhelpful to younger early psychosis patients. Examples of this include the nature, dose, and sequence of drug therapies (McEvoy, Hogarty & Steingard, 1991; McGorry & Kulkarni, 1994), the content and style of psychological approaches (Jackson et al., 1996, 1998; McGorry et al., 1998), and the approach with relatives and peers. More detail on the rationale and content of these therapeutic interventions is provided in the comprehensive *Early Psychosis Training Pack* (McGorry & Edwards, 1997).

It must be acknowledged that there is relatively little definitive evidence for the above contentions to date, apart from the data reported in McGorry et al. (1996). In this paper, significant improvements in outcome were reported over the first year following entry into treatment with a first episode of psychosis for patients treated with an enhanced phase-specific programme of intervention. Patients were carefully matched on key variables known to influence outcome with historical controls treated in an earlier but less specialized programme. The weaknesses of this study relate to the lack of randomly assigned or concurrent controls and, hence, the findings are not definitive; however the magnitude of the effects were substantial. This study has also demonstrated substantial improvements in cost-effectiveness for the new model over the former one (McGorry, Mihalopoulos & Carter, 1998). The improved outcomes appeared more likely to derive from more intensive and specific treatment after entry (McGlashan, 1996) rather than reductions in DUP, which were relatively modest and difficult to interpret. Clearly, however, more rigorous testing of the notion that such specific phase-related interventions are more effective is required, and this should occur via a combination of specific efficacy-oriented RCTs and broader 'real world' effectiveness studies including a mandatory focus on cost-effectiveness.

Delayed remission...? Treatment resistance...? – Why not wait and see?
A series of authors dating back to the time of Kraepelin concur that

1 PREVENTIVE STRATEGIES IN EARLY PSYCHOSIS

a plateau of impairment and disability is reached on average around 2–3 years following illness onset (Birchwood & Macmillan, 1993; McGlashan & Johannessen, 1996). While this may still vary from patient to patient, and such variation is enhanced by a lack of clarity concerning the timing of illness onset, some patients may have reached this plateau by the time of first treatment. For others, there is still a time window, labelled by Birchwood the 'critical period', in which at least prevention of further damage and, for some, at least a partial reversal of the process may occur (Birchwood & Macmillan, 1993). This could be conceptualized as a blend of, first, turning around a declining situation through aggressive biopsychosocial treatment – in other words, a short-term 'rescue operation' – and, secondly, over a longer period, maybe several years, mounting a stable 'holding operation' in relation to the person's lifestyle, relationships, and vocational future.

It has been argued (Edwards et al., 1998) that it is important not to withhold, either by neglect or design, the full spectrum of effective treatments until treatment resistance has been confirmed and even entrenched, and the plateau of disability reached. This includes the early use of the newer anti-psychotics, and, following these, much earlier use of clozapine (Lieberman, 1996), and of the emerging cognitively oriented forms of psychological intervention, which appear to be able to accelerate recovery from acute psychosis (Drury et al., 1996) and to reduce treatment resistance (Fowler, Garety & Kuipers, 1995). While the latter interventions will also need to be modified for use at this phase of illness, there seems to be little logic in withholding them from patients who are slow to respond, and no logic at all in those with a clear-cut treatment resistance. It may also be worthwhile to broaden the definition of treatment resistance at this phase to include protracted or slow recovery, and also persistent neurocognitive impairments and negative symptoms, rather than focusing exclusively on persistent positive symptoms. We have termed this treatment endeavour 'recovery plus' to avoid stigmatization and minimize early pessimism for clinicians and patients. One could well argue on ethical grounds that the question 'why not wait and see?' should be replaced by an opposite one, i.e. 'why wait?'. Lieberman (1996) has put these contentions in the form of hypotheses which are helpful from a research standpoint. However, I would suggest that the onus of proof should be such that those advocating delays in more aggressive intervention should provide evidence that such an approach can be clinically and ethically justified. In any event, this is a rich arena for future efficacy studies using careful yet inclusive RCT methodology; however, it will probably require a multi-centre approach, given the low prevalence of treatment-resistant cases, even broadly defined, in first-episode samples.

Relapse prevention – is it vital?

Elsewhere, I have argued that to pursue the prevention of relapse as the *sole* goal of treatment, rather than as a key intervening variable influencing the overall quality of life of the patient and his or her family, can be limited and counterproductive (McGorry, 1995). Many treatment studies have adopted such a narrow approach, the logical extension of which would be to overtreat all patients with high-dose neuroleptics and excessively restrictive clinical practices. Indeed, such a pattern of treatment is all too common in routine clinical care. The trade-off between maintenance neuroleptic dosage-relapse prevention and quality of life has recently been illustrated in the 'treatment strategies in schizophrenia' study (Schooler et al., 1997). On the other hand, based on the same logic as reducing the DUP, it is probably equally important to reduce the proportion of time following entry to treatment that the patient suffers from ongoing psychotic symptoms. This duration of psychosis during treatment is contributed to by the time period to initial remission, i.e. the degree of initial treatment resistance, the frequency of psychotic relapse, and the degree of subsequent or emergent treatment resistance.

Once again the frequency of relapse is another feature which appears to peak during the early years following onset (Eaton et al., 1992), particularly in those with a long DUP (Johnstone et al., 1992). Furthermore, there is also the clinical suggestion that those who relapse demonstrate an emerging resistance to treatment, as evidenced by an increasing time to remission with increasing episode number. Now this could be due to the fact that those with more severe treatment-resistant illness also have a higher vulnerability to relapse (and a long DUP); however, such emergent treatment resistance might be preventable by reducing the frequency of relapse (as well as the DUP – see above). Despite the increasing time to remission in later episodes than the initial one noted by Loebel et al. (1992), it is still not clear whether the fact that multi-episode patients require somewhat higher doses of neuroleptics for a response than first-episode patients (McEvoy et al., 1991) is due to the development of treatment resistance, the development of tolerance to neuroleptics, the concentration of the subsample of treatment-resistant patients in multi-episode samples over time, or a combination of these factors. Once again, all of these questions should be the focus of ongoing research.

It seems obvious that *frequent* relapse is likely to be deleterious to the outcome of psychotic disorder and relapses are inherently risky and undesirable, hence the question posed may once again seem like a paper tiger. However, determining whether the vulnerability to psychotic relapse is still present in the individual patient is an important task in the management of the early phases of psychosis, i.e. which patients can safely come off medication and when. Further, the patient who remains relapse-prone ideally needs to be convinced *personally* by whatever means that prophylactic or maintenance treatment is really necessary. In some cases this only occurs when relapse is directly experienced. In others, of course, even this fails to convince. In addition, future research needs to focus on the impact relapse has upon the illness process, the person and their families. Finally, other aspects of persistent or intermittent co-morbidity should be brought into the focus of research and treatment, which has hitherto focused largely upon positive psychotic relapse.

Conclusion

The burgeoning interest in the potential for early intervention in psychotic disorder has led to a series of seminal international conferences in recent years, a number of landmark publications, changes in structure of mental health service provision in some countries, extensive research, and even the establishment of an international association to promote and encourage further advances in this area of psychiatry. While it is most important not to inhibit rational enthusiasm, constrained for so long by corrosive scepticism, it is timely to sound a cautionary note. Many of the most potent and far-reaching changes in service provision have been driven by powerful peripheral forces, such as economic imperatives (managed care) or ideological policies (de-institutionalization), and these have had 'juggernaut' effects which continue to pose great risks to patient care. It is theoretically possible that early intervention, if implemented in 'bushfire' mode, could come to be seen in a similar light. One way in which it could become rapidly discredited is that, if not implemented in a planned, staged and targeted manner, it might not prove to be cost-effective, hence causing financial erosion of other valuable services. If this were to occur, the cause of prevention and early intervention would be greatly set back.

All of the exciting developments and the strategies which flow from them outlined above, ultimately must be based upon sound evidence which can only arise from well conducted clinical research. This kind of statement tends to have a pious ring to it and, certainly, in many of these areas the best evidence may follow rather than drive change. Some health care systems do not seem to realize this, and have been paralysed in mid-reform, obsessively waiting (in vain) for rock-solid evidence to support their reform agenda. Hence, on the one hand it is important to avoid such paralysing crises of confidence and *do something*! On the other hand, implementing changes at a pace whereby they can be evaluated and modified is sensible. Such a strategy does not need to paralyse, but may guide and provide escape routes from inappropriate pathways. This is especially so since it is becoming clearer that clinically based research, supported by neuroscientific advances, *can* strongly catalyse change in service delivery. This has certainly been our local experience.

The rise of the evidence-based paradigm is a welcome development, particularly if a range of evidence can be included to guide clinical practice. The potential of the early intervention strategy in turn creates additional responsibility on all of us to conduct sound research and evaluation and not to overstate or oversell the results. To do otherwise could jeopardize the strategy and potentially consign us all to a further era of pessimism. The stakes are very high. The rise of a new preventive paradigm in many parts of the world, particularly in Australasia, Scandinavia, Western Europe and Canada, is very encouraging. This paradigm is attracting the interest of established and highly competent researchers who have clearly laid out blueprints for future research (McGlashan, 1996; Wyatt, 1991; Wyatt, Pina & Henter, 1998). Large-scale intervention projects have been generously funded in Norway, Denmark, Sweden, the Netherlands, Australia, New Zealand and Canada, and should provide important new knowledge.

What will be required ultimately, however, is the development of funding models which support a dramatic increase in, and shift of resources to, the earlier phases of disorder, without disenfranchizing those with more established illness. This will ultimately depend on these preventive strategies proving genuinely cost-effective, and interim 'hump' funding being available to cover a transitional period. This will be difficult in the era of economic rationalism and 'first generation' managed care, the effects of which are being felt well beyond their epicentre in the United States. These policies have the capacity to become the new clouds to shut out the preventive sunshine. Paradoxically, if their originators and those responsible for implementing them have the skill and foresight to think beyond the bottom line of the single financial year, then what is currently a threat could be turned to a synergistic force. It is likely that resources expended during the early phases of illness will prove cost-effective not only in the short term (McGorry, Mihalopoulos & Carter, 1998), but over the long haul for those patients who do require long-term care. The danger with this argument is that it could be implemented prematurely across the board, and even misused to support cost cutting which resulted in extensive neglect in the context of deinstitutionalization. Clearly, patients with continuing vulnerability and or disability beyond the early phases of illness also require sophisticated and expert continuing care. This is one of the characteristics of this group, namely that effective treatment of some kind must be continued indefinitely (McGlashan & Johannessen, 1996). It is hoped that the size of this group and their level of disability and need for care could be substantially reduced by earlier and intensive intervention. Perhaps the intensity of treatment could ultimately be relaxed in many people after the critical period (Birchwood et al., 1997), but we do not know this yet.

If this is to occur it will need to be guided by extensive clinical research on at least two levels. The first of these is *efficacy* studies, essentially RCTs, to develop and refine strategies for early detection, and the various elements of treatment, namely drug therapies, psychological treatments and psychosocial interventions, as appropriate for the specific phase and developmental stage of the patients. The second is at the level of systems of care, including studies of *effectiveness*, which are intended to test the real world impact of efficacious treatments. RCTs have major limitations in this area of clinical research and need to be rethought and supplemented by a range of evidence (Aveline, 1997; Thorneycroft & Tansella, 1996). Research and evaluation will also be crucial to enable effective systems for a range of societies and cultures to be developed. It is well known that many efficacious treatments prove less than optimally effective in 'real world' situations for a variety of reasons. Examples include lithium prophylaxis in bipolar disorder and family interventions in schizophrenia. Hence early intervention must also make sense to consumers, carers, to the average clinician, and to communities around the world, have a good 'reach', and be properly funded to enable better quality of life to be achieved for those vulnerable to psychotic disorders. This volume provides detailed coverage of the present state of knowledge of this emerging clinical paradigm.

References

Aveline, M. O. (1997). The limitation of randomized controlled trials as guides to clinical effectiveness with reference to the psychotherapeutic management of neuroses and personality disorders. *Current Opinion in Psychiatry*, **10**, 113–15.

Bachrach, L. L. (1994). Deinstitutionalization: What does it really mean? In *Schizophrenia: Exploring the Spectrum of Psychosis*, ed. R. J. Ancill, S. Holliday & J. Higenbottam, pp. 21–33. Chichester, UK: Wiley.

Bell, R. Q. (1992). Multiple-risk cohorts and segmenting risk as solutions to the problem of false positives in risk for the major psychoses. *Psychiatry*, **55**, 370–81.

Birchwood, M. & Macmillan, J. F. (1993). Early intervention in schizophrenia. *Australian and New Zealand Journal of Psychiatry*, **27**, 374–8.

Birchwood, M., McGorry, P. & Jackson, H. (1997). Early intervention in schizophrenia. *British Journal of Psychiatry*, **170**, 2–5.

Bleuler, E. (1908). The prognosis of dementia praecox: the group of schizophrenias. In *The Clinical Roots of the Schizophrenia Concept*, eds. J. Cutting & M. Shepherd (1987), pp. 59–74. Cambridge: Cambridge University Press.

Bleuler, E. (1911). *Dementia Praecox or the Group of Schizophrenias*. Translated by J. Zinkin (1950). New York: International Universities Press.

Boyle, M. (1990). *Schizophrenia: A Scientific Delusion?* London: Routledge.

Cameron, D. E. (1938). Early schizophrenia. *American Journal of Psychiatry*, **95**, 567–78.

Cohen, P. & Cohen, J. (1984). The clinician's illusion. *Archives of General Psychiatry*, **42**, 1178–82.

Curson, D., Hirsch, S., Platt, S., Bamber, R. & Barnes, T. (1986). Does short term placebo treatment of chronic schizophrenia produce long term harm? *British Journal of Psychiatry*, **293**, 718–26.

Derogatis, L. R., Della Pietra, L. & Kilroy, V. (1992). Screening for psychiatric disorder in medical populations. In *Research Designs and Methods in Psychiatry*, ed. M. Fava & J. F. Rosenbaum, pp. 170–245. Elsevier: Amsterdam.

Drury, V., Birchwood, M., Cochrane, R. & Macmillan, F. (1996). Cognitive therapy and recovery from acute psychosis: a controlled trial. I. Impact on psychotic symptoms. *British Journal of Psychiatry*, **159**, 593–601.

Eaton, W. W., Bo Mortensen, P., Herrman, H., Freeman, H., Bilker, W., Burgess, P. & Wooff, K. (1992). Long-term course of hospitalisation for schizophrenia: Part 1. Risk for rehospitalisation. *Schizophrenia Bulletin*, **18**, 217–28.

Eaton, W. W., Badawi, M. & Melton, B. (1995). Prodromes and precursors: Epidemiologic data for primary prevention of disorders with slow onset. *American Journal of Psychiatry*, **152**, 967–72.

Edwards, J., Francey, S. M., McGorry, P. D. & Jackson, H. J. (1994). Early psychosis prevention and intervention: evolution of a comprehensive community-based specialized service. *Behaviour Change*, **11**, 223–33.

Edwards, J., Maude, D., McGorry, P. D., Harrigan, S. M. & Cocks, J. T. (1998). Prolonged recovery in first-episode psychosis. *British Journal of Psychiatry*. (Supplement) In Press.

Fallon, I. R. H. (1992). Early intervention for first episode of schizophrenia: a preliminary exploration. *Psychiatry*, **55**, 4–15.

Fallon, I. R. H., Kydd, R. R., Coverdale, J. H. & Laidlaw, T. M. (1996). Early detection and intervention for initial episodes of schizophrenia. *Schizophrenia Bulletin*, **22**, 271–82.

Fowler, D., Garety, P. & Kuipers, E. (1995). *Cognitive Behaviour Therapy for Psychosis. Theory and Practice*. Chichester, UK: Wiley.

Gordon, R. (1983). An operational classification of disease prevention. *Public Health Reports*, **98**, 107–9.

Häfner, H., Maurer, K., Löffler, W., Bustamante, S., an der Heiden, W., Reicher-Rössler, A. & Nowotny, B. (1995). Onset and early course of schizophrenia. In

Search for the Causes of Schizophrenia, Vol. III, ed. H. Häfner & W. F. Gattaz, pp. 43–66. New York: Springer-Verlag.

Helgason, L. (1990). Twenty years' followup of first psychiatric presentation for schizophrenia: what could have been prevented. *Acta Psychiatrica Scandinavica*, **82**, 231–5.

Jackson, H. J., McGorry, P. D., Edwards, J. & Hulbert, C. (1996). Cognitively orientated psychotherapy for early psychosis (COPE). In *Early Intervention and Prevention in Mental Health*, ed. P. Cotton & H. Jackson, pp. 131–54. Melbourne: Australian Psychological Society.

Jackson, H. J., McGorry, P. D., Edwards, J., Hulbert, C., Henry, L., Francey, S., Cocks, J., Power, P., Harrigan, S. & Dudgeon, P. (1998). Cognitively oriented psychotherapy for early psychosis (COPE): Preliminary results. *British Journal of Psychiatry* (Supplement). In Press.

Johnson, D. A., Pasterski, G., Ludlow, J. M., Street, K. & Taylor, R. D. (1983). The discontinuance of maintenance neuroleptic therapy in chronic schizophrenic patients: drug and social consequences. *Acta Psychiatrica Scandinavica*, **67**, 339–52.

Johnstone, E. C., Crow, T. J., Johnson, A. L. & Macmillan, J. F. (1986). The Northwick Park Study of first episode schizophrenia: I. Presentation of the illness and problems relating to admission. *British Journal of Psychiatry*, **148**, 115–20.

Johnstone, E. C., Frith, C. D., Crow, T. J., Owens, D. G. C., Done, D. J., Baldwin, E. J. & Charlette, A. (1992). The Northwick Park 'Functional' Psychosis Study: diagnosis and outcome. *Psychological Medicine*, **22**, 331–46.

Jones, P. B., Bebbington, P., Foerster, A., Lewis, S. W., Murray, R. M., Russell, A., Sham, P. C., Toone, B. K. & Wilkins, S. (1993). Premorbid social underachievement in schizophrenia: results from the Camberwell Collaborative Psychosis Study. *British Journal of Psychiatry*, **162**, 65–71.

Kraemer, H. C., Kazein, A. E., Offord, D. R., Kessler, R. C., Jensen, P. S. & Kupfer, D. J. (1997). Coming to terms with the terms of risk. *Archives of General Psychiatry*, **54**, 337–43.

Kraepelin, E. (1896). Dementia praecox. In *The Clinical Roots of the Schizophrenia Concept*, ed. J. Cutting & M. Shepherd (1987), pp. 13–24. Cambridge: Cambridge University Press.

Lader, M. (1997). High-dose antipsychotic treatment – boon or bane? *Current Opinion in Psychiatry*, **10**, 69–70.

Larsen, T. K., McGlashan, T. H. & Moe, L. C. (1996). First episode schizophrenia: I. Early course parameters. *Schizophrenia Bulletin*, **22**, 241–56.

Lieberman, J. A. (1996). Atypical antipsychotic drugs as a first-line treatment of schizophrenia: a rationale and hypothesis. *Journal of Clinical Psychiatry*, **57** (Supplement), 68–71.

Lieberman, J. A., Jody, D., Alvir, J. M. J., Ashtari, M., Levy, D. L., Bogerts, B., Degreef, G., Mayerhoff, D. I. & Cooper, T. (1993). Brain morphology, dopamine, and eye-tracking abnormalities in first-episode schizophrenia: prevalence and clinical correlates. *Archives of General Psychiatry*, **50**, 357–68.

Loebel, A. D., Lieberman, J. A., Alvir, M. J., Mayerhoff, D. R., Geisler, S. H. &

Szymanski, S. R. (1992). Duration of psychosis and outcome in first-episode schizophrenia. *American Journal of Psychiatry*, **149**, 1183–8.

May, P. R., Tuma, A. H. & Dixon, W. J. (1976). Schizophrenia – a follow-up study of results of treatment methods. *Archives of General Psychiatry*, **33**, 474–8.

McEvoy, J. P., Hogarty, E. E. & Steingard, S. (1991). Optimal dose of neuroleptic in acute schizophrenia: a controlled study of the neuroleptic threshold and higher haloperidol dose. *Archives of General Psychiatry*, **48**, 739–45.

McGlashan, T. H. (1996). Early detection and intervention in schizophrenia: Editor's introduction. *Schizophrenia Bulletin*, **22**, 197–9.

McGlashan, T. H. & Johannessen, J. O. (1996). Early detection and intervention with schizophrenia: rationale. *Schizophrenia Bulletin*, **22**, 201–22.

McGorry, P. D. (1992). The concept of recovery and secondary prevention in psychotic disorders. *Australian and New Zealand Journal of Psychiatry*, **26**, 32–4.

McGorry, P. D. (1995). Psychoeducation in first episode psychosis: a therapeutic process. *Psychiatry*, **58**, 313–28.

McGorry, P. D. & Edwards, J. (1997). *Early Psychosis Training Pack*. Cheshire, UK: Gardiner–Caldwell Communications.

McGorry, P. D. & Kulkarni, J. (1994). Prevention and preventively oriented clinical care in psychotic disorders. *Australian Journal of Psychopharmacology*, **7**, 62–9.

McGorry, P. D. & Singh, B. S. (1995). Schizophrenia: risk and possibility. In *Handbook of Studies on Preventive Psychiatry*, ed. B. Raphael and G.D. Burrows, pp. 491–514. Amsterdam: Elsevier Science Publishers.

McGorry, P. D., Copolov, D. L. & Singh, B. S. (1990). Current concepts in functional psychosis. The case for a loosening of associations. *Schizophrenia Research*, **3**, 221–34.

McGorry, P. D., McFarlane, C., Patton, G., Bell, R., Jackson, H., Hibbert, M. & Bowes, G. (1995). The prevalence of prodromal symptoms of schizophrenia in adolescence: a preliminary survey. *Acta Psychiatrica Scandinavica*, **92**, 241–9.

McGorry, P. D., Edwards, J., Mihalopoulos, C., Harrigan, S. M. & Jackson, H. J. (1996). EPPIC: An evolving system of early detection and optimal management. *Schizophrenia Bulletin*, **22**, 305–26.

McGorry, P. D., Phillips, L., Henry, L. & Maude, D. (1998). Preventively-orientated psychological interventions in early psychosis. In *Cognitive Psychotherapy of Psychotic and Personality Disorders*, ed. C. Perris & P. McGorry. Chichester, UK: Wiley. In Press

McGorry, P. D., Mihalopoulos, C. & Carter, R. C. (1998). Is early intervention in first episode psychosis an economically viable method of improving outcome? In *Proceedings of the Xth World Congress of Psychiatry*, Madrid, August 23–28, 1996.

Meares, A. (1959). The diagnosis of prepsychotic schizophrenia. *Lancet*, **I**, 55–9.

Mrazek, P. J. & Haggerty, R. J. (eds.) (1994). *Reducing Risk for Mental Disorders: Frontiers for Preventive Intervention Research*. Washington, DC: National Academic Press.

Murray, R. M. (1987). Is schizophrenia a neurodevelopmental disorder? *British*

Medical Journal, **295**, 681–2.
Sachdev, P. & Sachdev, J. (1997). Sixty years of psychosurgery: Its present status and its future. *Australian and New Zealand Journal of Psychiatry*, **31**, 457–64.
Sacks, O. (1982). *Awakenings*. London: Pan Books.
Schooler, N. R., Keith, S. J., Severe, J. B., Matthews, S. M., Bellack, A. S., Glick, I. D., Hargreaves, W. A., Kane, J. M., Ninan, P. T., Frances, A., Jacobs, M., Lieberman, J. A., Mance, R., Simpson, G. M. & Woerner, M. G. (1997). Relapse and rehospitalization during maintenance treatment of schizophrenia. *Archives of General Psychiatry*, **54**, 453–63.
Scull, A. (1979). *Museums of Madness: The Social Organisation of Insanity in Nineteenth Century England*. London: Allen Lane.
Sullivan, H. S. [1927] (1994). The onset of schizophrenia. *American Journal of Psychiatry*, **151**(Supplement 6), 135–9.
Thorneycroft, G. & Tansella, M. (eds.) (1996). *Mental Health Outcome Measures*. Berlin: Springer-Verlag.
Vaglum, P. (1996). Earlier detection and intervention in schizophrenia: unsolved questions. *Schizophrenia Bulletin*, **22**, 347–51.
Valenstein, E. S. (1986). *Great and Desperate Cures: The Rise and Decline of Psychosurgery and Other Radical Treatments for Mental Illness*. New York: Basic Books.
Weinberger, D. R. (1987). Implications for normal brain development for the pathogenesis of schizophrenia. *Archives of General Psychiatry*, **44**, 660–99.
Wyatt, R. J. (1991). Neuroleptics and the natural course of schizophrenia. *Schizophrenia Bulletin*, **17**, 325–51.
Wyatt, R. J. (1995). Early intervention for schizophrenia: can the course of the illness be altered? *Biological Psychiatry*, **38**, 1–3.
Wyatt, R. J., Green, M. F. & Tuma, A. H. (1997). Long-term morbidity associated with delayed treatment of first admission schizophrenic patients: a re-analysis of the Camarillo State Hospital data. *Psychological Medicine*, **27**, 261–8.
Wyatt, R. J., Pina, L. M. & Henter, I. D. (1998). First-episode schizophrenia: early intervention and medication discontinuation in the context of course and treatment. *British Journal of Psychiatry* (Supplement). In Press
Yung, A. R. & McGorry, P. D. (1996). The prodromal phase of first-episode psychosis: past and current conceptualizations. *Schizophrenia Bulletin*, **22**, 353–70.
Yung, A. R., McGorry, P. D., McFarlane, C. A., Jackson, H. J., Patton, G. C. & Rakkar, A. (1996). Monitoring and care of young people at incipient risk of psychosis. *Schizophrenia Bulletin*, **22**, 283–303.
Yung, A. R., Phillips, L. J., McGorry, P. D., McFarlane, C. A., Francey, S., Harrigan, S., Patton, G. C. & Jackson, H. J. (1999). The prediction of psychosis: A step towards indicated prevention of schizophrenia. *British Journal of Psychiatry* (Supplement). In press

Part II

Onset and detection of psychosis

2

The onset of psychotic disorder: clinical and research aspects

ALISON R. YUNG AND HENRY J. JACKSON

The births of all things are weak and tender, and therefore we should have our eyes intent on beginnings. (Montaigne *Of Managing the Will* Essays (1580–1588))

Introduction

Clinicians dealing with patients with schizophrenia and other psychotic disorders know the frustration of being able only to provide partial treatment and palliative care. As McGlashan (1996, p. 198) wrote of managing such cases: 'I remained convinced that with them I came upon the scene too late; most of the damage was already done.' This echoes the sentiments of Harry Stack Sullivan who wrote in 1927 (Sullivan, 1994, p. 135): 'The psychiatrist sees too many end states and deals professionally with too few of the pre-psychotic ... I feel certain that many incipient cases might be arrested before the efficient contact with reality is completely suspended, and a long stay in institutions made necessary.' Sullivan's idea of treating cases of incipient schizophrenia is an example of *indicated prevention*, as described in Chapter 1. As Sullivan's quote suggests, the patients to be treated are symptomatic as they have signs of impending psychosis ('incipient cases'), but are not yet psychotic (have not yet lost 'contact with reality'). What is needed for such a preventive approach is the identification of the features around the time of the onset of the disorder, before it becomes established, as well as some indication of the likelihood and timing of the onset of frank psychosis. This chapter focuses on the onset phase of psychotic disorders. It has its 'eyes intent on beginnings' and aims to explore the following issues: What is meant by onset? What are the characteristic onset features? What precedes frank psychosis? How can psychosis be predicted? Can it be prevented or modified?

Underlying conceptual issues and definition of terms

Defining onset

Before the onset of a disorder can be defined it is necessary first to discuss what we mean by 'disorder' itself. Current nosological systems define several different psychotic disorders, all with the commonality of having 'positive' psychotic symptoms (usually meaning hallucinations and/or delusions) at some time in their course. Thus, in most current diagnostic systems, psychosis is a necessary but not sufficient criterion for making a diagnosis of a particular psychotic disorder. Other defining features must be present as well. For example, affective or mood psychoses require the presence of mood-related symptoms and signs in addition to psychotic features. The additional defining features of schizophrenia will depend on the model used. For example, DSM-IV schizophrenia requires the presence of a chronic course (six months or greater) and psychosocial decline, in addition to characteristic positive psychotic features (American Psychiatric Association (APA) 1994). Bleulerian schizophrenia requires the presence of certain fundamental symptoms, generally thought of today as 'negative' symptoms, including blunted affect, autistic withdrawal, loose associations, ambivalence and asociality, and 'positive' psychotic symptoms are thought of as being secondary to these primary disturbances (Bleuler, 1911). In addition, ICD-10 recognizes a category of 'simple schizophrenia', which consists of negative symptoms and a deteriorating course, but without the presence at any time of positive psychotic features (World Health Organization, 1994).

These nosological issues have implications for determining when onset is said to occur. Since our current classificatory systems focus on the presence of psychosis, and then subclassify the syndromes into different psychotic disorders, 'onset' is generally thought of as being the time when psychotic symptoms first appear (Haas & Sweeney, 1992). For instance, DSM-IV only diagnoses schizophrenia once positive psychotic features have become manifest. It leaves simple schizophrenia out of the psychotic disorders and classifies it under the personality disorders as schizotypal personality disorder (APA, 1994).

A complicating factor however, is that there is a significant degree of diagnostic instability at the time of the first psychotic episode

(McGorry, 1994). Even Kraepelin acknowledged this (1987, p. 60), stating: 'I was forced to realise that in a frighteningly large number of patients, who at first seemed to have the syndrome of mania, melancholia, insanity, amentia or madness, the syndrome changed fairly quickly into a typical progressive dementia and in spite of some differences, the syndromes became increasingly similar. I soon realised that the abnormalities at the beginning of the disease had no decisive importance compared to the course of the illness leading to the particular final state of the disease'. Thus, in having 'our eyes intent on beginnings', we must acknowledge that we are examining the onset of *psychosis*, which forms part of a heterogeneous group of disorders, including schizophrenia. The final diagnosis may not be able to be made for some time.

It is important to highlight at this point that delay in definitive diagnosis, necessary in many cases because of diagnostic instability, need not mean delay in treatment. This is true obviously for cases of first-episode psychosis, which require treatment regardless of what diagnosis is given. This thinking can also be applied around the concept of recognizing and intervening in patients who seem to be 'incipient cases'. The idea of identifying features leading up to frank psychosis and intervening in these cases, i.e. indicated prevention, will be discussed in the remainder of this chapter.

The concept of the prodrome in psychotic disorders

Frank psychotic symptoms rarely arise 'out of the blue', with no prior mental state changes at all. In schizophrenia in particular, many writers hold that the disorder begins before the onset of psychosis (Haas & Sweeney, 1992; Häfner et al., 1992a, 1993, 1994, 1995; Jones et al., 1993; Olin & Mednick, 1996), at least in some cases. Häfner and his associates distinguish 'illness onset' from 'episode onset' in schizophrenia, defining illness onset as the first (non-specific) sign of mental disturbance, and episode onset as the first first-rank symptom (specific sign) or the first point in time when the operationalized criteria of a diagnostic system are fulfilled (Häfner et al., 1992a, 1993, 1994, 1995; Larsen, McGlashan & Moe, 1996). Regardless of when onset of the disorder is thought of as occurring, it is useful to consider the stages leading up to the onset of frank psychosis, which is seen to define the disorder. The 'prodrome' refers to the time period characterized by mental state features which represent a change from a person's pre-morbid functioning, up until the onset of frank psychotic features (Beiser et al., 1993; Keith & Matthews, 1991; Loebel et al., 1992; Yung & McGorry, 1996a). Figure 2.1 illustrates these phases.

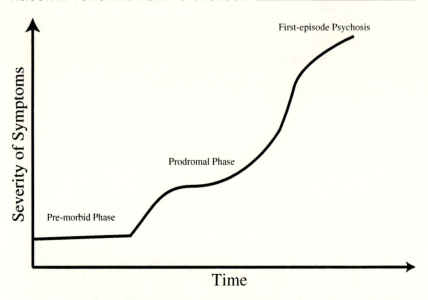

Figure 2.1. The transition from pre-morbid phase through prodrome to first-episode psychosis.

As is highlighted by Figure 2.1, the pre-morbid phase blends into the time of the first non-specific psychiatric symptoms – the prodrome – which, in turn, blends into the onset of first-episode psychosis. This latter continuity exists because it is difficult to say precisely when a person has slipped into a psychosis. Is this defined by the presence of one hallucination or a transiently abnormal idea? The degree of deviation from normal, the frequency of the experience and the length of time for which it has been present, must all be taken into account (Larsen et al., 1996; Yung et al., 1996). We have illustrated this issue with case examples in a previous paper (Yung & McGorry, 1996a). There is also continuity between the pre-morbid state and the prodromal phase; that is, it may be difficult to pinpoint when psychiatric symptoms begin in a person who is evolving over time with each developmental phase. For example, an individual may have always been shy and avoidant as an infant and young child; this may become more pronounced as greater demands are placed on the young person in secondary school years, especially with regard to dating, and could reach the threshold for a diagnosis of social phobia in the late teen years.

Thus, the point at which the prodromal phase would be said to begin (Häfner's 'illness onset') may be difficult to define exactly, and the point at which the first episode of psychosis is said to begin ('episode onset') may be similarly difficult to define. This difficulty is compounded because the prodrome is a retrospective concept, diagnosed only after the first episode of psychosis is recognized. With the benefit of hindsight, those changes noted in the person are then attributed to the onset of the 'prodrome' (Eaton, Badawi & Melton, 1995; Yung & McGorry, 1996a). This inherently retrospective reconstruction of changes which make up the prodrome, gives rise to a number of factors affecting the accuracy of such descriptions which must be considered.

Issues in retrospective description

Obviously, asking patients and informants to recall events from the past relies on their memories of these events. Memory is fallible – it does not operate analogous to a computer storage model (Loftus, 1993). Rather, memories are reconstructed with each retrieval, being generally modified to fit with a person's core schemas about themselves and their life (Singer & Salovey, 1993). A number of factors influence what is recalled and the accuracy of recall time since the onset of the prodrome is one such factor. The longer the time since onset, the more probable inaccuracies are likely to arise. In addition, asking patients who have been ill for a long time to reconstruct the changes which led up to the first episode, introduces confounding influences such as the effects of treatments, psychosocial difficulties, and disease progression (Haas & Sweeney, 1992). Similar influences may operate for informants. 'Effort after meaning' may come into play. This refers to the situation where patients and families look for an event which seemed to precipitate the changes, and date their histories from this point (Fava & Kellner, 1991; Henderson, 1988; Hirsch, Cramer & Bowen, 1992; Tennant, 1985). The lack of salience and novelty of at least some of the prodromal symptoms may make them difficult to recall accurately (Baddeley, 1993).

The degree of 'sealing over' similarly will influence what is recalled (Levy, McGlashan & Carpenter, 1975; McGlashan, Levy & Carpenter, 1975). The patient may not wish to recall this period of his or her life. The family may feel similarly. In other words, the coping style of both patients and informants will affect a retrospective description of the prodrome. These aforementioned self-serving biasing processes are described in the extensive clinical judgement literature with other terminology, such as: (*a*) the search for illusory correlations; (*b*) hindsight bias – in which the significance of the 'symptom' is only accorded importance in retrospect; and (*c*) confirmatory bias (Arkes, 1981; Basic Behavioral Science Task Force of the National Mental Health Council, 1996; Dawes, 1994; Turk & Salovey, 1985). Additionally, when the patient is asked to reflect on his or her experience, the current mental state may affect what is revealed or remembered.

Priming symptoms, for example by using semi-structured interviews, may help patients to recognize symptoms (as opposed to recall them), but this does not guarantee their accuracy (note here the work of Dawes (1994) on prediction, and Loftus (1993) on false memories and eye witness testimony). All in all, the most accurate retrospective descriptions of prodromal symptoms leading up to a first episode of psychosis would be gained by interviewing recovering first-episode psychosis patients and their families soon after the initial episode, using a semi-structured interview method (see below).

Descriptions of onset features

We recently reviewed the literature (Yung & McGorry, 1996a) on prodromal symptoms of schizophrenia and other psychotic disorders, the work describing 'early symptoms' of these conditions and some of the epidemiological data on onset features, particularly the reports from the Mannheim group (Häfner, 1989; Häfner et al., 1992a,b, 1993, 1994, 1995; Hambrecht, Häfner & Löffler, 1994). A brief summary of the pertinent findings follows.

Early literature

There is a body of literature from the 1960s, 1970s and earlier, which describes prodromal and early symptoms of schizophrenia. Most of the reports are anecdotal, relying on small numbers of cases in which patients are requested to recall the events leading up to a first psychotic episode. We reviewed this work in more detail elsewhere (Yung & McGorry, 1996a) and arrived at the following conclusions.

(1) There is a wide diversity of signs and symptoms found in the prodrome. These include: so-called 'neurotic' symptoms, such as anxiety, irritability and anger; mood-related symptoms, e.g. depressed mood, anhedonia, guilt, suicidal ideas, and mood swings; changes in volition such as apathy and loss of drive, boredom and loss of interest, fatigue and lack of energy; cognitive changes including disturbances of attention and concentration, and preoccupation and reduced abstraction; physical symptoms such as somatic complaints, loss of weight and appetite, and sleep disturbance; other symptoms, including obsessive compulsive phenomena, dissociative phenomena, increased interpersonal sensitivity, delusional mood, change in motility, speech abnormalities, suspiciousness, and changes in affect; and behavioural changes, e.g. deterioration in role functioning, social withdrawal, im-

Table 2.1. *Prodromal features in first-episode psychosis most commonly described in first-episode studies*

Prodromal features
Reduced concentration, attention
Reduced drive, motivation, anergia
Depressed mood
Sleep disturbance
Anxiety
Social withdrawal
Suspiciousness
Deterioration in role functioning
Irritability

pulsivity, odd behaviour, and aggressive, disruptive behaviour (Bleuler, 1911; Bowers, 1965, 1968; Bowers & Freedman, 1966; Cameron, 1938; Chapman, 1966, 1967; Conrad, 1958; Docherty et al., 1978; Donlon & Blacker, 1973; Fish, 1976; Huber et al., 1980; Kraepelin, 1919/1971; McGhie & Chapman, 1961; Meares, 1959; Offenkrantz, 1962; Stein, 1967; Varsamis & Adamson, 1971).

(2) There is a wide variability between patients with respect to which symptoms are manifest. The most commonly occurring symptoms and signs found in the most methodologically sound studies are shown in Table 2.1.

(3) Some authors suggested that certain symptoms had some specificity for the prediction of subsequent psychosis. For example, Cameron suggested that symptoms such as suspiciousness, feeling 'dazed or confused' and odd somatic experiences, have some predictive power (Cameron, 1938). Chapman believed that disorders of attention, particularly selective attention, and perception (e.g. illusions) were specific and were manifestations of the underlying abnormality in schizophrenia (Chapman, 1966, 1967). Huber's group have suggested that subjective deficits (the subjective equivalents of negative symptoms), including abnormal somatic sensations, represent the fundamental abnormality in schizophrenia but, rather confusingly, also state that they may be found in other disorders (Huber et al., 1980).

In marked contrast to the literature focused on the prodrome in schizophrenia, there are relatively few studies dealing with the prodromal features of affective psychoses. No reports have examined prodromes in *first-episode patients with affective disorders*. Hypomanic features such as increased activity, irritability and sleeplessness have been recorded in the prodromes of patients with multiple episodes of bipolar disorder (Carlson & Goodwin, 1973; Kraepelin, 1987; Molnar, Feeney & Fava, 1988; Winokur, 1976). Depressed mood, anxiety, and reduced energy were noted in the unipolar depression prodrome (Fava & Kellner, 1991; Hays, 1964; Murphy et al., 1989).

Most of these early reports can be criticized for: (*a*) their reliance on small sample sizes; (*b*) their failure to use standardized measures, and the consequent lack of inter-rater reliability data; (*c*) their lack of rigorous diagnostic assessment; and (*d*) their complete reliance on cross-sectional examination of symptomatology. In addition, it is unclear as to how representative the patients were, and at times it is unclear as to at which phase of disturbance they were formally assessed or observed. All these studies were retrospective and most used convenience samples.

DSM descriptions

Perhaps because of the reasons cited above, and in an attempt to use a more systematized approach, the 'case study' form of assessing prodromal and onset features was superseded by a series of studies using the DSM-III (APA, 1980) and DSM-III-R (APA, 1987) operationalized descriptions of the schizophrenia prodrome. The DSM-III defined eight features as making up the prodrome, and the DSM-III-R defined nine. The nine items which make up the DSM-III-R criteria are set out in Table 2.2.

A brief study of these items quickly reveals a number of concerns. First, they are mainly behavioural abnormalities, which could result from a number of underlying psychopathological conditions, importantly including frank psychosis itself. Secondly, many of the commonly described prodromal features, such as 'neurotic' symptoms and other non-specific sounding symptoms such as mood-related symptoms, are omitted, ignoring the fact that these are common even in typical (and subsequent) schizophrenia. Both of these factors are probably intentional with the aim of increasing the reliability and specificity of the assessment. However, several investigations of these items have been carried out and most cast doubt on the reliability of their measurement (Andreasen & Flaum, 1991; APA, 1992; Endicott et al., 1982; Jackson, McGorry & McKenzie, 1994; Jackson et al., 1996).

As we have pointed out elsewhere (Jackson et al., 1994), two of these studies examined prodromes of people who have had more than one episode, i.e., they examined relapse prodromes (e.g. Andreasen & Flaum, 1991; Endicott *et al.*, 1982). We maintain that in such cases it is difficult to know if one is studying true prodromes, with the clinical

2 THE ONSET OF PSYCHOTIC DISORDER

Table 2.2. *DSM-III-R prodromal symptoms for schizophrenia*

Prodromal symptoms
1. Marked social isolation or withdrawal
2. Marked impairment in role functioning
3. Markedly peculiar behaviour
4. Marked impairment in personal hygiene and grooming
5. Blunted or inappropriate affect
6. Digressive, vague, overelaborate, or circumstantial speech, or poverty of speech, or poverty of content of speech
7. Odd beliefs or magical thinking
8. Unusual perceptual experiences
9. Marked lack of initiative, interests or energy

picture in relapse prodromes possibly being complicated by residual positive symptoms, negative symptoms, patients' and families' different explanatory models for the phenomena, altered reactions to the symptoms by patients and families, and the effects of medication. One study included separate data for first – versus multiple – episodes (APA, 1992), and therefore permits some degree of comparison. The inter-rater reliability kappas for first-episode patients were unacceptable, whilst the multiple-episode patients were higher, and mostly, but not inevitably, acceptable (i.e. kappas of 0.5 or better). The findings (and readers seeking more details can be referred to the Table contained within Jackson et al., 1996) can be summarized as follows: first, there are no discernible patterns in the findings when the range of studies is considered collectively. In some investigations, symptoms attained high kappas, but the same symptoms were accorded low kappas in other studies; secondly, a comparison of patient ratings of prodromal symptoms, informant ratings, and ratings which blended these two sources of information plus file data, revealed that there was little agreement amongst the three sets of ratings (Jackson et al., 1994). The ratings varied markedly, and the choice of structured instrument used to index these symptoms appeared to have influenced the reliability of the ratings (Jackson et al., 1994, 1996).

A further study of the DSM-III-R schizophrenia prodrome symptoms by our group (Jackson, McGorry & Dudgeon, 1995) examined the specificity of these symptoms for schizophrenia as opposed to other psychotic disorders. The study focused on 313 first-episode psychosis patients (94 with schizophrenia, 62 schizophreniform psychosis, 43 schizoaffective disorder, 49 bipolar disorder, 16 delusional disorder, 28 psychotic depression, 21 psychotic disorder not otherwise specified).

Prodromal symptoms were found to be ubiquitous across all DSM-III-R (APA, 1987) categories of psychotic disorders, and symptoms by themselves were not specific to schizophrenia, although they had a higher loading for that disorder. Their specificity for schizophrenia increased once drug use and depression were excluded and a temporal component (six months) was added; nevertheless, they were clearly not pathognomonic for schizophrenia. This study, however, does not include patients with other non-psychotic disorders or persons with no pathology at all. Thus, it is highly likely that these symptoms would perform even more poorly in a wider, non-clinical context.

Another relevant study examining the DSM-III-R conceptualization of schizophrenia prodrome was conducted by our group (McGorry et al., 1995), as part of a wider epidemiological survey performed in Victoria, Australia, covering 657 year 11 school children (see Patton et al., 1996). Large percentages of students (mean age = 16.5 years) endorsed these prodromal symptoms. The prevalence of DSM-III-R prodromes, defined as the presence of two or more of the nine symptoms (APA, 1987) ranged from 10–15% to 50%, depending on the duration specified. There are a number of possible reasons for this high endorsement rate. One is that the symptoms may be non-specific and be rated as positive by adolescents in situational crises or experiencing other non-psychotic problems or disorders, as well as being endorsed by those adolescents with actual prodromes of schizophrenia. Substance abuse is another possible 'cause' for the high endorsement of these symptoms but it is unlikely to be the whole explanation, given that marijuana abuse only correlated 0.25 (accounting for only about 6% of the variance) with the total number of prodromal symptoms. A third possibility is that an unknown number of students may have been actively psychotic at the time. Furthermore, a number of students may have been experiencing 'outpost syndromes', or syndromes which resemble prodromes but which resolve spontaneously. These have been found to occur in a percentage of individuals who ultimately do progress to manifest schizophrenia (Huber *et al.*, 1980; Yung & McGorry, 1996a). Alternatively, if the symptoms had been present at an early age, some students may have been evidencing schizotypal personality traits which resemble attenuated forms of psychosis. Finally, students may have been endorsing the symptoms because of social desirability factors. Whatever the explanations, in the absence of direct follow-up interviews, it is difficult to determine accurately the relative validity of each of these explanations for the high prevalence of these prodromal symptoms in this study.

All in all, the reliability and validity of the specific DSM-III and DSM-III-R (APA, 1980, 1987) prodromal symptoms for schizophrenia appear to be poor, and subsequently this list has been dropped from the DSM-IV (APA, 1994). We believe that there is little point in pursuing further investigations of this particular collection of features.

Other recent studies

Recognizing the limitations of the DSM-III-R conceptualization of the prodrome, we set out to examine this period again from first principles, using a retrospective semi-structured interview method in a consecutive series of 21 patients with first-episode psychosis (Yung & McGorry, 1996b). Unconstrained by the DSM-III/R (APA, 1980, 1987) conceptualizations and criteria sets, we identified a diversity of prodromal phenomena reported by these patients. Consonant with the other non-DSM investigations we recorded three general groupings of prodromal symptoms: (1) attenuated psychotic symptoms, such as perceptual changes, perplexity, suspiciousness and delusional mood; (2) non-specific neurotic and mood-related symptoms, some of which were reactions to other symptoms, e.g. sleep disturbance, anxiety, irritability, poor motivation, and depressed or elevated mood; and (3) behavioural changes, which were frequently in response to other experiential phenomena, both neurotic and attenuated psychotic symptoms. These included impaired role functioning, social withdrawal, aggressive behaviour and self-neglect. The non-specific symptoms and behavioural signs were the most commonly occurring features. Allowing for the small numbers, mania was found to be frequently preceded by a hypomanic prodrome of elevated mood, increased energy, increased activity and disinhibition. Conversely, the features more commonly reported in the group with diagnoses of schizophrenia or schizophreniform psychosis were poor concentration, suspiciousness, lack of motivation, low energy, loss of interests and indecisiveness. We concluded that the extent of pre-psychotic phenomena found in this sample demonstrated that the prodromal period was likely to be associated with a high level of disability and this has since been confirmed by our ongoing work in other areas (Yung & McGorry, 1996a).

The other main sections of literature which require examination are several impressive studies by the German group led by Häfner (Häfner, 1989; Häfner et al., 1992a,b, 1993, 1994, 1995; Hambrecht et al., 1994) which retrospectively assess onset in schizophrenia using a structured interview schedule designed for this purpose – the Interview for the Retrospective Assessment of the Onset of Schizophrenia (IRAOS, Häfner et al., 1992b). The research is finely detailed and employs trained raters using standardized instrumentation which is rigorously and systematically applied. However, like all studies of the initial psychotic prodrome, it is necessarily retrospective. These studies found that negative-type symptoms tended to occur first and were common in the 2–6 years preceding admission. Non-specific neurotic-type symptoms, such as anxiety, restlessness, and depression, also occurred early. Positive symptoms were a relatively late phenomenon.

Further information on the psychopathology preceding the onset of positive symptoms of schizophrenia can be gathered from the Epidemiologic Catchment Area (ECA) program data. This large-scale project studied all adults aged 18 years and over in five cities in the USA: New Haven, Connecticut; Baltimore, Maryland; Durham, North Carolina; St Louis, Missouri; and Los Angeles, California. Subjects were assessed twice with a one-year interval between assessments using the Diagnostic Interview Schedule (DIS, Robins et al., 1981). It was found that obsessive compulsive disorder and social phobia were strongly associated with increased risk for schizophrenia, i.e. these diagnoses were made at baseline, and at subsequent interview a high incidence of schizophrenia was found, suggesting some longitudinal temporal relationship. Panic attacks and simple phobias at baseline were also found to be associated with increased risk of schizophrenia at follow-up (Tien & Eaton, 1992).

The duration of the prodromal period

In our review of the prodromal literature (Yung & McGorry, 1996a), we found that duration of the initial psychotic prodrome was extremely variable, ranging from a few days to many years and, in a minority of cases, no prodromal period was found at all, and this is allowing for the rather approximate and diverse way in which it was measured in the various reports. If one accepts only studies with superior methodologies, then prodromal periods for schizophrenia appear to be in the order of magnitude of 1–2 years. For example, Beiser et al. (1993) reported median prodrome lengths of 52.7 weeks and 51.4 weeks for schizophrenia and bipolar disorder, respectively. Loebel et al. (1992) recorded a mean of 98.5 weeks in their first-episode study of patients with first-episode schizophrenia and schizoaffective disorder (but not bipolar disorder). Surprisingly, in both studies the time intervals were not significantly different between the stipulated diagnostic groupings. This is unusual in the sense that it is not consistent with clinical folklore which avers that the duration of the manic prodrome is brief (a matter of days only) (Carlson & Goodwin, 1973; Kraepelin, 1987; Winokur, 1976). Other more recent researchers, on the other hand, have confirmed this result, describing prodromes lasting weeks to even years in affective disorders (Molnar et al., 1988). Häfner's group report 'time

2 THE ONSET OF PSYCHOTIC DISORDER

lags' between onset of negative symptoms and onset of positive symptoms in their samples, and note that negative symptoms begin on average 4.6 years before admission, whereas positive symptoms occur within two years of admission; however, estimation of prodrome length is not actually stated (Häfner et al., 1992a, 1993, 1994).

In summary, from our examination of the literature on prodromes and onset in psychotic disorders, we can draw the following conclusions: first, there is a wide variety of symptoms and signs which can occur, leading up to the development of positive psychotic symptoms. Negative symptoms and non-specific symptoms, including anxiety, depressed mood, and obsessive compulsive phenomena, tend to occur early, and are followed by more frank deviations from normal, such as attenuated forms of positive symptoms. The mean time period between first mental symptoms and onset of psychosis seems to be about two years (the median is one year). How then can we apply this knowledge in the detection of those with impending psychosis? The next section deals with some of the conceptual issues involved in this, and Chapter 4 examines some of the practical issues involved in case finding and intervention in these individuals.

Towards indicated prevention

The previous section summarized the current state of knowledge about prodromal features leading up to a first episode of psychosis. The reason this was done in detail was in order to be able to identify psychotic prodromes prospectively. This strategy has been used in the relapse prevention literature, in which symptoms and signs which have been found frequently to precede relapse are identified prospectively and trigger early targeted intervention. This aims to avert a further relapse or to modify the relapse (Birchwood et al., 1989; Heinrichs & Carpenter, 1985; Heinrichs, Cohen & Carpenter, 1985; Herz & Melville, 1980; Herz et al., 1989; Malla & Norman, 1994). Can we apply this strategy in identifying the prodrome of a first-ever psychotic episode? Could this lead to prevention of the onset of psychotic disorders, i.e. effect a reduction in the incidence of these disorders? Or could their onset be modified, attenuated (i.e. made less severe) or delayed? All of these would be worthy achievements indeed, and are the sorts of outcomes advocated by Sullivan at the beginning of this chapter (Sullivan, 1994). In other words, we return to the concept of indicated prevention. However, such a preventive approach requires the transformation of the retrospective concept of a 'prodrome' into a prospective form. There are several issues, therefore, which need to be taken into account.

Applying the 'prodrome' concept prospectively

Although we know the types of features which precede the onset of psychosis, it does not necessarily follow that we can predict psychosis from the presence of an apparent prodromal syndrome. As Eaton et al. point out, when discussing prodromes of mental disorders in general: 'At the present state of our knowledge, there are few signs and symptoms that predict the onset with certainty ... it is likely that many individuals with signs and symptoms that appear to have originated in disorder will not go on to develop the full-blown criteria' (Eaton et al., 1995, p. 968). In other words, false positives are likely – individuals who seem to be presenting with typical prodromal features may not go on to develop a psychotic disorder. There are several possible reasons for this. For example, the apparent prodromal syndrome was not that at all, but instead reflected another 'pathology' such as a situational crisis, or a transient drug-induced state. Secondly, the syndrome may have represented a prodrome of another psychiatric disorder, such as a depressive disorder, which followed it sequentially. Finally, the syndrome may have been in the process of developing into a full-blown psychotic disorder, but the psychotic episode was avoided due to some change in circumstance, such as increased social support, enhanced coping, or a therapeutic intervention of some kind. The first two examples can be seen as 'true false positives' and the third as a 'false false positive'. The term 'false false positive' is used because this group of patients would have the same vulnerability markers as the true positives, who do progress to psychosis, but they do not make such a transition due to the influence of certain resilience or protective factors. Conceptually, they may be thought of as having early manifestations of the disorder, but make a 'recovery' before the frank psychosis develops. The difficulty is that cross sectionally, these groups cannot be distinguished. This has implications when considering the measurement of markers. In true positives specific markers are present, and in false positives specific markers are absent. However, in false false positives specific markers are also present, yet their course over time was the same as that of the false positives, i.e. non-progression to frank psychosis (Yung & McGorry, 1996a). This issue is illustrated in Figures 2.2 to 2.5, and the implication for measurement of markers is shown in Table 2.3.

This discussion underlines the point made previously, that a syndrome can only be labelled as a 'prodrome' in retrospect. Prospectively, it would be more accurate to call the cluster of psychopathological changes 'precursor signs and symptoms' (Eaton et al., 1995) or an 'at risk mental state' (McGorry & Singh, 1995; Yung & McGorry,

2 THE ONSET OF PSYCHOTIC DISORDER

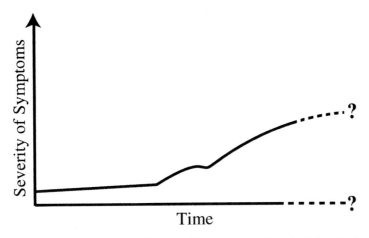

Figure 2.2. An 'at risk mental state'. Note: cross-sectionally it is not clear whether or not a 'prodrome-like syndrome' will develop into a psychotic episode. Hence, prospectively, this syndrome is best conceptualized as an 'at risk mental state'.

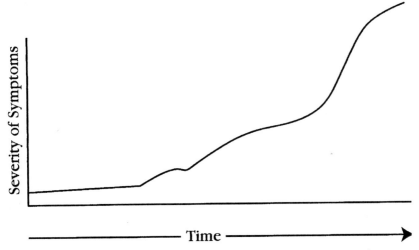

Figure 2.3. A true positive. Note: an 'at risk mental state' progresses into a psychotic episode.

1996a). This latter term, coined by our group, highlights the idea that the syndrome confers risk for the development of subsequent psychosis, but that psychosis is not inevitable. Thus, it is a 'state' (as opposed to a trait) risk factor for psychosis (Yung & McGorry, 1996a). Eaton et al. (1995) viewed precursor states similarly, and emphasized

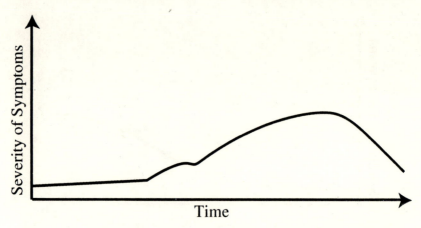

Figure 2.4. A false positive. Note: an 'at risk mental state' resolves without progression to psychosis.

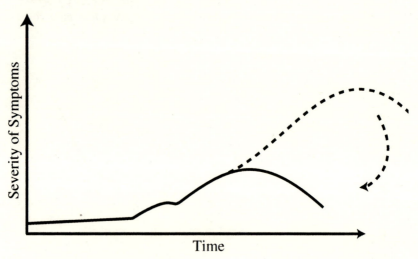

Figure 2.5. A 'false false positive'. Note: an 'at risk mental state' which would have developed into psychosis, but which resolved instead, due to reduction in stress, enhanced supports, coping, and so forth.

the importance of calculating the relative risk of precursor features including adding in a time factor, i.e. calculations aimed at estimating the relative risk of full-blown syndrome 'x' in follow up period 'y' conferred by precursor feature 'a'. This type of calculation would enable screening and identification of those at high risk and, if effective interventions were available, preventive treatment.

2 THE ONSET OF PSYCHOTIC DISORDER

Table 2.3. *Patient clinical status and the measurement of markers*

Clinical status	Markers
True positive	Specific markers present
False positive	Specific markers absent
False false positive	Specific markers present

The challenge of false positives for indicated prevention

It follows then that the major clinical difficulty in an indicated prevention approach is the issue of false positives. This is especially the case in psychotic disorders because, as we have seen, many of the characteristic prodromal features are non-specific. Falloon's (1992) pioneering work in attempting to identify and intervene in 'prodromal cases of schizophrenia' is reviewed more fully in Chapter 4. However, the point needs to be made that the issue of false positives arose in his project, and Falloon himself acknowledged that some individuals may have been treated unnecessarily (Falloon, 1992). As can be seen from some of the literature reviewed before, if all year 11 students in our survey (McGorry et al., 1995) presenting with DSM-III-R prodromal features of schizophrenia (APA, 1987) were treated, at least 10–15%, and up to 50%, of them could receive an intervention! Obviously, work needs to be done on refining risk factors for development of psychosis and examining the interplay of various state and trait risk factors.

Recently our group has developed a specialized clinic, the Personal Assessment and Crisis Evaluation (PACE) clinic (Yung et al., 1995; Yung & McGorry, 1996a) which aims to follow up possible 'prodromal' cases. Research taking place in the clinic aims to examine the 'natural history' of these putatively prodromal syndromes and to assess the relative risks and predictive powers of several variables in the 'at risk' group. The clinic is described in more detail in Chapter 4. Variables being measured include state markers such as various precursor symptoms and signs, and trait markers such as family history of psychotic disorder (Gottesman & Shields, 1982), structural brain abnormalities (Kelsoe et al., 1988; Lieberman et al., 1993; Rossi et al., 1994; Seidman et al., 1994), and abnormalities of cognitive functioning including attentional dysfunction as measured by the Continuous Performance Task (CPT) (Cornblatt & Keilp, 1994). Subjects are recruited via two different strategies: first, by using those psychopathological features which have been reported in the literature as having some specificity for subsequent transition to psychosis, including attenuated symptoms of psychosis (Cameron, 1938; Chapman, 1966, 1967) and transient self-limited psychotic symptoms (Yung & McGorry, 1996a); and, secondly, by combining risk factors to identify a group with enhanced risk of psychotic disorder. This is known as a 'close in' strategy (Bell, 1992). We combined the trait risk factors of family history of psychotic disorder (Gottesman & Shields, 1982) or schizotypal personality disorder (Meehl, 1962, 1989), with the state risk factor of mental state changes sufficient to result in a significant decline in functioning of greater than one month (full details of the inclusion criteria are included in Chapter 4). The additional risk factor of age was also added as an inclusion criterion, i.e. subjects are aged between 16 and 30 – the age of maximum risk for becoming psychotic (Kosky & Hardy, 1992). We are following cases for two years, recognizing that this is the mean duration of prodromal periods and therefore the time period likely to confer the maximum risk for emerging psychosis.

Our experience in the clinic to date suggests that we can identify a group at high risk of transition to psychosis in a brief (i.e. two year) follow-up period (Yung & McGorry, 1996a). We are aiming to further refine our predictive power by examination of the above risk factors but also intend to trial different interventions in an attempt to determine which treatments should be used with this group. We have chosen to focus on at-risk populations who have been strictly defined, sought by, and referred to our clinic, electing not to make any attempt to generalize our set of predictive variables beyond such a defined sample to the general community. We recognize that our ability to detect psychosis in the general community will be severely limited simply on statistical grounds, i.e. the low base rate of psychosis in the community and the error rate associated with our detection procedure (Dawes, 1994). To illustrate this, let us assume a hypothetical example whereby we have developed a screening based on a set of predictive variables derived in a 'clinical' sample. The detection procedure consists of an algorithm derived from a logistic regression comprising multiple risk factors and prodromal symptoms, all of which are accorded weightings. The sensitivity of the algorithm (the detection procedure) is 75%, and its specificity is 80%. Let us assume that the base rate of all psychosis is approximately 3 in 100 in the general community – a generous assumption, given that this is the prevalence and not the annual incidence. In our hypothetical community, the population numbers 10 000 persons. Using the formulae provided by Arkes (1981, p. 328), the probability that we will detect a psychotic person with our procedure is only approximately 8.5%. This result indicates the sheer magnitude of the detection task beyond the at-risk or pre-clinical samples. So, what is an apparently feasible task for a 'precursor' sample using a close follow-up strategy, becomes a totally non-feasible one when attempting to detect cases in the general community.

Conclusion

The prodromal phase of psychosis is an area of great potential in prevention and early intervention psychosis. The clinical features found in this phase have been described by reference to retrospective studies. It is possible to apply this knowledge prospectively in an attempt to intervene in high-risk young people before the advent of frank psychosis. However, these mental state changes need to be viewed as a state risk factor for psychosis rather than as inevitable precursors to the condition, and the possibility of false positives needs to be recognized. Ongoing research is needed, in particular the assessment of the predictive value of certain psychopathological features and identification of any specific phenomena, as well as examination of other trait markers for psychosis, such as neurobiological, neurochemical, and neuropsychological abnormalities. Such research has the potential to prevent, or at least minimize, a great deal of psychosocial disability associated with psychotic disorders such as schizophrenia, at least in those patients deemed in need of referral for their difficulties.

References

American Psychiatric Association (1980). *Diagnostic and Statistical Manual of Mental Disorders*, 3rd edn. Washington DC: American Psychiatric Association.

American Psychiatric Association (1987). *Diagnostic and Statistical Manual of Mental Disorders*, 3rd edn, revised. Washington DC: American Psychiatric Association.

American Psychiatric Association (1992). *Report from the DSM-IV Field Trial for Schizophrenia and Related Psychotic Disorders* (M. Flaum, MD, Field Trial Coordinator). Iowa City, Iowa: University of Iowa.

American Psychiatric Association (1994). *Diagnostic and Statistical Manual of Mental Disorders*, 4th edn. Washington DC: American Psychiatric Association.

Andreasen, N. C. & Flaum, M. (1991). Schizophrenia. The characteristic symptoms. *Schizophrenia Bulletin*, **17**, 27–49.

Arkes, H. R. (1981). Impediments to accurate clinical judgment and possible ways to minimise their impact. *Journal of Consulting and Clinical Psychology*, **49**, 323–30.

Baddeley, A. (1993). *Your Memory: A User's Guide.* Harmondsworth, Middlesex, UK: Penguin.
Basic Behavioral Science Task Force of the National Mental Health Council (1996). Basic behavioral science for mental health: thought and communication. *American Psychologist,* **51,** 181–9.
Beiser, M., Erickson, D., Fleming, J. A. & Iacono, W. G. (1993). Establishing the onset of psychotic illness. *American Journal of Psychiatry,* **150,** 1349–54.
Bell, R. Q. (1992). Multiple-risk cohorts and segmenting risk as solutions to the problem of false positives in risk for the major psychoses. *Psychiatry,* **55,** 370–81.
Birchwood, M., Smith, J., Macmillan, J. F., Hogg, B., Prasad, R., Harvey, C. & Bering, S. (1989). Predicting relapse in schizophrenia: the development and implementation of an early signs monitoring system using patients and families as observers, a preliminary investigation. *Psychological Medicine,* **19,** 649–56.
Bleuler, E. (1911). *Dementia Praecox or the Group of Schizophrenias.* New York: International Universities Press.
Bowers, M. (1965). The onset of psychosis – a diary account. *Psychiatry,* **28,** 346–58.
Bowers, M. B. (1968). Pathogenesis of acute schizophrenic psychosis. *Archives of General Psychiatry,* **19,** 348–55.
Bowers, M. B. & Freedman, D. X. (1966). 'Psychedelic' experiences in acute psychoses. *Archives of General Psychiatry,* **15,** 240–8.
Cameron, D. E. (1938). Early schizophrenia. *American Journal of Psychiatry,* **95,** 567–78.
Carlson, G. A. & Goodwin, F. K. (1973). The stages of mania. *Archives of General Psychiatry,* **28,** 221–8.
Chapman, J. (1966). The early symptoms of schizophrenia. *British Journal of Psychiatry,* **112,** 225–51.
Chapman, J. (1967). Visual imagery and motor phenomena in acute schizophrenia. *British Journal of Psychiatry,* **113,** 771–8.
Conrad, K. (1958). *Die Beginnende Schizophrenie.* Stuttgart: Georg Thieme Verlag.
Cornblatt, B. A. & Keilp, J. G. (1994). Impaired attention, genetics, and the pathophysiology of schizophrenia. *Schizophrenia Bulletin,* **20,** 31–47.
Dawes, R. M. (1994). *House of Cards. Psychology and Psychotherapy Built on Myth.* New York: The Free Press.
Docherty, J. P., Van Kammen, D. P., Siris, S. G. & Marder, S. R. (1978). Stages of onset of schizophrenic psychosis. *American Journal of Psychiatry,* **135,** 420–6.
Donlon, P. T. & Blacker, K. H. (1973). Stages of schizophrenic decompensation and reintegration. *Journal of Nervous and Mental Disease,* **157,** 200–9.
Eaton, W. W., Badawi, M. & Melton, B. (1995). Prodromes and precursors: epidemiologic data for primary prevention of disorders with slow onset. *American Journal of Psychiatry,* **152,** 967–72.
Endicott, J., Nee, J., Fleiss, J., Cohen, J., Williams, J. B. W. & Simon, R. (1982). Diagnostic criteria for schizophrenia: reliabilities and agreement between systems. *Archives of General Psychiatry,* **39,** 884–9.
Falloon, I. R. H. (1992). Early intervention for first episodes of schizophrenia: a

preliminary exploration. *Psychiatry*, **55**, 4–15.
Fava, G. A. & Kellner, R. (1991). Prodromal symptoms in affective disorders. *American Journal of Psychiatry*, **148**, 823–30.
Fish, F. J. (1976). *Fish's Schizophrenia*. Bristol: John Wright and Sons.
Gottesman, I. I. & Shields, J. (1982). *Schizophrenia: The Epigenetic Puzzle*. Cambridge: Cambridge University Press.
Haas, G. L. & Sweeney, J. A. (1992). Premorbid and onset features of first-episode schizophrenia. *Schizophrenia Bulletin*, **18**, 373–86.
Häfner, H. (1989). Application of epidemiological research toward a model for the etiology of schizophrenia. *Schizophrenia Research*, **2**, 375–83.
Häfner, H., Riecher-Rössler, A., Maurer, K., Fätkenheuer, B. & Löffler, W. (1992a). First onset and early symptomatology of schizophrenia. A chapter of epidemiological and neurobiological research into age and sex differences. *European Archives of Psychiatry and Clinical Neurosciences*, **242**, 109–18.
Häfner, H., Riecher-Rössler, A., Hambrecht, M., Maurer, K., Meissner, S., Schmidtke, A., Fätkenheuer, B., Löffler, W. & van der Heiden, W. (1992b) IRAOS: an instrument for the assessment of onset and early course of schizophrenia. *Schizophrenia Research*, **6**, 209–23.
Häfner, H., Maurer, K., Löffler, W. & Riecher-Rössler, A. (1993). The influence of age and sex on the onset and early course of schizophrenia. *British Journal of Psychiatry*, **162**, 80–6.
Häfner, H., Maurer, K., Löffler, W., Fätkenheuer, B., van der Heiden, W., Riecher-Rössler, A., Behrens, S. & Gattaz, W.F. (1994). The epidemiology of early schizophrenia. Influence of age and gender on onset and early course. *British Journal of Psychiatry*, **164** (Supplement 23), 29–38.
Häfner, H., Maurer, K., Löffler, W., Bustamante, S., an der Heiden, W., Riecher-Rössler, A. & Nowotny, B. (1995). Onset and early course of schizophrenia. In *Search for the Causes of Schizophrenia*, Vol III, ed. H. Häfner & W. F. Gattaz, pp. 43–66. Berlin: Springer-Verlag.
Hambrecht, M., Häfner, H. & Löffler, W. (1994). Beginning schizophrenia observed by significant others. *Social Psychiatry and Psychiatric Epidemiology*, **29**, 53–60.
Hays, P. (1964). Modes of onset of psychotic depression. *British Medical Journal*, **2**, 779–84.
Heinrichs, D. W. & Carpenter, W. T. (1985). Prospective study of prodromal symptoms in schizophrenic relapse. *American Journal of Psychiatry*, **142**, 371–3.
Heinrichs, D. W., Cohen, B. P. & Carpenter, W. T. (1985). Early insight and the management of schizophrenic decompensation. *Journal of Nervous and Mental Disease*, **173**, 133–8.
Henderson, A. S. (1988). *An Introduction to Social Psychiatry*. Oxford: Oxford University Press.
Herz, M. I. & Melville, C. (1980). Relapse in schizophrenia. *American Journal of Psychiatry*, **137**, 801–5.
Herz, M. I., Glazer, W., Mirza, M., Mostert, M. & Hafez, H. (1989). Treating prodromal episodes to prevent relapse in schizophrenia. *British Journal of Psychiatry*, **155**, (Supplement), 123–7.
Hirsch, S., Cramer, P. & Bowen, J. (1992). The triggering hypothesis of the role

of life events in schizophrenia. *British Journal of Psychiatry*, **161** (Supplement 18), 84–7.

Huber, G., Gross, G., Schuttler, R. & Linz, M. (1980). Longitudinal studies of schizophrenic patients. *Schizophrenia Bulletin*, **6**, 592–605.

Jackson, H. J., McGorry, P. D. & McKenzie, D. (1994). The reliability of DSM-III prodromal symptoms in first episode psychotic patients. *Acta Psychiatrica Scandinavica*, **90**, 375–8.

Jackson, H. J., McGorry, P. D. & Dudgeon, P. (1995). Prodromal symptoms of schizophrenia in first episode psychosis: prevalence and specificity. *Comprehensive Psychiatry*, **36**, 241–50.

Jackson, H. J., McGorry, P. D., Dakis, J., Harrigan, S., Henry, L. & Mihalopoulos, C. (1996). The inter-rater and test–retest reliabilities of prodromal symptoms in first-episode psychosis. *Australian and New Zealand Journal of Psychiatry*, **30**, 498–504.

Jones, P. B., Bebbington, P., Foerster, A., Lewis, S. W., Murray, R. M., Russell, A., Sham, P.C., Toone, B.K. & Wilkins, S. (1993). Premorbid social underachievement in schizophrenia. Results from the Camberwell Collaborative Psychosis Study. *British Journal of Psychiatry*, **162**, 65–71.

Keith, S. J. & Matthews, S. M. (1991). The diagnosis of schizophrenia: a review of onset and duration issues. *Schizophrenia Bulletin*, **17**, 51–67.

Kelsoe, J. R., Cadet, J. L., Pickar, D. & Weinberger, D. R. (1988). Quantitative neuroanatomy in schizophrenia. A controlled magnetic resonance imaging study. *Archives of General Psychiatry*, **45**, 533–41.

Kosky, R. & Hardy, J. (1992). Mental health: is early intervention the key? *Medical Journal of Australia*, **156**, 147–8.

Kraepelin, E. [1919] (1971). *Dementia Praecox and Paraphrenia*. New York: Robert E. Krieger Publishing Co.

Kraepelin, E. (1987). *Memoirs*. Berlin: Springer.

Larsen, T. K., McGlashan, T. H. & Moe, L. C. (1996). First-episode schizophrenia: I. Early course parameters. *Schizophrenia Bulletin*, **22**, 241–56.

Levy, S. T., McGlashan, T. H. & Carpenter, W. T. (1975). Integration and sealing over as recovery styles from acute psychosis. *Journal of Nervous and Mental Disease*, **161**, 307–12.

Lieberman, J. A., Jody, D., Alvir, J. M., Ashtari, M., Levy, D. L., Bogerts, B., Degreef, G., Mayerhoff, D.I. & Cooper, J. (1993). Brain morphology, dopamine, and eye-tracking abnormalities in first-episode schizophrenia: prevalence and clinical correlates. *Archives of General Psychiatry*, **50**, 57–68.

Loebel, A. D., Lieberman, J. A., Alvir, J. M., Mayerhoff, D. I., Geisler, S. H. & Szymanski, S. R. (1992). Duration of psychosis and outcome in first-episode schizophrenia. *American Journal of Psychiatry*, **149**, 1183–8.

Loftus, E. F. (1993). The reality of repressed memories. *American Psychologist*, **48**, 518–37.

Malla, A. K. & Norman, R. M. (1994). Prodromal symptoms in schizophrenia. *British Journal of Psychiatry*, **164**, 487–93.

McGhie, A. & Chapman, J. (1961). Disorders of attention and perception in early schizophrenia. *British Journal of Medical Psychology*, **34**, 103–15.

McGlashan, T. H. (1996). Early detection and intervention in schizophrenia: Editor's introduction. *Schizophrenia Bulletin*, **22**, 197–9.

McGlashan, T. H., Levy, S. T. & Carpenter, W. T. (1975). Integration and sealing over. Clinically distinct recovery styles from schizophrenia. *Archives of General Psychiatry*, **32**, 1269–72.

McGorry, P. D. (1994). The influence of illness duration on syndrome clarity and stability in functional psychosis: does the diagnosis emerge and stabilise with time? *Australian and New Zealand Journal of Psychiatry*, **28**, 607–19.

McGorry, P. D. & Singh, B. S. (1995). Schizophrenia: risk and possibility. In *Handbook of Preventive Psychiatry*, ed. B. Raphael & G. D. Burrows, pp. 492–514. Amsterdam: Elsevier.

McGorry, P. D., McFarlane, C., Patton, G.C., Bell, R., Hibbert, M.E., Jackson, H. & Bowes, G. (1995). The prevalence of prodromal features of schizophrenia in adolescence: a preliminary survey. *Acta Psychiatrica Scandinavica*, **90**, 375–8.

Meares, A. (1959). The diagnosis of prepsychotic schizophrenia. *Lancet*, **i**, 55–9.

Meehl, P. E. (1962). Schizotaxia, schizotypy, schizophrenia. *American Psychologist*, **17**, 827–38.

Meehl, P. E. (1989). Schizotaxia revisited. *Archives of General Psychiatry*, **46**, 935–44.

Molnar, G., Feeney, M. G. & Fava, G. A. (1988). Duration and symptoms of bipolar prodromes. *American Journal of Psychiatry*, **145**, 1576–8.

Montaigne (1580–1588). In *The International Thesaurus of Quotations*, ed. R. T. Tripp, p. 74. New York: Penguin (1970).

Murphy, J. M., Sobol, A. M., Olivier, D. C., Monson, R. R., Leighton, A. H. & Pratt, L. A. (1989). Prodromes of depression and anxiety. The Stirling County Study. *British Journal of Psychiatry*, **155**, 490–5.

Offenkrantz, W. (1962). Multiple somatic complaints as a precursor of schizophrenia. *American Journal of Psychiatry*, **119**, 258–9.

Olin, S. S. & Mednick, S. A. (1996). Risk factors of psychosis: identifying vulnerable populations premorbidly. *Schizophrenia Bulletin*, **22**, 223–40.

Patton, G.C., Hibbert, M., Rosier, M.J., Carlin, J.B., Caust, J. & Bowes, G. (1996). Is smoking associated with depression and anxiety in teenagers? *American Journal of Public Health*, **86**, 225–30.

Robins, L. N., Helzer, J. E., Croughan, J. & Ratcliff, K. A. (1981). National Institute of Mental Health Diagnostic Interview Schedule: its history, characteristics and validity. *Archives of General Psychiatry*, **38**, 381–9.

Rossi, A., Stratta, P., Mancini, F., Gallucci, M., Mattei, P., Core, L., D. Michele, V. & Casacchia, M. (1994). Magnetic resonance imaging findings of amygdala–anterior hippocampus shrinkage in male patients with schizophrenia. *Psychiatry Research*, **52**, 43–53.

Seidman, L. J., Yurgelun-Todd, D., Kremen, W. S., Woods, B. T., Goldstein, J. M., Faraone, S. V. & Tsuang, M.T. (1994). Relationship of prefrontal and temporal lobe MRI measures to neuropsychological performance in chronic schizophrenia. *Biological Psychiatry*, **35**, 235–46.

Singer, J. A. & Salovey, P. (1993). *The Remembered Self: Emotion and Memory in Personality*. New York: Free Press.

Stein, W. J. (1967). The sense of becoming psychotic. *Psychiatry*, **30**, 262–75.
Sullivan, H. S. (1994). The onset of schizophrenia. *American Journal of Psychiatry*, **151** (Sequicentennial Supplement), 135–9.
Tennant, C. C. (1985). Stress and schizophrenia. *Integrative Psychiatry*, **3**, 248–61.
Tien, A. Y. & Eaton, W. W. (1992). Psychopathological precursors and sociodemographic risk factors for the schizophrenia syndrome. *Archives of General Psychiatry*, **49**, 37–46.
Turk, D. C. & Salovey, P. (1985). Cognitive structures, cognitive processes, and cognitive-behavior modification: II. Judgements and inferences of the clinician. *Cognitive Therapy and Research*, **9**, 19–33.
Varsamis, J. & Adamson, J. D. (1971). Early schizophrenia. *Canadian Psychiatric Association Journal*, **16**, 487–97.
Winokur, G. (1976). Duration of illness prior to hospitalisation (onset) in the affective disorders. *Neuropsychobiology*, **2**, 87–93.
World Health Organization (1994). *Manual of the International Classification of Diseases, Injuries and Causes of Death*. Geneva, Switzerland: World Health Organization.
Yung, A. R. & McGorry, P. D. (1996a). The prodromal phase of first episode psychosis: past and current conceptualisations. *Schizophrenia Bulletin*, **22**, 353–70.
Yung, A. R. & McGorry, P. D. (1996b). The initial prodrome in psychosis: descriptive and qualitative aspects. *Australian and New Zealand Journal of Psychiatry*, **30**, 587–99.
Yung, A. R., McGorry, P. D., McFarlane, C. A. & Patton, G. (1995). The PACE Clinic: development of a clinical service for young people at high risk of psychosis. *Australasian Psychiatry*, **3**, 345–9.
Yung, A. R., McGorry, P. D., McFarlane, C. A., Jackson, H. J., Patton, G. C. & Rakkar, A. (1996). Monitoring and care of young people at incipient risk of psychosis. *Schizophrenia Bulletin*, **22**, 283–303.

3

Pathways to care in early psychosis: clinical and consumer perspectives

CLARE LINCOLN AND PATRICK D. MCGORRY

Introduction

This chapter explores various issues related to the access of young people with early psychosis to initial treatment, with studies having typically reported that these consumers experience delays in obtaining help (Lincoln & McGorry, 1995). The late presentation of these patients to services is associated with slower and less complete recovery (Helgason, 1977, 1990; Loebel et al., 1992; McGorry et al., 1996), and long-term follow-up studies confirm that disability develops during the early years (Bleuler, 1978; Carpenter & Strauss, 1991; McGlashan & Carpenter, 1988), with clinicians asserting that earlier intervention may reduce subsequent levels of disability (Birchwood & Macmillan, 1993; McGorry, 1992).

The notion of a 'pathway to care' has been advanced as a helpful concept (Gallo et al., 1995a,b; Goldberg & Huxley, 1980, 1992; Manktelow, 1994; Rogler & Cortes, 1993; Sheppard, 1993; Spicker et al., 1995). Examining the routes to initial treatment for individuals with an emergent psychosis may increase our understanding of the barriers to care, whilst understanding those pathways may assist clinicians in targeting better intervention strategies.

The experiences of young people with a psychotic illness are unique to the individual, and their personal narratives (Strauss, 1994) provide a different lens through which to view the pathways experience. Actively listening to lay experiences of help-seeking and help-receiving in a first contact group may raise awareness amongst clinicians that consumers have a complex and generally misunderstood 'discourse' or story-line, which needs to be 'given a voice' if service providers are to respond adequately to this patient group's needs. The ambivalent and contradictory views which consumers seem to hold about their experiences of the 'pathway to care' may help to explain why treatment delays have failed to be addressed.

While the potential of early intervention in psychotic disorders is becoming increasingly accepted by clinicians and researchers, our research data suggest that the wider community has yet to appreciate its value, although the need for early intervention is gaining recognition amongst the public in relation to some serious medical illnesses, notably hypertension and cancer. It appears that the notion of delay may be a clinician-centred concept 'resisted' by a significant proportion of patients who reluctantly seek treatment and view psychiatric services in a negative light. Nevertheless, clinicians are gradually turning their attention to developing innovative and more responsive services for young people with psychotic disorders. This could be relatively congruent with the challenges to the system posed by consumers contributing to a process of reform. Ultimately, consumer empowerment is the common theme (or strategy) which may facilitate secondary prevention and enhance young people's chances of recovery.

This chapter provides an overview of the key research into treatment delay in this population. Personal narratives are utilized to illuminate a 'topographical' view of the pathways, in which helping contacts prior to first treatment have been recorded as well as the nature of the experience itself. Discussion highlights how understanding a consumer combined with a clinical–epidemiological perspective sheds light on the contradictions involved and has implications for service delivery. A broader review of the literature is available elsewhere (Lincoln & McGorry, 1995).

Landscape of delay

There are two main areas of psychiatric research literature which are of particular relevance here: the first area includes studies which have examined pathways to care in common mental disorders such as depression and anxiety; the second area includes studies with a specific focus examining treatment delays in first-episode psychosis.

If the focus is not sharpened beyond the general literature, one might wonder whether treatment delay constitutes a problem. The relative intervals in time between the onset of problems and being seen by mental illness services, associated with various pathways to care, have been studied in a number of related studies (Gater et al., 1991). Goldberg & Huxley (1980, 1992) describe a number of filters which are selectively permeable to severe mental disorders and which ensure that those with schizophrenia and related disorders obtain treatment quickly. However, in a recent Italian study (Balestrieri et al., 1994), psychotic patients were shown to have a median interval before seeking any care, of more than three months, although specialist services were quickly accessed once the patient had decided to consult a professional. In contrast, in the United Kingdom, patients were shown to have a short median interval of two weeks between first experiencing psychotic symptoms and presentation to first carer (Gater & Goldberg, 1991). These patients were also rapidly referred to specialist mental health services. This pattern may only be true for known cases of psychotic disorders, in contrast to first-episode cases. Indeed, it seems probable that the general literature and first-episode studies are not readily comparable (Cole et al., 1995). Research covered by the former includes studies that focus on help-seeking pathways in a broad spectrum of 'newly referred patients'; only some of these will be psychotic patients accessing mental health services for the first time (Lincoln & McGorry, 1995).

A more specific examination of first-episode studies provides compelling evidence that treatment delay is a hallmark of early psychosis (Helgason, 1977, 1990; Johnstone et al., 1986; Loebel et al., 1992). This finding has surprised many, given the severity of the disorders involved; however, in other 'less severe' disorders, such as anxiety and depression, in addition to the problem of delay, there are higher proportions of individuals whose condition is never detected or remains untreated. Arguably, the majority of those experiencing a psychotic episode will reach services and be treated at some stage. Unfortunately, even when we confine our examination to first-episode studies only, comparisons between the studies constituting this domain are not easily made (Beiser et al., 1993; Docherty et al., 1978; Haas & Sweeney, 1992; Keith & Mathews, 1991; Keshavan & Schooler, 1992). Notwithstanding certain methodological limitations, which include the widely discrepant definitions and criteria used for the populations in the studies and difficulties measuring illness onset and durations (Keith & Mathews, 1991; Keshavan & Schooler, 1992), most studies report extensive delays and the negative impact of delayed or inadequate treatment (Lincoln & McGorry, 1995; McGorry et al., 1996).

Review of studies

The Northwick Park study is notable for its focus on pathways to initial treatment and highlighted delay as a major problem (Johnstone et al., 1986). In a cohort of 253 first-episode patients, this study established that the interval between onset of psychosis and hospital admission was often more than one year. Although in 73 cases (28.8% of the sample) admission was arranged after no more than three contacts, in 46 cases (18.2% of the sample) at least nine contacts were made before reaching a helper who arranged admission. The Northwick Park data and those of similar studies (Beiser et al., 1993; Gift et al., 1981; Loebel et al., 1992) demonstrate that individuals may live in the community for extended periods with untreated psychotic psychopathology. In a 20-year follow-up of patients first presenting with schizophrenia, Helgason (1977, 1990) recorded a mean delay of 6–7 years, this being measured from the time of onset of symptoms until initial contact with a psychiatrist. No patient sought treatment within the first year of the onset of their symptoms, with the majority of patients seeking treatment after 2.5 years of illness onset.

Loebel et al. (1992) measured treatment delay taking into account, amongst other variables, diagnostic and gender differences. For the sample, the total mean duration of psychotic symptoms before initial treatment was 52 weeks, with a mean duration of illness, from the onset of prodromal symptoms, of 151 weeks. Male patients were consistently younger at the onset of psychotic symptoms, and the duration of untreated psychotic symptoms was more than twice as long for males compared with females. Length of illness before psychiatric treatment was not correlated with age at onset, mode of onset, pre-morbid adjustment, or severity of illness at entry into the study.

Similarly, Beiser et al. (1993) established that for patients with schizophrenia, the interval between first psychotic symptoms and treatment seeking was, on average, more than one year. As in our own study (McGorry et al., 1996), the treatment lag time for patients with affective psychosis was much shorter. The prodromal period (defined as the period dated from the first noticeable signs to the first prominent psychotic symptoms) was highly variable in length. Unexpectedly, an insidious prolonged prodrome proved as characteristic of affective psychosis as of schizophrenia. The research by Beiser et al. highlights a difficulty in distinguishing retrospectively in this age group between stable (albeit compromised) pre-morbid functioning and true prodromal features in those cases with longer prodromes. The work of Häfner et al. (1992) has addressed this issue and has contributed to a clearer understanding of the patterns leading up to the onset of schizophrenia.

During the period 1989–92, we conducted a prospective follow-up study of 200 first-episode cases, in which patterns of delay, similar to those found elsewhere, were demonstrated in our own region (McGorry, Singh & Copolov, 1990; McGorry et al., 1990, 1996). For the 61 patients meeting criteria for schizophrenia, the mean duration of untreated psychosis was 508.9 days ($SD = 1035.0$), with a median of 122.0 days. The duration of the prodromal period in the 52 patients with schizophrenia who experienced a prodrome was 779.2 days ($SD = 1089.9$) with a median of 390.5 days. For the total sample including those in the non-schizophrenia group ($n = 139$), the mean duration of untreated psychosis was 193.7 days ($SD = 615.6$) while the median was 25.0 days.

Our findings indicate that, when median delays are relatively low, as they tend to be in affective disorders, a further reduction in the period of untreated psychosis may not be feasible. Conversely, our data highlights that there may be real scope for reductions in delay for those with schizophrenia. Longer recorded delays in the schizophrenia group are partly due to the six-month criterion but may also be due to the difficulty in recognizing psychosis in the context of an insidious onset. It is within this same group that one finds a significant subsample of 'outliers' who produced large standard deviations on duration variables, and who could be a target for early intervention strategies. There may also be a 'critical period' following the emergence of frank psychosis, during which treatment will have most impact on remission or recovery. As can be seen from Figure 3.1, our data suggest that more than one month of untreated psychosis but less than six months of psychosis may constitute the boundaries of such a 'critical period'. If the psychosis has been present for less than one month before treatment commences, then outcome is good anyway. Similarly, if the psychosis lasts for longer than six months before treatment begins, then the outcome is worse (McGorry et al., 1996).

Within the 1–6 month 'window', there may be an opportunity for early intervention, since if intensive treatment is offered during this phase, in contrast to earlier approaches, the outcome seems to be significantly better. The two curves in Figure 3.1 pertain to different models of service delivery with greater sophistication and more resources involved in the EPPIC sample when contrasted with the pre-EPPIC sample. There is a significant difference between the samples only between one and six months of untreated psychosis. (It seems possible that if delay is significant but not too protracted, there is an opportunity for a therapeutic 'rescue' to be mounted which, if intensive enough, can change the early course of the disorder.) Other explanations for these data are clearly possible, yet the pattern is intriguing.

Risk factors for delay

Age of onset, gender, and diagnosis, are all potentially interactive factors associated with delay. Deviant behaviour amongst adolescents

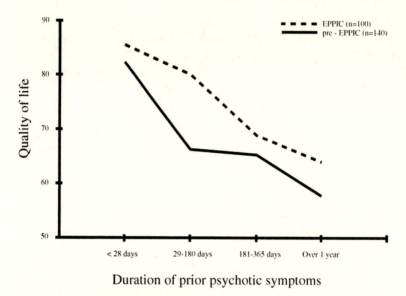

Figure 3.1. The relationship of duration of untreated psychosis (DUP) to 12-month outcome in first-episode psychosis.

may be tolerated by the community and young males may be at particular risk of their illness going undetected (Loebel et al., 1992). Psychopathology influences clinical presentation and similarly influences what attracts attention and leads to intervention (Beiser et al., 1993; Gift et al., 1981; Loebel et al., 1992). Although insidious onset is characteristic of both schizophrenia and affective psychosis, mood disturbance and a more florid symptom picture in affective psychosis, incorporating an effect similar to Berkson's bias (1946), may partly explain why the initiation of treatment seeking can be longer for schizophrenia than for affective psychosis (Beiser et al., 1993).

Gift et al. (1981) noted wide variation in the chronicity of psychotic symptoms prior to admission. In their first-admission study of individuals with schizophrenia, 20% of the patients had been symptomatic for more than two years. Furthermore, Gift and his colleagues reported that patients with high levels of paranoid symptoms tended to spend a long time in the community after the onset of psychotic symptoms, and prior to their being hospitalized. Interestingly, in our first-episode study we noted that symptoms such as social withdrawal and persecutory delusions were associated with delayed presentation, suggesting that these symptoms in particular, may confer a high risk for treatment delay (McGorry et al., 1996).

The impact of delay

Clinicians increasingly believe that failure to obtain early treatment is likely to have negative consequences (Lincoln & McGorry, 1995). The social consequences of early-onset psychotic disorder are just becoming apparent, with vocational and educational attainment being a major casualty (Kessler et al., 1995).

Delay has been associated with considerable difficulties for patients and families alike (Helgason, 1990; Humphreys et al., 1992; Johnstone et al., 1986; Mintz et al., 1989). For example, just becoming a patient may confer unintended negative consequences (Lally, 1989; McGorry et al., 1991), including stigma for consumers and carers (Fink & Tasman, 1992; Hatfield & Lefley, 1994).

However, if it is true that much of the psychosocial decline in schizophrenia occurs prior to initial treatment, as is suggested by Jones et al. (1993), then the stakes are raised when weighing up the benefits of early intervention alongside the potential disadvantages, namely the iatrogenic effects of being treated in the psychiatric system. This balance in favour of early commencement of treatment is further influenced by accumulating evidence that acute psychotic symptoms reflect an active morbid process, which, if not addressed by early neuroleptic treatment, may result in more tenacious and prolonged morbidity (Stahl, 1994; Wyatt, 1991a,b, 1998). In addition, it appears that people with schizophrenia presenting to services late incur double the health care costs in the three years subsequent to their first contact, as compared with a similar patient group presenting earlier (within six months) to treatment services (Moscarelli, Capri & Nerri, 1991).

Longitudinal studies have linked the period of untreated psychosis with prognosis and outcome. Helgason (1977, 1990) found that outcomes were better for those patients with schizophrenia who sought treatment earlier than for those with later presentations. Late-admitted patients were admitted more often and stayed longer than those admitted early.

In a study of 70 first-episode schizophrenia patients, Loebel et al. (1992) concluded that duration of psychotic symptoms before treatment was significantly associated with time to remission and level of remission. Longer duration of illness since onset of any prodromal symptoms was also associated with degree of remission. This was not a function of insidious onset, since mode of onset was not associated with time to remission nor significantly associated with level of remission. Loebel et al.'s finding provides support for delay having an independent effect on level and rate of recovery.

In a similar fashion to Loebel et al. (1992), we examined the relationship between the duration of untreated psychosis and outcome in a sample of 200 first-episode cases (McGorry et al., 1996). The duration of untreated psychosis was moderately correlated with duration of psychotic symptoms during the first hospitalization ($r = 0.33$, $p < 0.0001$) and with severity of symptoms for both BPRS and SANS scores, being $r = 0.26, p = 0.002$, respectively, at 12-month follow-up. Furthermore, the Quality of Life Scale (Heinrichs, Hanlon & Carpenter, 1984) scores were negatively correlated with the duration of untreated psychosis ($r = -0.38, p < 0.001$). In summary, there were better levels and rates of recovery in those patients with a shorter duration of untreated psychosis. Clearly, variables such as diagnosis and symptomatology could be correlated with duration of untreated psychosis, and help to explain the associations observed. We can speculate that more serious illnesses with poorer outcomes might be characterized by specific symptoms or patterns of symptoms, which in themselves might lead to delayed presentation. While the exact role that delays play in influencing outcomes is only likely to be clarified by an intervention study, it seems logical that illness duration can be viewed as a dynamic and relatively independent variable with a range of contributing factors, and with considerable influence upon short-term outcomes (McGlashan, 1996; McGorry et al., 1996).

Topography of the pathways

We now examine the 'topography' of the initial pathway, an approach which encompasses more than a mapping of key referral nodes or helper contacts, symptoms and helper response. By extension, it includes personal or contextual factors and allows for an appreciation of consumer experiences. What follows is descriptive but illuminates a paradox; namely, the barriers and inefficiencies in the pathways experienced by many patients, contrasting with the reluctance and resistance of other patients to follow them.

In a study carried out by one of the authors (CL), examining the nature and extent of delays in first-episode psychosis, 40 men and 22 women with a mean age of 22.8 years were interviewed in order to map the topography of the pathways. This sample was a subset of cases drawn from our larger samples of first-episode psychosis and the interview group ($n = 62$) and non-interview group ($n = 88$) were similar in terms of age, age of onset, education, and marital status. Diagnosis, duration of untreated psychosis, and duration of prodome were also not significantly different.

Within this sample, a total of 307 helping contacts with a variety of professionals and non-professionals was recorded. The mean number of contacts per person was 4.9 ($SD = 2.8$), with a range of 1–17 contacts. Just over half of the patients (55%) had 4–6 contacts, nearly one-third (29%) had 1–3 contacts, and 16% had more than six helper contacts. These figures are comparable with, although a little lower than, those reported in the Northwick Park study (Johnstone et al., 1986). Some of the differences may be explained by the way that, in our study and in this instance, the helping contacts were calculated. Each help-seeking contact was recorded solely on the basis of consumer self-reports; contacts which were part of an ongoing 'treatment' arrangement between the young person and helper, were not included when mapping the inital pathway.

Data indicate that general practitioners (GPs) have a potentially significant role in the recognition of psychosis, especially early on in the pathway. Thirty-six per cent of the patients' initial help-seeking contacts were with a GP, although some avoided their own GP. As many as 50% had consulted a GP and almost invariably this was prior to initial effective treatment. Contrary to what one might expect, there were no significant age differences among those consulting, or not consulting, GPs.

There appears to be a 'natural' progression from non-psychiatric to psychiatric services, so that only those who require specialist intervention receive it (Goldberg & Huxley, 1980, 1992). We can speculate that individuals initially look towards non-psychiatric sources of help to avoid contact with unfamiliar and stigmatizing services. To some extent this is appropriate, but it is consequently important that primary health care personnel are sensitized and appropriately trained to detect the occasional cases of potential serious mental illness that they encounter.

There appears to be enormous potential for delays, especially in reaching the first potential helper. According to criteria developed during our study to establish the absence or presence of symptoms and syndromes, 50% of those patients interviewed were psychotic by the time they first sought help, and a further 37% were manic or depressed and required treatment. Given our knowledge that the onset of psychotic symptoms is a relatively late phenomenon for many patients (Häfner et al., 1992), who may experience a prolonged and potentially damaging pre-psychotic phase of illness (Jones et al., 1993), and that nearly 30% had initially visited a non-health professional with limited knowledge about mental illness, there is room for concern.

At this stage of the analysis, it is difficult to say how help-seeking behaviours relate to psychological or psychiatric symptoms. Our data more clearly show that pathways were diverse and experienced in different ways. Help-seeking was sometimes continuous, intermittent, concurrent or temporarily halted. In fact, individuals were not necessarily referred from one helping modality to another, nor were referrals or 'treatments' always acted upon. Data from families, not yet fully analysed, seem to tell a different story again, with their help-seeking strategies being independent or linked in a variety of ways to that of their ill relative.

Despite difficulties experienced by some patients in identifying the onset and offset of prodromal or psychotic symptoms, the findings correlate reasonably well with independently assessed data collected for the same patients ($n = 62$), and with a subset of 150 15 to 30–year-old patients from the full cohort of 347 patients (McGorry et al., 1996). For the 62 patients interviewed, the mean number of days between first symptoms and first help-seeking attempt was 112 days ($SD = 169.77$) with a median of 31 days. The mean number of days between first symptoms and initial treatment was 273 days ($SD = 510.02$) with a median of 121 days. The mean number of days between the onset of first symptoms and treatment at the Early Psychosis Prevention and Intervention Centre (EPPIC) Program was 405.03 days ($SD = 803.08$) with a median of 167 days.

Although commencement of treatment usually coincided with the patient contacting mental health services, what constituted treatment was not always clear-cut. What constitutes potentially effective treatment has recently been defined in a Norwegian study (Larsen, McGlashan & Moe, 1996). For some patients, the relatively long pathways may have been due to their receiving sporadic or ineffective help. If it is true that many people are very unwell before accessing any service, targeted health promotion activities in the community could be warranted in view of this finding. Similarly, what may be required is a strategy to enhance GP skills in recognizing the signs of other potentially serious mental illnesses such as depression, as well as a broad-based educational strategy amongst those working as helping professionals in the community.

Pathways as personal experiences

Consumer accounts can 'stand alone' and four are presented below to highlight how difficult the experience of psychosis can be for the individual patient. The analysis which follows, however, has adopted a more critical stance (Banton et al., 1985; Cook, 1995; Manktelow, 1994; Pearlin, 1992; Strauss, 1994; Thomas, 1993). This approach enables us to appreciate how consumer and clinician perspectives may differ, with

3 PATHWAYS TO CARE

the family perspective providing yet another viewpoint (Hatfield & Lefley, 1994) which, due to space limitations, cannot be addressed here.

> Jane is a single parent in her 20s living with her pre-school-aged child in rented accommodation. She believes she was unwell for at least six months before contacting EPPIC. Her voices were 'like angels' and initially were 'helpmates' and inhibited her seeking treatment. Jane recalls that the onset of illness was gradual and insidious. She went to her GP with symptoms suggestive of anxiety and depression. Jane did not disclose the full symptom picture, including voices. She says that she wanted help but she did not want to acknowledge that she was mentally ill. Although Jane had a family history of schizophrenia, the doctor failed to recognize the onset of her first psychotic episode. Over the following months, she sought support from neighbours, family, and a variety of professionals. The professionals Jane contacted did not appear to want to entertain the idea that she was becoming ill and needed treatment. On the day that Jane created a disturbance in the GP's surgery, her doctor finally recognized the severity of her mental state, and telephoned EPPIC. However, Jane recalls the period of initial treatment she received at home as a 'terrible experience'. For her, being acutely psychotic was frightening and overwhelming in her home environment; even twice-daily visits from psychiatric services were insufficient in her case to provide the reassurance and support she now feels she required at that time. Her medication gave her unpleasant side-effects and the symptoms were not easily controlled. For Jane, recovery from her first episode began on admission to the inpatient unit of EPPIC. Although Jane believes that her hospitalization indicated that she was a failure and had let others down, hospital was also perceived by her as a refuge where she could begin her own personal struggle for recovery. Jane states that she sometimes feels treatment has been helpful and is optimistic about keeping well. After a recent re-admission to hospital, her self-confidence is shaky, and she wonders if she can hope for a lasting recovery. The impact of her illness on her child is an ever-present concern. A description of Jane's pathway is depicted in Figure 3.2.

> George is in his late teens, is casually employed, and lives with his mother. He believes he was unwell two years before his emergency

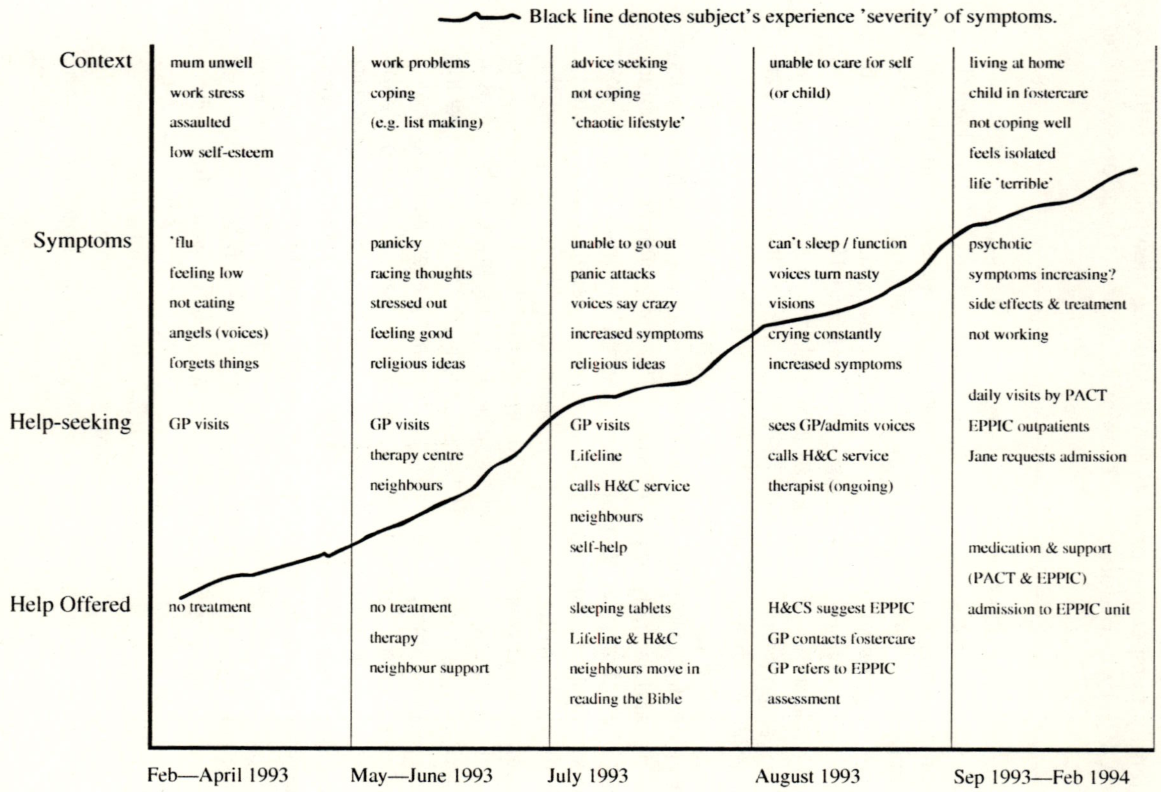

━━━ Black line denotes subject's experience 'severity' of symptoms.

	Feb—April 1993	May—June 1993	July 1993	August 1993	Sep 1993—Feb 1994
Context	mum unwell work stress assaulted low self-esteem	work problems coping (e.g. list making)	advice seeking not coping 'chaotic lifestyle'	unable to care for self (or child)	living at home child in fostercare not coping well feels isolated life 'terrible'
Symptoms	'flu feeling low not eating angels (voices) forgets things	panicky racing thoughts stressed out feeling good religious ideas	unable to go out panic attacks voices say crazy increased symptoms religious ideas	can't sleep / function voices turn nasty visions crying constantly increased symptoms	psychotic symptoms increasing? side effects & treatment not working
Help-seeking	GP visits	GP visits therapy centre neighbours	GP visits Lifeline calls H&C service neighbours self-help	sees GP/admits voices calls H&C service therapist (ongoing)	daily visits by PACT EPPIC outpatients Jane requests admission
Help Offered	no treatment	no treatment therapy neighbour support	sleeping tablets Lifeline & H&C neighbours move in reading the Bible	H&CS suggest EPPIC GP contacts fostercare GP refers to EPPIC assessment	medication & support (PACT & EPPIC) admission to EPPIC unit

Figure 3.2. Topography of the pathways: Jane's account. Note: H & SC=Health and Community Services; EPPIC=Early Psychosis Assessment and Community Treatment Team.

admission to hospital. He was using marijuana heavily and the voices would tell him to kill himself. George says he knew he was 'dead sick' but felt unable to tell anyone what was happening. The eight-month pre-admission period was agony for him. He was in emotional and physical pain, yet felt that no-one could help him. His friends thought he was a 'wacky bloke' and 'off with the fairies' and yet this gave him a peculiar sense of being accepted by the group. His mother attributed his strange behaviour to adolescence and socializing with 'off-beat' friends. His day and night cycle was reversed and so the family missed the signs that he was becoming very unwell. George had not appreciated that mental illness was treatable and so he could not envisage how a GP or psychiatrist would be of much use to him. The illness itself seemed to make it impossible for him to communicate with others and explain to them what was going on. George now regrets the delay in his obtaining help. He now says that perhaps it was a 'godsend' when he tried to harm himself at home as this forced him into treatment. Looking back, he believes his suicide attempt was a 'cry for help'. After 'the accident' he was taken to a local casualty department and later transferred to the inpatient unit of EPPIC. Unfortunately, on discharge from hospital the voices continued to squeal and laugh at him, and at times he has felt low and suicidal. George requested to be re-admitted to hospital as soon as he felt he was unable to cope back at home. Now discharged, the medication has been ineffective in stopping the voices; George wonders whether early treatment might have prevented him from being so sick now. His mother believes moving interstate will give him a chance to get away from everything, and allow him to make a new start. Similarly, other relatives believe moving away will help George and his mother to put the experience behind them.

Susan is a university student still living at home. She believes that she started to become unwell six months before approaching anyone for help. She couldn't motivate herself to get out of bed in the mornings, had strange and bizarre thoughts, felt paranoid, and wasn't able to concentrate or cope with her studies. Feeling tearful and 'stressed out' sent her to a GP a number of times, although visits didn't result in treatment. Susan realized that 'something was definitely wrong' but could no longer trust anyone and she didn't want to let go of experiences that she had come to 'own'. She had an inner fantasy world of her own and it fascinated her. But six months later, Susan felt as if she was dying and that close friends were out to kill her. The intensity and reality of these ideas pushed her to seek help from a University counsellor. Susan was immediately admitted to a local private hospital but discharged when she refused treatment. Several days later she was found by the police wandering the city streets in a psychotic state. Re-admission to the private hospital did not appear to offer a viable option. Family pressure led to the Early Psychosis Assessment and Community Treatment Team (EPACT) arranging for her admission to the EPPIC inpatient unit. Admission was short and symptoms disappeared rapidly once treatment began. Susan says that she did not feel stigmatized by her friends as many young people she has met have ended up in hospital because of drugs, including drug-related psychosis. However, since returning home, the thought of being 'mentally ill' is daunting and threatens her sense of self. Susan has dropped out of her studies and is unsure whether she'll get 'back on track' again. Not being understood by the family because they see her as 'crazy' is a terrible experience for her. And 'not being helped' once back in the community is the hardest thing for her to accommodate. She believes that talking to someone, not medication, can make her better, but she doesn't know where to turn to for help. Things seem a struggle now that she is back at home and expected to 'get back to normal'. She is trying to find a direction in life, something she used to take for granted.

Danni is single, in his 20s, unemployed, and living with a relative. He never realized there was anything wrong with him until his admission. Even today he isn't convinced that he was ill, although recently he was re-admitted to hospital following a second episode. His sister believes he first became ill five years ago when he broke up with a girlfriend. He was using drugs, his temper was out of control, and he took up with a 'bad crowd'. At the time his sister advised him 'to get himself sorted out and see a psychiatrist', although she knew no-one could get him to do anything he did not want to do. From then on, he became embroiled in disputes and arguments with his family and with the police. Danni didn't take any notice of the advice that his family members tried to give him. His sister recalls that she was the only person who could control or talk to him. By then, she had come to the conclusion that he was a 'crazy (bad) person' who could not be helped. In the 12 months prior to admission, Danni was eating, injecting and snorting amphetamines, and was irritable and moody for much of the time. In the six months prior to admission, he lost his job and was jailed for drink driving and assault. This period of time had become a 'nightmare' for Danni. He felt constantly paranoid and found it impossible to separate fantasy from reality. He thought everyone was out to kill him and that he had committed terrible criminal acts. When Danni threatened to shoot a relative, things reached crisis point and his sister managed to get him to see a GP. The same day, a referral to a community mental health centre was made and EPPIC arranged his admission. Danni says that hospital was 'a bit like a hotel' and gave him time out from all the hassles. He isn't sure whether he ever needed help but before discharge he was put on a 'community treatment order' so he has been forced to continue with his treatment. Yet Danni also states that if his difficulties had been discerned earlier, he might not have gone to jail. His sister says that the family tried to live with Danni's difficult behaviour as long as they could as they did not believe anyone could do anything about it. They can now appreciate how treatment has helped him, but are concerned for Danni, who denies that he is unwell and still doesn't recognize the signs of illness and when treatment is required.

Delay as a paradox

While reductions in delays are considered positively by clinicians, data from retrospective accounts suggest that the potential consumer's perspective is often out of step with this view. There seems to be a complex interplay between the two perspectives: on the one hand, there is a risk that clinical staff may fail sufficiently to take into account the perspective of the consumer and carers in their zeal to reduce treatment delay, and may be excessively paternalistic. On the other hand, consumers may be said to have an 'antipsychiatry' perspective, which is naïve and based on 'myth' and heresay, since in general they genuinely lack knowledge about services available to them, and opportunities for informed choices about treatments and care options. The potential consumer is generally unaware that current developments promise to deliver less restrictive and more humane treatments to service users; however, getting the timing of the intervention and the quality of service right, as well as the right service mix, is an enormously complex affair which often eludes even state-of-the-art preventive programs (Lincoln, 1996). Clinicians need to become more aware that the goal of reducing treatment delay is critically dependent upon the perceptions that individual consumers have of mental health services, their personal attitudes to seeking help for themselves from such services, and their ultimate experiences and interactions with services and clinicians.

For mental health professionals, the common descriptor 'pathways to psychiatric care' conjures up a picture of relatively visible, organized and defined routes to the varied providers who possess the mandate to treat and care responsibly for the mentally ill. From a consumer perspective (and although there might be great variability in this perspective), the pathway may seem unfamiliar and impersonal, invisible, even mysterious or frightening. Based on widespread negative stereotypes, the ideal of care may be pushed aside by biases and fears associated with involuntary hospital treatments – 'strait jackets', 'chemical restraints' and social control (Goffman, 1961; McGorry et al., 1991). Resisting treatment or a diagnosis of 'mental illness' can be entirely comprehensible and reasonable.

Below, a tentative analysis is made from a consumer angle, conceptualizing delay as a process characterized by ambivalence, confusion, contradictions and resistance. The key message here is that the 'professional voice' and 'consumer voice' express different concerns about the context and process of treatment which need to be examined when considering new and innovative directions in service delivery. If the goal of early intervention is to be achieved, clinicians need to respond to the consumers' range of experiences as well as the experiences of family members, ensuring the 'pathways experience' is a more palatable one.

Illness recognition

Consumers' retrospective accounts vary, with some patients identifying symptoms in the pre-treatment period. Others deny current or past awareness of problems, their families possibly having played a key role in recognizing the first signs (Birchwood et al., 1992). Lack of insight, together with the impaired capacity of a patient to understand that he or she has a problem, has been associated with severe psychopathology, postponed treatment-seeking and barriers to being helped (Amador & Strauss, 1993; Amador et al., 1991; Greenfeld et al., 1989; Loebel et al., 1992).

Recent research suggests that insight should be conceptualized as a relative and multidimensional construct involving psychological defences mediated through or influenced by social and cultural factors (Amador & Strauss, 1993; Amador et al., 1991; Birchwood et al., 1994; Johnson & Orrell, 1995; Kleinman, 1980; O'Mahony, 1982). First-episode studies suggest that illness recognition is partly determined by lay stereotypes. Denial may be a particular feature of early psychosis, individuals viewing symptoms as trivial or fleeting, perceiving an 'episode' as an isolated event. Generally, young adults feel invulnerable and are likely to protect their self-esteem from stigma (Greenfeld et al., 1989; McGorry et al., 1991; O'Mahony, 1982).

Personal accounts provide a contradictory picture as to how individuals recognize 'something isn't quite right' or 'something is definitely wrong'. Consumer recall of events leading to an initial admission, suggests, in line with research on insight in psychosis, that individuals do *and* don't recognize they are unwell. Consumers' stories capture the ambivalence of individuals or society to acknowledge the reality of mental illness. 'Naïve' consumers may demonstrate 'resistance' to recognizing symptoms for differing reasons which largely remain obscure. We ultimately need to develop a common language between consumers and clinicians in order to understand the complexity of the issues involved.

In the cases we cited, George and Susan claimed that they knew they were ill but failed to act. George talks poignantly of the emotional and physical agony that accompanied the awareness of 'being mad', unable to 'break out of the self' and obtain assistance. In contrast, Susan reported her fascination with the 'good and crazy bits' of being unwell and her unwillingness to give up experiences to professionals who she felt would 'devalue', 'misunderstand', and take these experiences away.

As two members of the immediate family had suffered psychotic episodes, Jane was sensitized to the 'early warning signs'. Despite this, Jane speculated that growing up with a parent with schizophrenia made it hard to distinguish 'normal' from 'abnormal' behaviour. Whereas Jane put off acknowledging she was unwell, her sister was able to use her knowledge of psychosis to identify what was happening. Jane reports that as her symptoms intensified, her reluctance to accessing help diminished. No longer able to cope, 'nasty voices' and concern for the welfare of her child, particularly the latter, increased her motivation to seek assistance. However, resistance to involvement in the psychiatric system influenced the effectiveness of her efforts and those of the professionals from whom she sought help. Paradoxically, Jane had overcome her resistance to seeking help, because she was concerned that her changed mental state might lead to her harming her child, when 'well-meaning' professionals inhibited the process. Jane was relatively isolated and unsupported as a single parent at the time of her initial illness and, as a consequence, some of the professionals whom Jane contacted along the pathway were keen to provide her with support in her role as a mother with a view to keeping the family intact. It appears that the definition of her behaviour as seriously disturbed (and as a sign of serious mental illness) was avoided by these same professionals as long as possible (Manktelow, 1994).

Help-seeking

For secondary prevention to be effective, people with a psychotic illness and their relatives must be educated to seek help (Helgason, 1990). Yet patients and families may resist seeking assistance, hoping that the patient's symptoms are temporary aberrations which can be tolerated or managed without external help. Even when a problem is identified as serious and requiring action, knowing what to do and how to obtain access to care may constitute significant barriers to care.

Although in some areas of prevention and treatment, such as breast cancer and hypertension, individuals have become proactive in seeking help early, the community at large still needs to appreciate that early intervention makes a difference for psychotic disorders. Cook (1995) argues that various factors influence the utilization of mental health services, including the beliefs of the day as to whether mental illness is seen as a treatable condition and how sufferers are evaluated. Greater acceptance of treatments and services may also reduce the stigma surrounding serious mental illness and promote help-seeking. As attitudes in the community shift, the response of professionals (who weigh up what they should do when individuals present with varying degrees of psychopathology) might also change. Anecdotal evidence from our research suggests that at least some professionals are loathe to refer their clients or patients to the psychiatric system as they do not perceive it as preventive or effective in nature.

In the meantime, lay stereotypes about mental illness and 'bad press' about treatment, loom large in the minds of some first-time service users. Late-presentation consumers in particular do not appear to reconstruct help-seeking as a consequence of rational choice and decision-making. Utilizing mental health services, especially inpatient facilities, may seem to be a last resort option. Contacting services in crisis is particularly common, at times leading to emergency admission. Paradoxically, service systems developed to respond better to emergency and crisis situations may, if they are gate-keepers to the service, discourage referrals at a less severe stage or phase, thereby increasing delays and late presentations. In the case of Danni, his sister knew her brother needed treatment but she had no idea to whom she should turn for help. She lacked confidence in what professionals could do for him, and so the family learned to live with his bizarre behaviour until

Danni's threatening behaviour pushed them into action. After a couple of years, an invisible threshold was crossed which precipitated the family into seeking help. This decisive action led to Danni's immediate and compulsory admission to hospital and illustrates a late presentation with consequent failure of early intervention. Although for some individuals, like George, diagnosis legitimizes suffering and gives them a sense of control over their illness, Danni currently denies that he is unwell and is loathe to utilize services he feels he does not require.

Symptoms and coping
Symptoms may inhibit or promote help-seeking in complex ways (Romme & Escher, 1989). Susan reports that psychosis was such a personal experience she did not want anyone to remove her symptoms. Jane's voices came to her as 'angels' and acted as 'helpmates'. Their benevolent role puts a new complexion on understanding the interactive effects between illness and treatment-seeking. Jane's contact with professionals increased as the voices 'turned against her'. However, help-seeking was ineffectual, because Jane was frightened of disclosing the nature of her symptoms.

The relationship between coping and help-seeking remains obscure. Coping appears to be about actively managing symptoms, attributing them to other sources, or resisting the consequences of disclosure. Resistance to discovery is common in stigmatizing illness as it is bound up with 'avoiding public awareness' (Brown, 1995), and a variety of strategies have been developed as a device to 'cover' stigma. As the examples we have cited demonstrate, families are not immune from accommodating disturbed behaviour, as enlisting professional help may seem like a betrayal or dishonouring of family allegiances (Goffman, 1961; Manktelow, 1994). There is a degree of awareness that, whereas physical illness usually elicits sympathy, mentally ill persons are negatively valued and discriminated against (Cook, 1995; Fink & Tasman, 1992; Goffman, 1963).

George recalls that as his illness developed he cultivated a 'wacky personality' so as to fit in and provide him with a sense of identity. Susan and Danni tried 'self-medication' through drug use, which initially seemed to attenuate the voices. Susan decided to avoid help-seeking until there was a point at which her study and life problems could no longer go unnoticed by others, such as staff and students, family and friends. Jane began reading the Bible, tried list-making, and labelled items in her home. In the early stages of illness, her family attempted to 'hold things together' through a process of reciprocal 'support and strain' (Cook, 1995), until external circumstances changed. The capacity of Jane's and Susan's social network was suddenly compromised when, in each case, a family member travelled away, acting as a catalyst for seeking help from outside the network.

Referral pathways

Diagnosis by health professionals

Referral involves organizing 'unprocessed' illness over time (Balint, 1957), behaviour being normalized or pathologized, depending on who individuals approach for help. Gender, race, age and class are all factors which will influence this process (Zola, 1973). Consumers may feel that they lose control when they utilize specialist services, although views may differ about this experience, depending on treatment outcome.

Diagnosis is the 'voice of medicine' (Brown, 1990, 1995; Mishler, 1984) and is powerful. In psychiatry it has been a process laden with controversy as diagnosis and the prescriptions for medical intervention have been reified (Brown, 1987). Diagnosis places doctors in the 'expert' role although it may be hard for medical professionals to live up to consumer idealizations of them (Banton et al., 1985). Patients may want doctors to be all-knowing, yet inevitably discover they cannot always effectively treat psychosis. Misdiagnosis is common and the labelling of symptoms and behaviour, useful for recognizing syndromes and indicating groups for effective treatment, have iatrogenic effects. Social relationships with others, and housing and employment opportunities may be affected, as well as a person's sense of identity and future possible selves (Farina & Felner, 1973; Lally, 1989; Markus & Nurius, 1986; Page, 1983).

At a micro-level, help-seeker and service-provider are engaged in a complex exchange. What may take place is a series of events or occurrences, in which behaviours or actions are interpreted and reinterpreted by professionals and significant others over a period of time. There is a process of action and reaction which contains a feedback effect on the behaviour in question. Although this decision-making process may barely attract our attention, the final entry to treatment may be dramatic to say the least (Manktelow, 1994). It appears that families may, or may not, 'join' with professionals when assessing options and the acceptability of alternatives. Professionals will have disparate views as to their role (Brown, 1987; Goffman, 1961), and the resistance of at least some professionals to construe symptoms as indicators of mental illness influences their service response (Lincoln & McGorry, 1995). Professionals may collude with consumers or families to explain away strange behaviours so that specialists play a role late in the pathway.

Our findings suggest that those who have presented early to services have often received an inadequate response from that service. Community-based professionals may not detect mental illness, nor view the 'early warning signs' as significant. The clinical picture in psychosis may be vague, confusing and unstable (Weiner, 1992), and problems emerge if patients and doctors fail to communicate adequately (Roberts, 1985).

It may be unclear to professionals as to what constitutes the most appropriate treatment response. Some professionals empathize with consumers by avoiding psychiatric labels and services that they consider may be 'damaging' (Fink & Tasman, 1992; Goffman, 1963). It seems that those crossing the boundary from a medical to a psychiatric setting, as a consequence of referral, may experience guilt or shame.

The pathways experience

It is through consumer accounts that we can appreciate that the 'pathway to care' is inseparable from the treatment experience. For Jane and Susan, easy access and non-specific symptoms made consulting a GP a 'natural' first port of call. Yet both consumers were frustrated that their GPs failed to detect that they were ill. Jane received no treatment from her doctor despite an evolving symptom picture and several consultations. Once symptoms intensified, Jane sought assistance with more frequency, but with professionals outside the medical profession. These professionals, in turn, provided an inadequate response, thereby increasing delay. Jane contacted a therapist who was reluctant to acknowledge that Jane was mentally ill or refer her on for psychiatric assessment. Unfortunately, once her GP called in EPPIC, Jane claims that her 'nightmare' still continued. Although community treatment, when initiated early, frequently offers a more acceptable option, Jane asserts that, in her case, avoiding hospital involved a high personal cost as the EPACT was unable to provide sufficient intensive support at home. Being ill at home made a familiar environment an uncomfortable one; treatment felt intrusive as illness became a public affair.

Similarly, Susan says her GP initially didn't take her symptoms seriously and failed to ask relevant questions. Susan eventually sought help via a counsellor who referred her to a private hospital, as a strategy to avoid stigma and allow Susan to retain some control. Ironically, once admitted, being categorized as a 'voluntary patient', signalled to Susan that she was different from other patients, and staff were able to discharge her when she refused medication! Discharged whilst psychotic, a crisis situation developed involving the police, and this led to Susan's involuntary admission via the public sector. Susan says that it is her family, rather than the community or psychiatric system, which has labelled her 'mentally ill'. This has undermined her confidence in her recovery and rendered her return to studies a particular challenge.

All four patients experienced delays and all of them, except Susan, have had readmissions, with recovery being slow. Patients and families have mixed and contradictory feelings about what has happened. Danni and his family appear to have no notion of either 'early intervention', nor of the risks associated with treatment delay. Susan believes patients make informed choices not to approach services and does not believe that treatment delay has made a difference to her getting back to normal. George and Jane wonder whether earlier treatment may have made a difference to their chances of recovery.

Three out of these four families have asked themselves whether their ill relatives will become chronically unwell. Thinking in this manner, however, is overwhelming as illness is then viewed as beyond one's control and as unpredictable. Undoubtedly, to cope with the stresses of illness, experiences have been redefined by Jane, George, Susan and Danni. People formulate new personal biographies and engage in narrative reconstructions on the basis of their experiences and illness (Williams, 1984). These accounts may be protective or promote healing, or serve a purpose as yet not understood.

Discussion

This chapter provides a tentative framework for understanding issues related to access to care in early psychosis. Reviewing the available evidence suggests that delays in obtaining early treatment is a major problem. Despite the fact that there will be those for whom earlier intervention may not provide significant benefits, clinicians are increasingly convinced that the evidence for the benefits of early intervention is indisputable. Our outcome data requires further examination, but gives impetus to the twin important notions of promoting early presentation to services, *and* adopting a proactive treatment response.

However, solely presenting data from a 'clinical–epidemiological' perspective places constraints on how we explore issues and think about service delivery. Personal narratives have been collected as a way of eliciting meaningful stories (Lincoln & McGorry, 1995; Strauss, 1994) so we can encourage consumers to contribute to discussion. These 'pathways experiences' enhance our understanding, particularly when examining barriers to implementing early intervention strategies.

Examining the topography of the pathways has demonstrated that there are ample opportunities for delay, especially in reaching the first helper. Mapping the pathways has shown that the GP has a key mediating role in the initial pathway, although further delays may still occur once contact with a GP or helping professional has been made, as the first encounter does not necessarily lead to action or an adequate response. One of the key tasks which remains, therefore, is to develop an explanatory model which goes beyond examining service utilization and predicts the adequacy of various pathways to treat effectively without delay, and with a general positive effect on quality of life.

Our research suggests that the notion of delay – associated with secondary prevention – is primarily a clinician's concept in the field of psychosis. This is despite the fact that in other medical domains early intervention has credibility and broad acceptance. What has become clear is that consumers, families, and sometimes professionals, may be ambivalent, confused, resistant and have contradictory views about utilizing mental health services. Specialist workers need to acknowledge and respond to the 'consumer voice' to bring about change.

From a service provider perspective, the challenge appears to be promoting early access to services by making the pathways accessible and user-friendly. Clinicians believe that the psychiatric system as a destination may be seen in a more positive light if community-based options are able to complement hospital care. There is considerable support for initiatives which promise to meet people's needs more humanely and effectively.

Case material allows us a glimpse of how future service developments could be relatively congruent with current challenges posed to the system by consumers. Improved services, education and consumer empowerment have to be key aspects to make early intervention as a strategy work. Service linkages need to be effective and efficient for those who require specialist treatment. Pathways need to be rapid or slow depending on consumer need, with there being non-stigmatizing accessible routes to treatment and care (see Chapter 4). Quality services need to be available to the patient – ones which involve choice, and are flexible, varied and comprehensive.

Improving psychiatric services alone will not be sufficient to encourage treatment-seeking. Until the stigma of mental illness is reduced it seems unlikely that treatment delay will be reduced beyond a certain point. Educating the community and professional training are necessary components of any initiative to enhance the pathways.

It is not surprising that individuals report their reluctance to set out on the pathway to treatment, as becoming a patient can be a threatening and disempowering event. Earlier treatments may make consumer empowerment a reality so 'everybody wins'. Empowering consumers may have untapped potential for assisting the recovery process itself. To respond to their challenge, we need to acknowledge that the perceived cost to some first-time consumers remains high. Future consumers may be more open to hear about the value of early intervention as others experience for themselves a social climate of change and, in keeping with this, radical service change.

Acknowledgements

We are grateful to our colleague from the Department of Psychiatry, University of Melbourne, Susy Harrigan, for statistical input and advice, and for the provision of Figure 3.1. The authors wish to thank the consumers and families who agreed to be interviewed and shared their personal experiences with us, and who have also assisted with their comments as findings have been reported.

References

Amador, X. F. (1994). Insight in psychosis: state or trait? Reply. Letter. *American Journal of Psychiatry*, **151**, 789.

Amador, X. F. & Strauss, D. H. (1993). Poor insight in schizophrenia. *Psychiatric Quarterly*, **64**, 305–18.

Amador, X. F., Strauss, D. H., Yale, S. A. & Gorman, J. M. (1991). Awareness of illness in schizophrenia. *Schizophrenia Bulletin*, **17**, 113–32.

Asai, K. (1984). Pathways of help-seeking of psychiatric patients in Japan: a research study in Togane City. *American Journal of Social Psychiatry*, **42**, 38–44.

Balestrieri, M., Bon, M. G., Rodriquez-Sacristan, A. & Tansella, M. (1994). Pathways to psychiatric care in South Verona, Italy. *Psychological Medicine*, **24**, 641–9.

Balint, M. (1957). *The Doctor, His Patient and the Illness*. New York: International Universities Press.

Banton, R., Clifford, P., Frosh, S., Lousada, J. & Rosenthall, J. (1985). *The Politics of Mental Health*. Oxford: Macmillan.

Beiser, M., Erickson, D., Fleming, J. A. E. & Iacono, W. G. (1993). Establishing the onset of psychotic illness. *American Journal of Psychiatry*, **150**, 1349–54.

Berkson, J. (1946). Limitations of the applications of fourfold table analysis to hospital data. *Biometrics Bulletin*, **2**, 47–53.

Birchwood, M. & Macmillan, F. (1993). Early intervention in schizophrenia. *Australian and New Zealand Journal of Psychiatry*, **27**, 374–8.

Birchwood, M., Cochrane, R., Macmillan, F., Copestake, S., Kucharska, J. & Cariss, M. (1992). The influence of ethnicity and family structure on relapse in first-episode schizophrenia. A comparison of Asian, Afro-Caribbean and White patients. *British Journal of Psychiatry*, **161**, 783–90.

Birchwood, M., Smith, J., Drury, V., Healy, J., Macmillan, F. & Slade, M. (1994).

A self-report insight scale of psychosis: reliability, validity and sensitivity to change. *Acta Psychiatrica Scandinavica*, **89**, 62–7.

Bleuler, M. (1978). *The Schizophrenia Disorders: Long Term Patient and Family Studies*, translated by S. M. Clemens. New York: International Universities Press.

Brown, P. (1987). Diagnostic conflict and contradiction in psychiatry. *Journal of Health and Social Behavior*, **28**, 37–50.

Brown, P. (1990). The Name Game: toward a sociology of diagnosis. *Journal of Mind and Behavior*, **11**, 385–406.

Brown, P. (1995). Naming and framing: The social construction of diagnosis and illness. *Journal of Health and Social Behavior*, **36** (Extra Issue), 34–52.

Carpenter, W. T. & Strauss, J. S. (1991). The prediction of outcome in schizophrenia. IV: Eleven-year follow-up of the Washington IPSS Cohort. *The Journal of Nervous and Mental Disease*, **179**, 517–25.

Cheung, F. K. & Snowden, L. R. (1990). Community mental health and ethnic minority populations. *Community Mental Health Journal*, **26**, 277–91.

Clausen, J. A., Pfeffer, N. & Huffine, C. (1982). Helpseeking in severe mental illness. In *Symptom, Illness Behaviour, and Helpseeking*, ed. D. Mechanic, pp. 135–55. New York: Prodist.

Cohen, S. & Wills, T. A. (1985). Stress, social support, and the buffering hypothesis. *Psychological Bulletin*, **98**, 310–57.

Cole, E., Leavey, G., King, M., Johnson-Sabine, E. & Hoar, R. (1995). Pathways to care for patients with a first episode of psychosis. A comparison of ethnic groups. *British Journal of Psychiatry*, **167**, 770–6.

Cook, J. A. (1995). Medical sociology and the study of severe mental illness: reflections on past accomplishments and directions for future research. *Journal of Health and Social Behavior*, **36** (Extra Issue), 95–114.

Crow, T. J., Macmillan, J. F., Johnson, A. J. & Johnstone, E. C. (1986). The Northwick Park study of first episodes of schizophrenia. II. A randomised controlled trial of prophylactic neuroleptic treatment. *British Journal of Psychiatry*, **148**, 120–7.

Denzin, N. K. (1989). *The Research Act: A Theoretical Introduction to Sociological Methods*, 3rd edn. Chicago: Aldine Publishing.

Docherty, J. P., Van Kammen, D. P., Siris, S. G. & Marder, S. R. (1978). Stages of onset of schizophrenic psychosis. *American Journal of Psychiatry*, **135**, 420–6.

Edwards, J., Francey, S. M., McGorry, P. D. & Jackson, H. J. (1994). Early psychosis prevention and intervention: evolution of a comprehensive community-based specialised service. *Behaviour Change*, **11**, 223–33.

Estroff, S. (1981). *Making It Crazy*. Berkeley, California: University of California Press.

Estroff, S. E. (1989). Self-identity and subjective experiences of schizophrenia. *Schizophrenia Bulletin*, **15**, 189–96.

Farina, A. & Felner, R. D. (1973). Employment interviewer reactions to former mental patients. *Journal of Abnormal Psychology*, **82**, 268–72.

Fink, P. J. & Tasman, A. (eds.) (1992). *Stigma and Mental Illness*. Washington, DC: American Psychiatric Press.

Gallo, J. J., Marino, S., Ford, D. & Anthony, J. C. (1995a). Filters on the pathway to mental health care. I. Incident mental disorders. *Psychological Medicine*, **25**, 1135–48.

Gallo, J. J., Marino, S., Ford, D. & Anthony, J. C. (1995b). Filters on the pathway to mental health care. II. Sociodemographic factors. *Psychological Medicine*, **25**, 1149–60.

Gater, R. & Goldberg, D. (1991). Pathways to psychiatric care in Manchester. *British Journal of Psychiatry*, **159**, 90–6.

Gater, R., De Almeida, E., Sousa, B., Barrientos, G., Caraveo, J., Chandrashekar, C. R., Dhadphale, M., Goldberg, D., Al Kathiri, A. H., Mubbashar, M., Silhan, K., Thong, D., Torres-Gonzales, F. & Sartorius, N. (1991). The pathways to psychiatric care: a cross-cultural study. *Psychological Medicine*, **21**, 761–74.

Gift, T. E., Strauss, J. S., Harder, D. W., Kokes, R. F. & Ritzler, B. A. (1981). Established chronicity of psychotic symptoms in first admission schizophrenic patients. *American Journal of Psychiatry*, **138**, 779–84.

Goffman, E. (1961). *Asylums: Essays on the Social Situation of Mental Patients and Other Inmates*. New York: Doubleday Anchor.

Goffman, E. (1963). *Stigma: Notes on the Management of Spoiled Identity*. Englewood Cliffs: Prentice Hall.

Goldberg, D. & Huxley, P. (1980). *Mental Illness in the Community: The Pathway to Psychiatric Care*. London: Tavistock.

Goldberg, D. & Huxley, P. (1992). *Common Mental Disorders*. London: Routledge.

Greenfeld, D., Strauss, J. S., Bowers, M. B. & Mandelkern, M. (1989). Insight and interpretation of illness in recovery from psychosis. *Schizophrenia Bulletin*, **15**, 245–52.

Guba, E. G. & Lincoln, Y. S. (1989). *Fourth Generation Evaluation*. Newbury Park, California: Sage Publications.

Haas, G. L. & Sweeney, J. A. (1992). Premorbid and onset features of first-episode schizophrenia. *Schizophrenia Bulletin*, **18**, 373–86.

Häfner, H., Riechler-Rössler, A., Maurer, K., Fötkenheuer, B. & Löffler, W. (1992). First onset and early symptomatology of schizophrenia. A chapter of epidemiological and neurobiological research into age and sex differences. *European Archives of Psychiatry and Clinical Neurosciences*, **242**, 109–18.

Hatfield, A. B. & Lefley, H. P. (1994). *Surviving Mental Illness: Stress, Coping and Adaption*. New York: Guilford Press.

Heinrichs, D. W., Hanlon, T. E. & Carpenter, W. T. (1984). The Quality of Life Scale: an instrument for rating the schizophrenia deficit syndrome. *Schizophrenia Bulletin*, **10**, 388–98.

Helgason, L. (1977). Psychiatric services and mental illness in Iceland: incidence study (1966–1967) with 6–7 year follow-up. *Acta Psychiatrica Scandinavica*, **268** (Supplementum), 111–37.

Helgason, L. (1990). Twenty years follow-up of first psychiatric presentation for schizophrenia: what could have been prevented? *Acta Psychiatrica Scandinavica*, **81**, 231–5.

Humphreys, M. S., Johnstone, E. C., Macmillan, J. F. & Taylor, P. J. (1992).

Dangerous behaviour preceding first admissions for schizophrenia. *British Journal of Psychiatry*, **161**, 501–5.

Jackson, H. J. & Edwards, J. (1992). Social networks, social support and schizophrenia. In *Schizophrenia: An Overview and Practical Handbook*, ed. D. Kavanagh, pp. 275–92. London: Chapman & Hall.

Johnson, S. & Orrell, M. (1995). Insight and psychosis: a social perspective. *Psychological Medicine*, **25**, 515–20.

Johnstone, E. C., Crow, T. J., Johnson, A. L. & Macmillan, J. F. (1986). The Northwick Park study of first episodes of schizophrenia: 1. Presentation of the illness and problems relating to admission. *British Journal of Psychiatry*, **148**, 115–20.

Jones, P. B., Bebbington, P., Foerster, A., Lewis, S. W., Murray, R. M., Russell, A., Sham, P. C., Toone, B. K. & Wilkins, S. (1993). Premorbid social underachievement in schizophrenia: results from the Camberwell Collaborative Psychosis Study. *British Journal of Psychiatry*, **162**, 65–71.

Keith, S. J. & Mathews, S. M. (1991). The diagnosis of schizophrenia: a review of onset and duration issues. *Schizophrenia Bulletin*, **17**, 51–67.

Keshavan, M. S. & Schooler, N. R. (1992). First-episode studies in schizophrenia: criteria and characterisation. *Schizophrenia Bulletin*, **18**, 491–513.

Kessler, R. C., Foster, C. L., Saunders, W. B. & Stang, P. E. (1995). Social consequences of psychiatric disorders. I. Educational attainment. *American Journal of Psychiatry*, **152**, 1026–31.

Kleinman, A. (1980). *Patients and Healers in the Context of Culture*. Berkeley, California: University of California Press.

Lally, S. J. (1989). Does being in here mean there is something wrong with me? *Schizophrenia Bulletin*, **15**, 253–65.

Larsen, T. K., McGlashan, T. H. & Moe, L. C. (1996). First-episode schizophrenia: I. Early course parameters. *Schizophrenia Bulletin*, **22**, 241–56.

Lincoln, C. V. (1996). Pathways to where? For young people with a mental illness. *Parity: Victorian Council to Homeless Persons*, **1**, 8–9.

Lincoln, C. V. & McGorry, P. D. (1995). Who cares? Pathways to psychiatric care in early psychosis. *Psychiatric Services*, **46**, 1166–71.

Lincoln, Y. S. & Guba, E. G. (1985). *Naturalistic Inquiry*. Beverly Hills, California: Sage Publications.

Loebel, A. D., Lieberman, J. A., Alvir, J. M. J., Mayerhoff, D. I., Geisler, S. H. & Szymanski, S. R. (1992). Duration of psychosis and outcome in first-episode schizophrenia. *American Journal of Psychiatry*, **149**, 1183–8.

Manktelow, R. (1994). *Paths to Psychiatric Hospitalisation. A Sociological Analysis*. Aldershot: Avebury Press.

Markus, H. & Nurius, P. (1986). Possible selves. *American Psychologist*, **41**, 954–69.

McGlashan, T. H. (1996). Early detection and intervention in schizophrenia: research. *Schizophrenia Bulletin*, **22**, 327–45.

McGlashan, T. H. & Carpenter, W. T. (1988). Long-term follow-up studies of schizophrenia. *Schizophrenia Bulletin*, **14**, 497–500.

McGorry, P. D. (1992). The concept of recovery and secondary prevention in psychotic disorders. *Australian and New Zealand Journal of Psychiatry*, **26**, 3–17.

McGorry, P. D. (1993). Early Psychosis Prevention and Intervention Centre. *Australasian Psychiatry*, **1**, 32–4.

McGorry, P. D. & Singh, B. S. (1995). Schizophrenia: risk and possibility. In *Handbook of Studies on Preventive Psychiatry*, ed. B. Raphael & G. D. Burrows, pp. 491–514. Amsterdam: Elsevier Press.

McGorry, P. D., Singh, B. S. & Copolov, D. L. (1990). Royal Park Multidiagnostic Instrument for Psychosis: Part I: Rationale and review. *Schizophrenia Bulletin*, **16**, 501–15.

McGorry, P. D., Singh, B. S., Copolov, D. L., Kaplan, I., Dossetor, C. R. & Van Riel, R. J. (1990). Royal Park Multidiagnostic Instrument for Psychosis: Part 2: Development, reliability and validity. *Schizophrenia Bulletin*, **16**, 517–36.

McGorry, P. D., Chanen, A., McCarthy, E., Van Riel, R., McKenzie, D. & Singh, B. S. (1991). Post-traumatic stress disorder following recent-onset psychosis. An unrecognised postpsychotic syndrome. *Journal of Nervous and Mental Disease*, **179**, 253–8.

McGorry, P. D., Edwards, J., Mihalopoulos, C., Harrigan, S. M. & Jackson, H. J. (1996). The Early Psychosis Prevention and Intervention Centre (EPPIC): an evolving system of early detection and optimal management. *Schizophrenia Bulletin*, **22**, 305–26.

Mintz, L. I., Nuechterlein, K. H., Goldstein, M. J., Mintz, J. & Snyder, W. S. (1989). The initial onset of schizophrenia and family expressed emotion: some methodological considerations. *British Journal of Psychiatry*, **154**, 212–7.

Mishler, E. (1984). *The Discourse of Medicine.* Norwood, New Jersey: Ablex.

Moscarelli, M., Capri, S. & Nerri, L. (1991). Cost evaluation of chronic schizophrenia patients during the first three years after the first contact. *Schizophrenia Bulletin*, **17**, 421–6.

O'Mahony, P. D. (1982). Psychiatric patient denial of mental illness as a normal process. *British Journal of Medical Psychology*, **55**, 109–18.

Page, S. (1983). Psychiatric stigma: Two studies of behavior when the chips are down. *Canadian Journal of Community Mental Health*, **2**, 13–9.

Pearlin, L. I. (1992). Structure and meaning in medical sociology. *Journal of Health and Social Behavior*, **33**, 1–9.

Roberts, H. (1985). *The Patient Patients. Women and Their Doctors.* London: Pandora Press.

Rogler, L. H. & Cortes, D. E. (1993). Help-seeking pathways: a unifying concept in mental health care. *American Journal of Psychiatry*, **150**, 554–61.

Romme, M. A. & Escher, A. D. (1989). Hearing voices. *Schizophrenia Bulletin*, **15**, 209–16.

Sheppard, M. (1993). GP and informal group referrals to a community mental health centre: an examination of the pathway to psychiatric care. *Social Work and Social Sciences Review*, **4**, 232–54.

Spicker, P., Anderson, I., Freeman, R. & McGilp, R. (1995). Pathways through psychiatric care: the experience of psychiatric patients. *Health and Social Care in the Community*, **3**, 343–52.

Stahl, S. M. (1994). New therapeutic advances in schizophrenia. In *Exploring the*

Spectrum of Psychosis, ed. R. Ancill, S. Holliday & J. Higenbottam, pp. 137–52. New York: John Wiley.

Strauss, J. S. (1994). The person with schizophrenia as a person. II: Approaches to the subjective and complex. *British Journal of Psychiatry*, **164** (Supplement 23), 103–7.

Thomas, J. (1993). *Doing Critical Ethnography: Qualitative Research Methods Series 26*. Newbury Park, California: Sage Publications.

Weiner, I. B. (1992). *Psychological Disturbance in Adolescence*, 2nd edn. New York: Wiley Interscience.

Williams, G. (1984). The genesis of chronic illness: narrative re-construction. *Sociology of Health and Illness*, **6**, 176–200.

Wyatt, R. J. (1991a). Neuroleptics and the natural course of schizophrenia. *Schizophrenia Bulletin*, **17**, 325–51.

Wyatt, R. J. (1991b). The effect of early neuroleptic intervention on the course of schizophrenia (abstract). *Schizophrenia Research*, **4**, 297.

Wyatt, R. J. (in press). Early intervention for schizophrenia: can the course of illness be attenuated? *Biological Psychiatry*.

Zola, I. K. (1973). Pathways to the doctor – from person to patient. *Social Science and Medicine*, **7**, 677–89.

4

Promoting access to care in early psychosis

ALISON R. YUNG, LISA J. PHILLIPS AND LORELLE T. DREW

Introduction

Paying attention to referral networks and the initial contact that a young person and his or her family have with psychiatric services can play a major role in improving outcome in early psychosis. While prospective consumers will continue to be ambivalent about seeking help, the initial contact with psychiatric services can be shaped to better address the needs of this patient population, and to overcome some of the barriers to care identified in Chapter 3. This chapter will examine ways in which access to effective intervention can be promoted and will describe two service models. The first, the Early Psychosis Assessment Team (EPAT) has as its goal *secondary prevention* in first-episode psychosis, aiming both to attenuate the period of untreated psychosis, and to reduce the secondary morbidity associated with becoming engaged with psychiatric services in general. The second model, the Personal Assistance and Crisis Evaluation (PACE) Clinic, has as its goal *indicated prevention* (see Chapter 1), aiming to deliver a service to young people who find themselves possibly in the prodromal phase of psychosis. The philosophy underpinning each of these service models will be described, and a description of the services provided. Some salient data from each service will also be presented.

Service access in the acute phase of first-episode psychosis

> Maybe Johnathon doesn't have schizophrenia, I thought hastily. But how the hell could I find out if Johnathon refused to go to the doctors and the doctors wouldn't come to him? (Deveson, 1991, p. 28)

4 PROMOTING ACCESS TO CARE

The difficulties in accessing appropriate treatment for a person experiencing a first psychotic episode, and the impact that this delay can have on outcome, have been described in previous chapters. This section draws on the 'pathways to care' literature to examine ways in which services can be structured to promote service access in first-episode psychosis. Case detection and promotion of early engagement in treatment are two important areas which need to be considered.

Case detection

The route to psychiatric services involves help-seeking by the individual, recognition of psychosis by the agency from which help is sought, and subsequent referral to psychiatric services. There is a potential for disruptions to occur at each of these stages, which will now be considered in turn.

Help-seeking

The general psychiatric literature indicates that most psychiatrically ill patients present to their primary carer at some stage in their illness (Goldberg & Huxley, 1980; Weissman, Myers & Harding, 1978). However, this help-seeking may be impaired in individuals with recent onset psychosis for several reasons. First, there are some factors which may have specificity for psychosis, such as suspiciousness and persecutory ideas, social withdrawal and lack of insight (Kissling, 1994) – all of which may inhibit help-seeking. This is illustrated in the vignettes presented in Chapter 3. Secondly, psychotic disorders usually manifest for the first time in adolescence and early adulthood (Kosky & Hardy, 1992). Young people may have difficulty understanding and interpreting psychotic experiences and their mental health problems (Lincoln & McGorry, 1995), and perceptions of adolescent 'invulnerability' may also delay help-seeking. This is often compounded by the family's lack of knowledge about psychosis, the ignorance of the wider community in general, and the stigma which is still associated with accessing care for mental health problems. Further, comorbid problems such as homelessness (Mundy, Robertson & Robertson, 1990), and substance use (Ridgely, Goldman & Willenbring, 1990), may render help-seeking difficult. A fuller discussion of these issues is presented in Chapter 3.

How can the situation be improved to enhance help-seeking amongst psychotic young people? Clearly, both the health behaviours of individuals alone, and attitudes towards mental health held by society in general, need to be challenged. Health promotion strategists have noted the need to reduce the stigma of mental illnesses via community education programmes, and by raising mental health on the political agenda

(Vlais, 1993). Highlighting the potential for recovery from psychotic disorders – a potential improved by the availability of newer medications with fewer side effects – forms one strategy for changing attitudes towards treatment. Additionally, promoting community treatment, as an alternative to hospitalized treatment, and focussing on the patient's ability to function adequately in the community, forms another strategy for changing community attitudes towards the mentally ill (Peterson, 1986). Services should also be developed which are sensitive to the needs of the young, the homeless, and to those who use substances. These changes will require broad shifts in government policy and community attitudes, and are likely to be difficult to achieve, especially in the short term. Mental health professionals and mental health service providers have a part to play in facilitating these changes at both policy and community levels.

Recognition
Recognition of psychiatric disorders by general practitioners (GPs) and other primary health workers is the next important step in the path to psychiatric care. Often, however, primary health carers do not correctly identify mental health problems (Goldberg & Huxley, 1980; Weissman et al., 1978). Possible reasons for this failure to detect psychiatric disorders have been suggested (Dunn, 1983; Goldberg & Huxley, 1980; Shepherd et al., 1966). Parenthetically, one should note that all of these studies are based on the detection of non-psychotic psychiatric disorders, such as anxiety and depression. One conclusion drawn from these studies was that patients often report somatic complaints to their family doctors rather than psychological or psychiatric symptoms (Shepherd et al., 1966), this being due perhaps to the patient misinterpreting his or her symptoms, the stigma associated with psychiatric disorders, or because of the patient's belief that physical symptoms are what the doctor expects to be consulted about (Goldberg & Huxley, 1980). One implication of this practice is that GPs need to be able to detect psychiatric symptoms in the midst of physical complaints – a skill that has been associated with the degree of interest in psychiatry held by the GP and the academic qualifications of individual GPs, as well as the level of concern for the patient in general (Goldberg & Huxley, 1980; Millar & Goldberg, 1991). In association with this, Goldberg & Huxley (1980) also found that interview techniques – in particular the asking of clarifying questions and interpreting verbal and non-verbal cues – was associated with both the tendency, and accuracy, of GPs to diagnose psychiatric illnesses.

Another factor which may make recognition of recent onset psychosis difficult is that in the early stages symptoms may be subtle (Weiner,

1992; Yung & McGorry, 1996a,b), and GPs need to be able to maintain an 'index of suspicion' for these disorders (Weiner, 1992). Educating GPs to increase their awareness of psychotic disorders and the various presentations of the same, is an important goal. Knowledge of mental health services also needs to be increased. The reluctance of some GPs to diagnose a serious, or potentially serious, mental illness, due to their own negative and pessimistic attitudes, also needs to be challenged. Of course, these educational measures should be expanded to include not just GPs, but also other groups of people likely to have contact with significant numbers of young people at risk for a range of psychiatric disorders, including teachers, youth workers, ethnic community workers, welfare workers, and university counsellors (Vlais, 1993).

Referral

Even after a psychiatric disorder has been recognized, many patients are still not referred to appropriate mental health services (Orleans et al., 1985; Shepherd et al., 1966). The literature suggests that psychotic patients are more likely to be referred than patients with other disorders, but referral is still not inevitable (McNamara & Lewin, 1989). Reasons for non-referral have been examined and include the belief that patients will be upset or stigmatized by psychiatric referral (Shepherd et al., 1966; Steinberg, Torem & Saravay, 1980), the view that care of the emotionally ill is the family doctor's job (Shepherd et al., 1966), and a belief that psychiatry cannot help (Steinberg et al., 1980). This may be the case with psychotic disorders, in particular, given the wide perception that these conditions are not treatable (McGorry, 1995).

Difficulties accessing mental health services comprise another factor in non-referral (McNamara & Lewin, 1989; Shepherd et al., 1966). Possible sources of this difficulty can be hypothesized. Existing overloaded services are often more comfortable dealing with known patients than new referrals, especially as new referrals may take a long time to engage in a service and thus require assertive follow-up at the initial phase of contact. New patients also require intensive assessment, and the diagnosis may not be clear-cut initially. This, in turn, leads to delays in engagement in the service (Weiner, 1992). Additionally, a tension may be perceived to exist between the brief of managing patients with 'serious mental illness' (often thought to mean chronic psychotic disorders), and the role of assessment and intake of new cases. This conflict may lead to an 'antiprevention' effect of 'wait until it worsens' before implementing effective treatment. This practice can be likened to waiting until a cancer metastasizes or a new diabetic patient develops ketoacidotic coma before offering treatment!

Dissatisfaction with the treatment provided by mental health clinics, including poor communication between the mental health service and the referring agency, may also contribute to non-referral (McNamara & Lewin, 1989; Shepherd et al., 1966). Inadequate liaison between referrer and the service may be a result of overwork in mental health services. The implications of these findings are that, notwithstanding the need to educate GPs, changes in psychiatric service structures and practices must also be made in order to facilitate referrals.

Engagement in treatment

Engagement in psychiatric treatment is the other important factor necessary for ensuring that patients receive appropriate help early in the course of illness. The body of literature examining compliance of psychotic patients with treatment suggests factors which may also pertain to early engagement in treatment. First, this research indicates that providing a community-based service, as opposed to a hospital-based service, improves both follow-up rates and outcome, probably because the former is more acceptable to patients and families alike (Burns et al., 1993; Merson et al., 1992).

Additionally, factors such as geographical access and the cultural appropriateness of services may promote treatment compliance (Gjerris, 1994; Royal College of Psychiatrists, 1987). Some provision for a collaborative approach between service providers and consumers has also been noted to be helpful in making a psychiatric service more acceptable to consumers (Gjerris, 1994), including tailoring treatment to the individual rather than incorporating the patient within existing programmes (Taube et al., 1990). Extending the hours of operation of both outpatient centres (Gjerris, 1994) and home visits (Taube et al., 1990), has also been associated with more rapid engagement and increased compliance of consumers. Although these studies have largely assessed the compliance of long-term patients with psychiatric services, it is felt that these factors may also promote the early engagement of individuals with recent-onset psychosis.

A further relevant finding is that the level of engagement of a patient with a service is improved if the same clinician is seen at all appointments (Gjerris, 1994). Thus, continuity of care is another important service factor for promoting engagement (Meltzer et al., 1991).

Attitudinal factors in psychotic patients, such as denial of illness, and the belief that medication is not needed or is ineffective, are often associated with non-compliance (Amador et al., 1994; Kane et al., 1982; Kissling, 1994). These attitudes tend to be more common in patients with first-episode psychosis than in multiple-episode patients (Kane et al., 1982). Non-compliance of patients may be further reinforced by families, only 20% of whom, in a recent study, considered that medication was suitable for the treatment of schizophrenia (Angermeyer & Matschinger, 1994). Thus, another important strategy for enhancing engagement in psychiatric services is the provision of psychoeducation to patients and families early in the contact with a psychiatric service (Kissling, 1994).

Psychotic patients with comorbid problems, including depression, low self-esteem, and substance misuse, have been found to be at increased risk of non-compliance and early drop-out from treatment (Mulaik, 1992). Hence, early attention to the possibility of such comorbid problems may also promote engagement in psychiatric services.

This section highlights the fact that various issues pertaining to psychiatric services need to be attended to, in order to enhance the engagement of first-episode patients in treatment. Many of these issues relate to the structure and practice of the psychiatric service. The provision of a community-based, and especially a home-based, service, complete with flexible hours and continuity of care is important. The ability to be both informal and to provide a collaborative and supportive approach tailored to the needs of the individual and the family, may enhance the rate of acceptance of psychiatric services by consumers. The provision of early psychoeducation may also enhance the engagement process. Training mental health workers both in the early recognition and treatment of comorbid problems, and to be assertive in the follow-up process, are other strategies aimed at increasing the acceptability of psychiatric contact and retention in the service.

Summary – promoting access to care in the acute phase

The pathway to effective intervention for a patient with early psychosis involves the complex interaction of a number of factors across a number of systems which affect help-seeking, recognition, referral and engagement. Strategies to facilitate the patient's access to care have been considered in relation to each of these variables. These are briefly summarized in Table 4.1. One service model which aims to address these issues is described below.

The Early Psychosis Assessment Team

The Early Psychosis Assessment Team (EPAT) is part of the Early Psychosis Prevention and Intervention Centre (EPPIC). EPAT functions as the entry point into EPPIC and aims to decrease the period of untreated psychosis and to reduce the trauma and secondary morbidity

Table 4.1. *Strategies to facilitate patient access to care*

Case detection	
Help seeking	Increase knowledge and recognition of symptoms by patients and families
	Reduce stigma and fear of psychiatric services
	Make services accessible and acceptable
Recognition by primary carers	Increase awareness of psychiatric disorders and psychiatric services
	Increase knowledge
	Enhance communication skills
Referral to psychiatric services	Make services accessible and provide high quality feedback to referring agencies
Engagement in treatment	Make services accessible and flexible
	Provide continuity of care
	Provide a comprehensive service for patients and families

which is often associated with engagement in psychiatric services. Several of the factors described above have been incorporated into the team's functioning in order to achieve these aims. Initially conceived with purely an assessment focus, EPAT was staffed by a multidisciplinary team and operated between the hours of 9.00 am and 5.00 pm, after which a local 24-hour psychiatric service responded to crises. Since August 1995, however, EPAT's hours of operation were expanded to 8.30 am to 10.00 pm daily, with an on-call recall system after those hours. A home-based treatment component, with 24-hour accessibility, has also been implemented. The operation of the team consists of three components, each of which is considered in turn.

The intake system

The intake system aims to provide an accessible point of contact for referring agencies, families, and young people. Referrals are accepted from any source, including young people and their families, with the majority received via the telephone. Naturally, the criteria for inclusion in the service are the same as those of the parent EPPIC programme, i.e. the young person must be aged between 15 and 30 years, reside in the Western Metropolitan region of Melbourne (population

4 PROMOTING ACCESS TO CARE

800,000), and be experiencing recent-onset psychosis. Basic details are ascertained over the telephone from the referral agent and, if there is a reasonable suspicion that the individual is experiencing recent-onset psychosis, then that young person is accepted for further assessment with EPAT. EPAT's philosophy is inclusive, rather than exclusive. In other words, we prefer to assess all young people who may have a psychosis in order to identify all true cases, even if this means seeing large numbers of patients with other psychiatric disorders, or who, for other reasons, are not appropriate for EPPIC. Some potential cases are monitored and assessed longitudinally over time, sometimes up to several weeks, where doubt about the presence of a psychosis exists. In addition, young people who may be in the prodromal phase of psychosis are referred to a specialized clinic designed to manage this group, PACE, which is also linked with EPPIC (described later in this chapter). Care is taken at the initial contact stage to be approachable and helpful to the referring agent. Referrers of inappropriate cases (i.e. persons who reside out of the area or do not fulfil other intake criteria), are given advice as to alternative services. EPAT workers will sometimes make these follow-up inquiries for the referring agents, particularly if they are young people referring themselves, or families referring a member, in order to reduce the trauma of gaining access to care. After the initial assessment of the young person is completed, EPAT team members give feedback to referring agents. This practice may encourage further referrals from the same source in the future.

Community education

EPAT aims to increase awareness of, and knowledge of, psychotic disorders; to promote the recognition of psychosis; and to provide information about available services and how to access them. These education activities are targeted at primary care health professionals such as GPs, and other people in the community who have contact with young people, such as school and university counsellors and youth workers. EPAT workers have also been involved in more general community education forums, such as appearing on national radio and television to discuss psychosis and participation in nationwide and statewide community-organized activities such as 'Schizophrenia Awareness Week' and 'Mental Health Week'. A series of educational videos has also been made, including two suitable for GPs and one for the general public. Education strategies targeting the general population are intended to increase knowledge and awareness of psychotic disorders, but also to reduce stigma and decrease fear of mental health workers and services. One strategy aimed at enhancing the general knowledge about psychosis was the introduction of an EPPIC home page on the Internet in 1995.

The clinical service

The clinical task of EPAT is to provide a comprehensive and readily accessible service for assessment of young people referred with a possible problem of recent onset, or untreated/never previously treated, psychosis. The team aims to incorporate the practices identified above which enhance referral and promote engagement in treatment. An additional aim is to reduce the trauma which may be associated with initial contact with psychiatric services, including minimizing the use of police and involuntary admission. The extended hours offered by EPAT, together with flexibility in the site of assessment (home, school or workplace, or other community environments), reduces the amount of stress experienced by the patient and family at this initial contact. EPAT aims to provide a rapid response, with urgent referrals being seen as soon as possible, often within two hours (averaging one hour), and always on the same day of referral. The EPAT team was separated from the case management system of EPPIC, in order to reduce or-organizational barriers which may inhibit the passage of new referrals into the service, such as the overloading of the case management system. As a result, a very open or porous entry channel can be assured. The disadvantage of this approach is that discontinuities in care arise when ongoing management of the young person is transferred to the case manager after the assessment phase. In order to minimize this problem, attempts are made to engage case managers early in the assessment process, and a gradual transfer of care is arranged.

The engagement in treatment itself is another major focus for EPAT. We acknowledge that it may take some young people several weeks at least, to be able to recognize the need for treatment, and to become sufficiently motivated to attend regular outpatient appointments. In such circumstances, rather than resorting to inpatient admission for these patients, EPAT can provide some home-based treatment and help transport the young person to the outpatient centre. The designated case manager is introduced and involved at an early stage, thus facilitating engagement with the service and enhancing continuity of care. This cautious and unobtrusive approach is not always appropriate, however, especially in cases where there is a likelihood of danger to the young person or others (see Case 3 below).

Finally, EPAT has a role in working with families at the time of initial contact (see Chapters 8 and 14). Often this is a time of crisis for families, who may be distressed at the changes in their family member and at finding themselves involved with psychiatric services. The EPAT team is aware of the potential trauma experienced by families at this time and provide both psychoeducation and support for families and patients at this early stage.

It is believed that recent changes to EPAT, including the expansion to include a home-based treatment component, will aid young peoples' retention within the service. It also increases our ability to provide a less stigmatizing treatment environment. It will be important, however, to ensure that the educational and assessment functions are not compromised by the change.

Illustrative data

Total referrals

In the 12 months from October 1993 to October 1994, EPAT dealt with 496 referrals, of which 314 were clinically assessed and 250 were accepted into the EPPIC programme (i.e. 50% of all referrals and 80% of those assessed). A number of other referrals were accepted after hours. This is consistent with the expected incidence of psychosis in the general population of 10–28 per 100,000 per year (Eaton, 1985; Jablensky et al., 1992). The most recent figures for the 12 months from March 1995 to March 1996 show an increased referral rate – perhaps due to the introduction of the 24-hour service in August 1995. During this time period, 231 patients were accepted into the EPPIC programme (Power et al., 1998). This slight reduction in accepted referrals may indicate that we are missing some cases, or might suggest that the 'backlog' of previously non-referred cases may have been largely cleared. An additional 45 referrals in this 12-month period were directed to the PACE Clinic.

Referral sources

Evaluation of our sources of referral reflects the effectiveness of community education and networking. In the first six months of operation 49.8% of referrals came from outside psychiatric services. This had increased to 57.0% in the last six months (i.e. January to June 1996). Family and friends comprised 9.8% of referrals in the first six months, and this had increased to 23.0% in the last six months (from January to June 1996).

Of some concern has been the low rate of referrals directly from GPs. This was constant at about 5% of referrals for the first two years of operation. Steps were taken to improve the liaison between EPAT and GPs by appointing a GP liaison officer – a GP who has had experience working with EPAT. Seminars and workshops targeted at GPs in the EPPIC catchment area are thought to be at least partly responsible for the increase in GP referrals from 9% of all referrals in 1995 to 14% in the last six months (from January to June, 1996).

Response time

Mean response time for urgent referrals to EPAT was 68.1 minutes in the first 12 months. This reflects EPAT's capacity to respond rapidly to potential emergency situations and is also indicative of EPPIC's large geographical catchment area, with some suburbs lying over an hour's drive away from EPAT's base. The response time to non-urgent referrals was 3.1 days, reflecting a complementary capacity to arrange assessments at a time convenient for the young person and his or her family.

Outcome of accepted referrals

Of the young people accepted into the EPPIC programme in the 12 months from March 1995 to March 1996, 85 (36.7% of accepted referrals) were treated in the community during the first six weeks, either by the mobile team or in the outpatient centre, and 146 (63.2%) were admitted to the inpatient unit at some stage during their first three months of involvement with EPPIC (Power et al., 1998). This compares to 85% of 51 cases hospitalized during the first year of operation of EPPIC (1993). Although the time frames are somewhat different, this suggests that there has been an increase in our ability to manage patients in the community as EPAT has developed and its role has changed, particularly with the advent of the 24-hour EPPIC mobile team.

Police involvement

As part of EPAT's objective to minimize the trauma associated with initial psychiatric contact, data about police involvement with transporting a young person to hospital were also collected. Nine cases in the last six months required police involvement. This represents 9.5% of all accepted referrals and 22.5% of all admissions – a substantial reduction from the early years of EPPIC's operation. Police involvement is avoided, if possible, because it might convey to the patient the confusing message that he or she has done something wrong, rather than being unwell. Additionally, police involvement has been found to be an index of late presentation to the service.

Duration of untreated psychosis

This outcome measure is a major determinant of the effectiveness of EPAT. Comparison was made with a historical control sample, the 'pre-EPPIC' group, which comprises a matched sample of first-episode patients recruited prior to the establishment of the full EPPIC programme, including EPAT. Comparison shows that the duration of untreated psychosis (DUP) in the EPPIC group was reduced from a mean of 193.7 days to 157.4 days. However, the median duration of DUP increased in the EPPIC sample from 25.0 days to 42.0 days. Further analysis of the data reveals that the reduction in the mean DUP is due to the decrease in the number of outliers with very long DUP. However, there were also fewer patients with very short DUP in the EPPIC sample compared to the pre-EPPIC sample (for further discussion of this see Chapter 3). It is noted that the DUP of EPPIC groups is very short (even in the 'pre-EPPIC' sample) compared with overseas data (e.g. Larsen, McGlashan & Moe, 1996; Loebel et al., 1992) indicating perhaps, that we have reached a ceiling effect of shortening the DUP – especially for the average patient presenting to EPPIC. Most effort now is being focussed on reducing the outliers (i.e. those patients with a DUP of greater than 6–12 months), particularly since it seems that more intensive treatment has less effect on outcome on such cases (see Chapter 3).

Case examples

The following case vignettes illustrate different aspects of EPAT's functioning.

Case 1

LC was a 25-year-old single woman of Mediterranean background, born in Australia. She lived with her mother in an outer suburb of Melbourne. Her 31-year-old sister lived in a neighbouring street and was in daily contact with LC and her mother. LC had been unemployed for the last five years prior to contact with psychiatric services, since the death of her father from heart disease. At the time of his death she was working as a factory process worker, but was unable to function in this role after the death. Over the last five years she had become increasingly withdrawn and unmotivated but, on questioning by the family, continued to deny that her decline was in any way related to the loss of her father. She put on weight and seemed increasingly less concerned by her appearance. She became irritable and moody. The family themselves were grieving and were unsure of what action to take. They arranged for LC to visit relatives in Europe for an extended stay, and she returned six months later, and 18 months prior to psychiatric contact, essentially unchanged.

Over the next 18 months she continued to deteriorate, and the family noticed that she exhibited some odd behaviour, including talking to herself, swearing at the pet dog, and dismantling various household items such as a clock and an exercise bicycle. When she started to throw valuables such as jewellery and credit cards in the garbage, and to physically assault the dog, the family became extremely worried and sought help.

LC's sister contacted their GP who had known the family for many years. He assessed LC and was suspicious that a psychotic disorder might be developing based on the above history, but was unable to elicit any psychotic phenomena on inquiry. He started LC on a low dose (10 mg) of thioridazine and, as he had heard of EPAT through an educational seminar, telephoned the team to discuss the case. The EPAT clinician who took the referral agreed with the doctor that the history was indicative of a psychosis. The clinician then telephoned the sister to discuss the case further and to organize an assessment plan.

LC's sister was concerned that LC would refuse to attend a mental health clinic as she did not believe that she was mentally ill and was reluctant to leave the house at all. A home visit by the EPAT psychiatrist and social worker was arranged. LC's sister felt that the best option was to refrain from informing LC of the appointment until the workers arrived, at which point she casually introduced them and stated that they had 'come for a visit'. In this case the EPAT workers agreed to this strategy.

The initial appointment was kept rather informal as LC was obviously guarded and suspicious of the EPAT clinicians. At one point this even included LC giving the workers a guided tour of the house. The GP's treatment was reinforced by the EPAT team and an early follow-up appointment at home was arranged. At this first contact family psychoeducation was conducted. This included the provision of written material and a video about psychosis.

Feedback was given to the GP after this first contact. The psychiatrist suggested that the medication should be increased as there was a strong suspicion of a psychotic disorder, and the GP was happy for EPAT to arrange this. The GP also stated that he was willing to continue to be involved in collaboration with the team.

The same EPAT clinicians returned the next day and continued the assessment. Again the contact was informal and rapport with the patient increased. LC disclosed that she had been under stress and sometimes felt 'uncomfortable'. This presented a rationale for increasing the medication.

This strategy of informal home visits continued for a further three weeks, essentially with the same clinicians. Over this time LC admit-

> ted to several frankly psychotic symptoms including thought broadcasting, thought insertion and auditory hallucinations. The thioridazine was slowly increased to 150 mg per day. After three weeks the EPAT clinicians introduced the outpatient case manager (OCM), and continued to visit LC at home accompanied by this case manager. LC's mental state improved, and as she became engaged with the OCM, the EPAT team gradually withdrew.

This case highlights a number of issues. First, there was quite a long DUP, probably at least 18 months, and possibly longer. This was due to various factors including the insidious onset of symptoms, the patient's guardedness and the family's difficulty in recognizing the signs of mental illness. This was compounded by the family grief over the loss of LC's father, possibly leading to the family experiencing difficulty both in coping and mobilizing treatment. The family might also have attributed some of LC's abnormal behaviour to grief.

The referral to psychiatric services was aided by the GP's skill in recognizing a possible psychosis and his knowledge of appropriate mental health services. Thus, multiple referrals were avoided. His long-standing relationship with the family would have been important in enabling him to evaluate the longitudinal history of the patient's condition as well as her mental state. Additionally, he was in a good position to rationalize the use of medication with LC. The ability of the EPAT team to see the patient in her own home and at a time convenient to the family was also important. This informal, friendly and unhurried approach to assessment was acceptable to LC and her family, and talking to the family about psychosis and options for treatment resulted in LC's mother and sister encouraging her to form a relationship with the EPAT workers. The establishment of a relationship between LC and EPAT workers was enhanced by EPAT's policy of ensuring continuity of care (i.e. the family and patient are seen by the same EPAT workers as much as possible, rather than seeing different workers on each visit). Finally, the introduction of the OCM on a home visit, and the gradual handover process, aided in the continued engagement of LC in the service, thus enabling her recovery to be assisted by access to the full range of EPPIC interventions and services.

Case 2

> PL was a 26-year-old single man who lived with his parents in the inner suburbs of Melbourne. He had a family history of chronic

schizophrenia in a paternal uncle; the latter had spent many years in a psychiatric hospital. For the last six years prior to referral PL had been living in his bedroom at home, rarely leaving it at all. PL's parents contacted their GP about him as they were experiencing financial difficulties in supporting him and wondered if there was anything that could be done to increase his motivation to work. The GP referred him to the local community mental health clinic which, in turn, referred him to EPAT.

The EPAT duty worker spoke to PL's mother on the telephone to gain further information. He discovered that PL had always been shy with few friends at school and was a student of below average aptitude. He left school at the age of 16, and for four years had worked intermittently at various unskilled jobs such as factory work. The longest he spent at any one workplace was three months. At the age of 20 he was accused of stealing some factory products by a manager. He was distressed by this, left the job, and had remained at home without attempting to seek work since then. His unemployment benefits had been ceased as he had not produced any evidence of seeking employment. On further questioning, PL's mother recalled that a few months ago he had shaved off all his body hair without explanation. There were no other examples of odd behaviour recalled by PL's mother.

After gaining this information, the EPAT clinician was suspicious that PL might be psychotic because of the history of psychosocial deterioration, the poor premorbid functioning and the family history of schizophrenia. It was thought that a clinical assessment should be conducted. This was suggested to PL's mother but she was anxious about this suggestion. She claimed that PL would be unlikely to agree to be seen, and stated that her son was 'not a danger to the community'. She requested that the team not visit the home, and assured the duty worker that she would contact EPAT if she became worried about her son.

At the EPAT team meeting it was decided to contact the GP and discuss the case with him further. He agreed to contact the family again with the intention of emphasizing to them the need for an assessment of PL. A few days later the original EPAT duty worker contacted PL's mother again and suggested that she should come to the centre to further discuss her concerns. One week later she arrived with her husband to speak to EPAT workers.

This proved to be a valuable family meeting. It became apparent that the family had a negative view of psychiatric services developed largely through their experiences in the 1970s and 1980s with their mentally ill relative. They were apprehensive that PL would be hospitalized for a lengthy period in a large psychiatric institution. They were afraid that he would be stigmatized and 'drugged', and they felt that psychiatric services could not help anyway. Additionally, they stated that their son could not have schizophrenia as he did not act violently or say odd things.

Over two sessions with PL's parents a number of these issues were discussed. The family's fears and misapprehensions regarding psychotic illnesses and mental health services were addressed. They were given written literature to read, shown a video describing treatment of psychosis, and given a tour of the outpatient facility. These sessions also enabled the family to get to know some of the EPAT clinicians. Eventually they felt comfortable, thus permitting EPAT to undertake an assessment of their son at home.

A similar process to that described in Case 1 then ensued in the assessment and engagement of PL in the service, with home visits by, wherever possible, the same clinicians. He admitted that his life was 'not normal', but justified his isolation by saying he was 'working out what to do'. This explanatory model was used by the team who suggested that he attend some group activities available at EPPIC which might help him decide on a career path. His case manager was introduced to him at one of these groups, and she encouraged him to take medication on the grounds that it may help him to think more clearly, and hence aid his decision making.

This case illustrates how ignorance and fear of mental health services may contribute to delayed help-seeking by potential patients and families. In this case, the previous experience of psychiatry and the psychiatric systems of over a decade ago compounded these anxieties. The EPAT team expended considerable effort demystifying the role of EPPIC clinicians and this seemed to be of benefit. Another factor which may have contributed to the delay in referral was the insidious onset of the disorder in this case, particularly in the context of a poorly functioning premorbid personality. Again, a friendly, unhurried and flexible approach was used in the assessment procedure, and the use of the patient's own explanatory model was a strategy to enhance engagement. Unfortunately, it is not always possible to have such an unhurried approach to referrals. This is the case with situations which are potentially dangerous for the patient or others.

Case 3

RW was a 19-year-old single university student who lived in shared accommodation in the inner city area. He was referred to EPAT by the local CMHC which had been telephoned by his mother. She was concerned about his erratic behaviour over the last few weeks, and the night prior to her seeking assistance he was found by his friends walking along a railway track. He claimed that he was trying to prove that he was more powerful than a train.

RW's mother was clearly distressed by the situation, and while one EPAT worker telephoned RW's house another worker spent time talking with her and assuring her that action would be taken. RW was not at his home when the duty worker telephoned, but information from his housemate confirmed that he had been acting oddly for several weeks. For example, he threw away all of his books or burnt them, praying loudly in his room (he was not previously known to be religious), and staying up until the early hours of the morning writing in a diary. As well as walking on the railway tracks, he had been found lying on the road the previous day saying he could defeat trucks and cars. Luckily, he had been seen by another of the house mates and dragged away. She had assumed that he was intoxicated.

The EPAT clinicians were concerned for RW's safety. Instructions were left both with the housemate and RW's mother for them to telephone the team if he were sighted. In these telephone interactions, care was taken to assure RW's mother and housemate that we were worried about RW, and had his interests in mind in attempting to assess and manage him. Premature labelling (such as saying RW probably had schizophrenia) was avoided, and the clinicians emphasized that it seemed that RW was ill and in need of help.

Later that afternoon RW's housemate phoned from a public telephone to say that RW had arrived home. EPAT clinicians attended immediately. RW presented as psychotic with some manic features including grandiose delusions. He stated that he knew he was not his normal self but felt better than he had ever felt before. The EPAT clinicians were unable to convince RW that he was unwell and needed treatment. In view of the risk he presented to himself if he were to remain untreated in the community, the decision was made to admit RW to hospital involuntarily. RW initially refused to be transported to hospital by the EPAT workers. However,after an ambulance arrived RW, seemingly confronted by the inevitability of his admission to hospital, agreed to be driven in the EPAT car.

Follow-up sessions were provided for RW's mother and his housemate. The aim was to 'debrief' them about RW's admission to hospital. Both the housemate and RW's mother were feeling guilty at not having recognized the problem or acting sooner. However, it was emphasized that they had both taken correct courses of action, and that RW was receiving the treatment he needed.

This was an urgent case of acute psychosis in which the young person was at risk due to the illness. In this situation it was unsafe to take a slow approach to assessment and management. However, it was still important to minimize trauma for the patient, for example, by avoiding police involvement, and treating him in a respectful manner, even at the time of compulsory hospitalization. Another issue this case highlights once again, is the importance of engaging the family and other significant persons in the management of the patient. The housemate and mother needed to be 'on side' in order to organize the assessment, and they also helped persuade RW to eventually be transported by EPAT to hospital. This case is also an example of how a patient's particular symptoms affect the ability to seek help. RW was enjoying his manic symptoms and did not want them to be removed. This proved to be a barrier to him requesting treatment for himself.

Accessing patients in the prodromal phase

Discussion thus far has dealt with strategies for reducing the delay between onset of psychosis and access to effective treatment. A still more ambitious aim, with an indicated prevention focus, is to access young people prior to the onset of frank psychotic disorder, during the prodromal phase. The conceptual issues which underlie this approach have been discussed in Chapters 1 and 2.

There are several difficulties in attempting to identify young people in the prodromal phase before a first episode of psychosis and subsequent intervention; these have been discussed in Chapter 2. To summarize briefly, these include doubts over which psychopathological features should be included in the concept of 'prodrome', how to measure these, and the non-specific nature of many of the putatively prodromal features which can lead to the identification of false positives.

Issues such as these have made the task of intervention in the prodromal phase seem almost impossibly difficult, despite calls for such a preventive approach being made earlier in this century (Cameron, 1938; Meares, 1959; Sullivan, 1927). One attempt was made by Falloon in Buckinghamshire, England (Falloon, 1992). In this project, the DSM-III-R (American Psychiatric Association, 1987) criteria for schizophrenic prodrome were used to identify putatively prodromal cases, and a combination of low-dose symptom-targeted neuroleptic medication and psychological interventions, such as stress management and individual and family psychoeducation about psychotic disorders, was implemented. Results were promising, with a reduction in the incidence of schizophrenia in that particular geographical region over a four-year follow-up period, compared to historical trends. A difficulty with this study is that it is not known how many of the cases identified as 'prodromal' were actually false positives, who would therefore have received unnecessary treatment. Falloon acknowledged this, and highlighted the preliminary nature of the research. Nevertheless, this study did illustrate that it might be possible, and appropriate, to access and treat people at the very earliest stage of illness, provided the risk: benefit ratio and the capacity of the clinician to inform the potential patient about such matters, could be enhanced through further research.

What can be done to minimize the false positives? One strategy is to sharpen the predictive focus by blending psychopathological changes which make up the potential 'prodrome' with other variables or potential risk factors, which would make transition to psychosis more likely, i.e. utilize a 'close-in' strategy (Bell, 1992). Potential risk factors for psychosis have been delineated in Chapter 2 and include age, family history, personality and life event features, and putative biological and cognitive markers (Adams et al., 1993; Cornblatt & Keilp, 1994; Lieberman et al., 1993; O'Callaghan et al., 1992). The degree of risk conferred by each of these factors is not yet known, and this would need to be investigated further. Nonetheless, some of these risk factors could be combined with the presence of a possibly prodromal syndrome to identify a group at high risk of transition to psychosis within a brief follow-up period.

Identification of putatively prepsychotic (high-risk) individuals in the community

A major practical issue involved in the indicated prevention focus is that of how to identify high-risk individuals in the community and how to promote their passage into psychiatric services. It is now known that most people who develop a schizophrenic disorder will experience a prepsychotic phase, which is associated clearly with substantial disability (Häfner et al., 1993; Jones et al., 1993; Yung et al., 1996). Hence, there is ample scope and justification for the identification of such individuals. The 'filters' which may form barriers to engagement with psychiatric services, and which were described previously, obviously apply to this group (Goldberg & Huxley, 1980). Similar tactics to those described above in relation to facilitating service access for first-episode patients can be used for the high-risk group. For example, Falloon (1992) used a two-stage approach, first training all the GPs in the area to recognize and refer all patients with possible prodromal symptoms; and, secondly, setting up a readily accessible system for assessment by specialized mental health workers. Falloon reported promising results, both in the use of this strategy for case finding, and as regards the ability of his service to respond to referrals. Our approach to this issue has been similar and will be described below.

Interventions in the high-risk group

Once a high-risk group is identified, the question arises as to which interventions to offer. The schizophrenia relapse prevention literature provides a starting point. Stress management is one intervention which has been evaluated (Hogarty et al., 1991). Since it is known that not only can stress play a major role in precipitating relapse (Zubin & Spring, 1977), but also often precedes the first onset of schizophrenia (Brown & Birley, 1968), strategies which aim to reduce stress and promote a sense of control over perceived stressors may be important in decreasing the likelihood of progression to psychosis. The efficacy of social skills training and problem solving in relapse prevention, and disability reduction associated with schizophrenia, have also been evaluated (Hogarty et al., 1991). Improved functioning and fewer relapses have been reported. As many of the deficits targeted by this sort of intervention are present prior to the onset of frank psychotic symptoms (Jones et al., 1993), it is likely that using these techniques may also be of benefit in the high-risk group. Providing family education and support, and reducing family conflict (Leff et al., 1985), combined with strategies aimed at decreasing substance use, are other strategies that could be applied in the high-risk group. Finally, symptom monitoring and targeted medication is another treatment method used in relapse prevention which can be applied to the 'at-risk' population. This involves detection of mental state changes which could represent the prodrome of a relapse, and then reintroducing or increasing neuroleptic dose (Marder et al., 1994). This strategy could be modified to fit the high-risk group; mental state could be monitored and low-dose neuroleptic medication and psychosocial interventions could be used to avert the onset of psychosis, or modify the onset features if a change indicative of emerging frank psychosis is detected. Falloon's project used several of these treatments in the 'prodromal' group (Falloon, 1992).

The Personal Assistance and Crisis Evaluation clinic

Our group has attempted to identify, access, and intervene in a group of patients who are possibly in the prodromal phase, prior to a first episode of psychosis. The PACE (Personal Assistance and Crisis Evaluation) clinic has been established for this purpose. The development of this service has been possible due to the development of EPAT as described above. Through its extensive community networking, this team comes into contact with not only young people experiencing psychosis, but also some 'doubtful' cases who may be in the prodromal phase, or an 'at-risk mental state' (Yung et al., 1996) (see also Chapter 2). We have also been encouraged by Falloon's work which indicated that it is possible to access possibly prodromal cases by establishing links with primary care agencies (Falloon, 1992).

Intake criteria

The PACE clinic inclusion criteria aim to identify a group of people at high risk for developing a psychotic disorder in the near future. The criteria used in our pilot study are described in detail elsewhere (Yung et al., 1996). These criteria were revised in the light of a modest transition rate of 5 of 21 cases over 12 months, which suggested that many individuals identified as 'high risk' were in fact false positives. The second-phase intake criteria are described below. In designing these criteria, we drew on a more complete review of the psychosis prodrome literature, as well as those derived from our clinical experience with the pilot phase of the clinic's operation. Essentially, two different strategies were used for identifying this high-risk group.

The first broad strategy was a 'state' or symptomatic approach in which individuals presenting with psychopathological features of a possible 'prodrome' were recruited. In order to minimize false positives non-specific mental state changes, such as anxiety, depressed mood and poor role functioning were not included in this category. Instead, an attempt was made to use features which seemed to suggest a developing psychosis. To do this, we returned to the idea that psychotic symptoms occur on a continuum with normal functioning and that subthreshold or attenuated forms of frank psychotic features can be detected and measured (Strauss, 1969). Our impression from the pilot phase was that these symptoms tended to precede onset of frank psychosis in those patients making the transition. Using these principles, we defined the 'attenuated' group as characterized by attenuated or subthreshold forms of psychotic symptoms. Fully operationalized criteria are described elsewhere (Yung et al., 1996). The other group which seemed likely to make the transition to psychosis because of particular mental state changes, were those who had experienced transient psychotic symptoms. A past history of brief transient episodes of psychotic symptoms which spontaneously resolve has been described occasionally by patients presenting with 'full blown' psychotic disorders (Faergman, 1963; Jauch & Carpenter, 1988). Such transient psychotic symptoms are also known to occur in some people under the influence of certain psychoactive substances such as amphetamines and hallucinogens (Tsuang & Coryell, 1993; Vardy & Kay, 1983) and cannabis (McGuire et al., 1994), as well as being experienced by patients with some personality disorders such as borderline personality, particularly when under stress (Gunderson & Singer, 1975). These transient psychotic episodes might indicate increased risk of subsequent psychosis. Using these principles we defined the 'BLIPS' group (Brief Limited or Intermittent Psychotic Symptoms). Fully operationalized criteria are again described elsewhere (Yung et al., 1996).

The second broad approach utilized the sequential screening or 'close in' strategy (Bell, 1992). A trait risk factor of either a family history of a psychotic disorder in a first degree relative, or a schizotypal personality disorder, is the first identifying factor of this group. In addition to this proposed premorbid vulnerability, patients recruited to PACE in this group have also experienced a clear mental state change lasting longer than one month, and associated with significant deterioration in functioning. This group is referred to as the 'vulnerability' group. Fully operationalized criteria are described elsewhere (Yung et al., 1996). In addition to the three intake criteria strands outlined above, PACE clients must also be aged 15–30, as first-episode psychosis typically emerges in this adolescent-to-young adult age range. As we are attempting to identify young people at risk of first psychotic episode, clients must not have experienced a previous psychotic episode.

Case detection and engagement in treatment
Having defined the inclusion criteria for the clinic, we then faced the twin issues of how to identify these high-risk individuals in the community, and how to deliver appropriate clinical services to them. The PACE clinic's approach to identifying high-risk patients and promoting their engagement in treatment has been similar to that of Falloon (1992), i.e. GPs and primary care workers received education and training regarding identification of the 'at-risk mental state'. However, unlike the situation under the British health care system, in which the vast majority of the population is registered with a GP, in Australia many young people are not linked to a particular general practice, especially those living in cities, and consequently do not see a GP regularly. Hence, other primary care facilities and networks which frequently come into contact with young people, such as school counsellors, teachers and youth workers, were also targeted. The PACE clinic utilized the community education activities of EPAT which were expanded to incorporate education about the new service and about prodromal

states and other risk factors. This activity has become increasingly necessary as potential referrers have learnt from previous experience that public psychiatric services will not assess or manage someone unless they are considered 'seriously mentally ill'. In the case of PACE, as for EPAT, the idea that a young person is 'not sick enough' to be referred needed to be turned around, and the message changed so that individuals are referred to prevent later serious ill health.

The PACE clinic attempts to provide an accessible and acceptable service. The philosophy of being inclusive, rather than exclusive, in screening and assessing referrals, which is used in EPAT, is also used in PACE. However, since there are fewer resources, some of the features of the EPAT intake and clinical system could not be applied; for example, the service tends to be centre-based with only a limited capacity for home visits, and the clinic operates in office hours only.

Engagement issues in the PACE clinic are somewhat different from those of EPAT and other clinical services which deal with patients with diagnosed psychotic disorders. First, young people presenting to PACE tend to be a help-seeking group. They have not generally been referred because of disruptive or bizarre behaviour which may be the case with psychotic patients. They are distressed by their symptoms and are usually asking for some kind of intervention. As the service is centre-based, these individuals tend to be more motivated to attend than psychotic patients. Psychotic symptoms such as persecutory delusions, which can interfere with help-seeking, do not occur in the PACE group. Sometimes, young people present with subthreshold forms of these symptoms, but because they are not full blown, the individual often has insight into the abnormal nature of the symptom, or the symptom is only present intermittently. These factors increase the likelihood of help-seeking. Engagement is therefore often easier for this group. It is important to recognize that the group is therefore not representative of the whole population of people with 'at-risk mental states'.

These are, of course, generalizations and situations have occurred in which a young person is referred by someone else, usually a family member, and issues of accessing the patient and engagement arise. The clinical mandate of the PACE clinic is a somewhat controversial issue. As there is no diagnosed psychotic disorder, in the absence of clear evidence of risk of self harm or risk to others, there are no grounds for compelling a young person to attend the clinic. Despite our belief that the young person is at high risk of incipient psychosis, it would be difficult to enforce follow-up under the Mental Health Act. At times PACE staff have kept in touch with concerned family members so that the first signs of psychotic symptoms can be detected as early as possible and other risks to the young person identified. Some of these issues are illustrated in the case history (Case 4) which follows on pp. 107–108.

The clinical service

The clinic is located at the Centre for Adolescent Health, a generalist outpatient service and health promotion centre for adolescents. This site was chosen so that patients would not have to attend a psychiatric facility, with its inherent potentially stigmatizing effect. Staffing consists of one consultant psychiatrist, two clinical psychologists and one research assistant (all sessional). Continuity of care is provided through a case management system, with case managers providing regular feedback to referring agencies. The treatment component at this stage includes some of the interventions detailed above, such as stress management, family interventions and support. Drug education about the potential psychosis-inducing properties of certain substances is provided. Neuroleptics are generally withheld until the occurrence of frank psychotic features. Patients are monitored for the emergence of these, enabling the earliest possible specific intervention if a frank psychosis develops. Hence, the severity of, and disruption caused by, psychosis can be minimized.

Ethical issues

The need for a non-stigmatizing location for the clinic was noted. The name of the PACE clinic itself was chosen in order to avoid implying the inevitability of progression to psychosis (hence the name 'Prodrome Clinic' was not used). Related to this, the potentially stigmatizing effect of being involved in such a service needs to be acknowledged. Our initial position on this issue was that the belief that an individual is 'at risk' of becoming psychotic should not be highlighted, especially as the degree of risk to progression to psychosis is not yet known. However, recent communication with some North American colleagues raised the opposing viewpoint, that, in fact, there is a duty to inform subjects about their increased risk of psychosis. Our experience to date has been that the information given varies from patient to patient. Some young people are aware of their family history and the possibility of increased risk for psychosis. This issue then needs to be discussed frankly with them. In other cases a 'wait and see' strategy, without unduly alarming the patient, seems to the best approach.

Illustrative data

Total referrals

In the 16-month period from March 1995 to July 1996, 119 referrals were made to PACE. Telephone screening assessment of these referrals excluded 22 (18.5%) and the remaining 97 (81.5%) were offered a screening interview at the PACE clinic. Twenty-four of these failed to attend the appointment. The other 73 (61.3% of the 119 referred) were seen in the clinic by either the PACE consultant psychiatrist (ARY) or research psychologist (LJP/CM), or both. Of these, 49 (41.2% of the 119 referred) met the intake criteria and 24 (20.2%) did not. Forty-one of these young people attended the clinic, and 38 of them consented to involvement in the research project. This represents 31.9% of the total referrals and 77.6% of those meeting intake criteria. Only eight (16.3% of appropriate accepted referrals) refused any follow-up (clinical or research). Four subjects have subsequently dropped out of the research (10.8% of the research sample).

Referral sources

Analysis of the sources of referrals to PACE shows that in this 16-month period, 45 of the 119 (37.8%) referrals were from the Early Psychosis Assessment Team (EPAT). In many cases, EPAT did not directly assess the young person, but made a judgement over the telephone that PACE was likely to be the more appropriate service, thus minimizing contacts in the pathway to care. In addition, 17 referrals (14.3%) were received directly from other adult psychiatric services, 15 (12.6%) from adolescent services, 14 (11.8%) from private psychiatrists or psychologists, 9 (7.6%) from school and university counselling services, 6 (5.0%) from general hospitals, and 2 (1.7%) from GPs. Eight referrals (6.7%) were from the patient or patient's family. Most of these had been given information about PACE from another primary carer and had been advised to telephone the clinic. It should be noted that unlike EPPIC, the catchment area for the PACE clinic is the wider Melbourne metropolitan area and, to some extent, rural Victoria.

The PACE clinic's close association with an already established clinical service specializing in managing psychotic adolescents and young adults (EPPIC), was an important factor in our ability to generate referrals. The relatively low rate of direct referrals from other sources was attributed to EPAT's accessible intake system; referring agencies tend to refer even doubtful cases to EPAT in the knowledge that the service will be responsive and offer either direct assessment, or advice on other appropriate services, including PACE.

Reason for referral

Most patients had more than one reason for referral. The most common reasons for referral were suspiciousness ($n = 15$) or other magical ideas ($n = 15$), presence of perceptual abnormalities ($n = 13$), and transient psychotic symptoms ($n = 10$). This finding probably reflects these phenomena forming part of the inclusion criteria. Non-specific symptoms such as depressed mood ($n = 7$), anxiety ($n = 7$) and social withdrawal ($n = 9$), were other frequently reported reasons for being referred. Obsessive compulsive phenomena were noted by the referrer in three cases and odd affect in four cases.

Psychopathology and disability in the PACE sample
A subsample of 38 of the 49 (77.6%) young people who met the PACE intake criteria for the second study was recruited into the 'research sample'. Reasons for not being recruited included refusal to participate ($n = 9$), and being subsequently treated with neuroleptic medication by another clinician ($n = 2$).

Patients in the research sample were assessed using a number of instruments. The Brief Psychiatric Rating Scale (BPRS; Overall & Gorham, 1962), the Schedule for the Assessment of Negative Symptoms (SANS; Andreasen, 1982), and the Quality of Life Scale (QLS; Heinrichs, Hanlon & Carpenter, 1984), were used to assess psychopathology and disability. The PACE (putatively 'prodromal' or high-risk) group was compared with a first-episode psychosis sample at both initial presentation and six-month follow-up on the BPRS, SANS and QLS, in order to compare the levels of symptomatology and disability across these groups. The first-episode subjects were recruited from EPPIC during 1993 and six-month follow-up data were collected during 1993–94. The characteristics of this sample, including intake data, are described in more detail elsewhere (McGorry et al., 1996). Forty first-episode subjects were assessed at intake and 41 at follow-up. The mean age of the EPPIC first-episode sample was 22.0 years, compared with 19.1 years in the PACE sample. Although not statistically significantly lower, the lower mean age in the PACE sample would be expected if we really are identifying a group of individuals in the prepsychotic phase. Twenty-two (57.9%) of the PACE research sample were male and 16 (42.1%) female. The mean age of PACE males was 19.6 years and PACE females 18.3 years. There were no significant differences between the genders with regard to age or the number included in the study. Results of the comparison of measures of symptomatology and functioning are shown in Table 4.2.

Total scores on the BPRS indicated that PACE subjects had a significantly higher mean level of general psychopathology than the 'recovering' first-episode patient group, but there was no difference in general psychopathology between the PACE patients and the acute first-episode patients (entry cases). BPRS psychotic subscale scores of the PACE group were significantly lower than those of the acute first-episode group, but significantly greater than the first-episode group at

Table 4.2. *Comparison of mean measures of symptomatology and disability across PACE and first-episode samples (standard deviations in parentheses)*

Measures	PACE ($n = 38$)	First episode at entry ($n = 40$)	First episode at 6 months ($n = 41$)
BPRS	22.2 (8.3)	27.5 (8.1)	8.1 (6.0)
BPRS psychotic subscale[a]	5.8 (3.0)	10.4 (3.6)[c]	1.4 (2.1)[c]
SANS	26.9 (16.0)	34.5 (24.5)	17.7 (18.5)[b]
QLS	76.9 (21.1)[c]	–	82.7 (24.2)

[a] BPRS psychotic subscale consists of the following items: conceptual disorganization, hallucinations, suspiciousness and unusual thought content.
[b] Data from one subject are missing.
[c] Data from two subjects are missing.

six-month follow-up. This indicates that the level of psychotic symptomatology of the PACE group (positive symptoms) lies between that of an acute group and a recovering group of first-episode patients. No difference was found between the PACE and first-episode group at entry to EPPIC on the SANS. The PACE group did, however, have significantly higher SANS scores than the recovering first-episode group (indicating higher levels of negative symptoms recorded by the PACE group). The QLS was not used with the first-episode sample in the acute phase, but the PACE group had a lower mean level of functioning than the 'recovering' first-episode group. These findings indicate that the putatively high-risk group (PACE sample) is indeed symptomatic and displaying difficulty in functioning, justifying both their identification and intervention with this group. The data also suggest that, in terms of positive psychotic symptomatology, the prodromal phase lies midway in severity between the acute psychotic episode and the recovery phase. The level of disability and negative symptoms reported by the PACE group was comparable with that of the acute first-episode group.

Transition to psychosis
An important finding from the clinic was the high transition rate from 'at-risk mental state' to psychosis. Of the 38 subjects recruited to the research sample to date, 12 have become psychotic according to an operationalized definition (Yung et al., 1996). This represents a transition rate of 31.6%, higher than the rate using the original PACE intake criteria.

4 PROMOTING ACCESS TO CARE

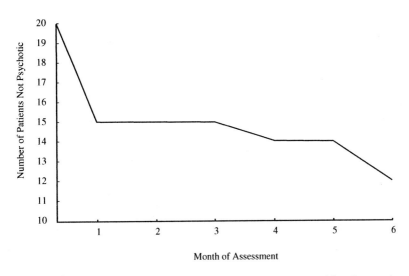

Figure 4.1. Transition to psychosis – PACE patients monitored for six months ($n = 20$).

Perhaps more informative is examination of the first 20 subjects recruited into the research sample who have been followed up at monthly intervals for six months or more, i.e. they have passed through a medium follow-up period. Of these, eight have become psychotic, representing a transition rate of 40%. Figure 4.1 shows a 'survival curve' for these first 20 subjects, indicating the timing of onset of psychosis.

As this figure indicates, five subjects became psychotic within the first month of follow-up. A further three developed psychosis between the fourth and sixth months. It is anticipated that the ultimate 12-month transition rate will be higher still. These preliminary findings indicate that we are identifying a group truly at high risk of imminent onset of psychosis. It is important to emphasize that PACE patients are not representative of the general population, but are a specific group of patients fulfilling strict criteria. Thus, the transition rate to psychosis is not representative of the general population, but of the identified high-risk population only. An example of a fairly typical PACE client and the referral and engagement process follows. This case highlights the need for an adaptable and accessible service for this high-risk population.

Case 4

FP was a 26-year-old single unemployed man who lived alone in the outer suburbs of Melbourne. He had a brother who had schizophrenia and who attended the local Community Mental Health Centre (CMHC) and received fortnightly depot neuroleptics.

FP presented to this same clinic stating that he was fearful he was 'going like my brother'. He had become suspicious of other people and thought they might harm him. This seemed to begin after he was assaulted and robbed by a group of youths near his home three months earlier. He had become reluctant to leave the house, and was anxious attending the clinic. In fact, he told the clinician that he had been trying to get help for some time but had been too nervous to attend the clinic until then. He was referred to PACE by the CMHC worker who thought that he was not actually psychotic but may be in the prodromal phase.

The CMHC clinician had already made a follow-up appointment with FP. Due to his obvious difficulty in attending, the PACE clinic worker arranged to see him at the CMHC with the other clinician in a joint session. He presented as described above, with attenuated psychotic symptoms of suspiciousness and persecutory ideas, although they were not of delusional intensity. He had marked social anxiety and withdrawal, and there was a consequent deterioration in functioning as he had been unable to seek work or even arrange for the ongoing payment of his unemployment benefits. His family history of psychotic disorder was another relevant risk factor.

FP was offered follow-up at the PACE clinic. His PACE case manager offered practical help such as arranging sickness benefit payments, and used a cognitive behavioural framework to deal with his post-traumatic symptoms and fears of other people. His persecutory ideas were challenged and he was able to see that he was catastrophizing from his experience of being assaulted. He attended regularly every two weeks. After two months of treatment a job rehabilitation course was organized for him and he was also able to attend this. His symptoms and functioning gradually improved, and at the time of this writing, ten months after initial PACE contact, he presents with some mild mistrust of strangers and still some social anxiety, but has not developed a psychotic disorder.

It is possible that FP represents a 'false positive' and is not at risk of becoming psychotic, even in the absence of treatment at PACE. The other possibility is that the PACE intervention has thus far averted the onset of psychosis, i.e. he is a 'false false positive'. Of course, he may still be at risk in the future, and this can only be discovered by long-term follow-up.

Future directions

EPAT and the PACE clinic are evolving services. A current aim of EPAT is to reduce the number of patients with long DUPs (over six months). It is hoped that this will be achieved by continuing community development and education activites to promote knowledge of psychosis and of services which are available, such as EPPIC.

At PACE, it is hoped that community development activities can increase the local knowledge of the service, particularly by referral sources, and that the number of young people referred to the service increases. It is proposed that PACE move to a two-stage screening process to enhance referral rates and to ensure that more young people are identified in the possible prodromal stage of a first-episode psychosis. The first stage would be to identify young people with social withdrawal and role function impairment manifesting as a change from premorbid functioning. The second stage would be to explore the more specific criteria outlined earlier, using a brief screening interview. In line with this change in the screening process, it is hoped that PACE can adopt more of EPAT's service principles, by becoming a more mobile and community-based service able to see patients at home, work, school, and so on.

This chapter has outlined some of the issues involved in promoting access to intervention in both first-episode patients and those possibly in the prodromal phase preceding a first-episode. Detection of mental state changes indicative of frank or emerging psychosis, by both the general population and primary health carers, is vital. Recognition by these groups of the significance of other risk factors, such as a family history of psychosis, has also been shown to be important. Reduction of the stigma associated with accessing psychiatric services must occur to further assist early preventive interventions. Additionally, services both for young people experiencing a first psychotic episode and those possibly in the prodromal phase, can be better structured to enhance engagement with potential patients and their families. An adaptable and accessible service must be provided. It can be seen that principles such as community education, particularly targeted to primary carers, and the development of service structures and practices conducive to referral and engagement in treatment, apply across both patient populations. These principles can be applied in most services and represent a step towards a preventive approach to psychotic disorders that is possible at the present state of knowledge. By adopting these measures we have the potential to improve outcome in psychotic disorders.

Acknowledgments

The authors would like to thank Colleen McFarlane (CM) for her role at the PACE clinic and other staff at the Early Psychosis Research Centre and the Early Psychosis Assessment Team for assistance in the research associated with this chapter. This research was made possible by the generous support of the Victorian Health Promotion Foundation, the Stanley Foundation and the Victor Hurley Medical Research Fund.

References

Adams, W., Kendell, R. E., Hare, E. H. & Munk, J. P. (1993). Epidemiological evidence that maternal influenza contributes to the aetiology of schizophrenia: an analysis of Scottish, English and Danish data. *British Journal of Psychiatry*, **163**, 522–34.

Amador, X. F., Flaum, M., Andreasen, N. C., Strauss, D. H., Yale, S. A., Clark, S. C., & Gorman, J. M. (1994). Awareness of illness in schizophrenia and schizoaffective and mood disorders. *Archives of General Psychiatry*, **51**, 826–36.

American Psychiatric Association (1987). *Diagnostic and Statistical Manual of Mental Disorders*, 3rd edn, revised: DSM-III-R. Washington DC: American Psychiatric Association.

Andreasen, N. (1982). Negative symptoms in schizophrenia: definition and reliability. *Archives of General Psychiatry*, **39**, 784–8.

Angermeyer, M. C. & Matschinger, H. (1994). Lay beliefs about schizophrenic disorder: the results of a population survey in Germany. *Acta Psychiatrica Scandinavica*, **89** (Supplement 382), 39–45.

Bell, R. Q. (1992). Multiple-risk cohorts and segmenting risk as solutions to the problem of false positives at risk for the major psychoses. *Psychiatry*, **55**, 370–81.

Brown, G. W. & Birley, J. L. T. (1968). Crisis and life changes and the onset of schizophrenia. *Journal of Health and Social Behaviour*, **9**, 203–14.

Burns, T., Raftery, J., Beadsmore, A., McGuigan, S. & Dickson, M. (1993). A controlled trial of home-based psychiatric services. 2. Treatment patterns and costs. *British Journal of Psychiatry*, **163**, 55–61.

Cameron, D. E. (1938). Early schizophrenia. *American Journal of Psychiatry*, **95**, 567–78.

Cornblatt, B. A. & Keilp, J. G. (1994). Impaired attention, genetics, and the pathophysiology of schizophrenia. *Schizophrenia Bulletin*, **20**, 31–47.

Deveson, A. (1991). *Tell Me I'm Here*. Ringwood, Australia: Penguin.

Dunn, G. (1983). Longitudinal records of anxiety and depression in general practice: the Second National Morbidity Survey. *Psychological Medicine*, **13**, 897–906.

Eaton, W. W. (1985). Epidemiology of schizophrenia. *Epidemiologic Reviews*, **7**, 105–26.

Faergman, P. (1963). *Psychogenic Psychoses*. London: Butterworths.
Falloon, I. R. H. (1992). Early intervention for first episodes of schizophrenia: a preliminary exploration. *Psychiatry*, **55**, 4–15.
Gjerris, A. (1994). The influence of community-based psychiatry in Copenhagen on the treatment of chronic psychoses. *Acta Psychiatrica Scandinavica*, **89** (Supplement 382), 71–3.
Goldberg, D. & Huxley, P. (1980). *Mental Illness in the Community: The Pathway to Psychiatric Care*. London: Tavistock.
Gunderson, J. G. & Singer, M. T. (1975). Defining borderline patients. *American Journal of Psychiatry*, **132**, 1–10.
Häfner, H., Maurer, K., Löffler, W., & Riecher- Rössler, A. (1993). The influence of age and sex on the onset and early course of schizophrenia. *British Journal of Psychiatry*, **162**, 80–6.
Heinrichs, D., Hanlon, T. & Carpenter, W. (1984). The Quality of Life Scale: An instrument for rating the schizophrenia deficit syndrome. *Schizophrenia Bulletin*, **10**, 388–98.
Hogarty, G. E., Anderson, C. M., Reiss, D. J., Kornblith, S. J., Greenwald, D. P., Ulrich, R. F. & Carter, M. (1991). Family psychoeducation, social skills training, and maintenance chemotherapy in the aftercare treatment of schizophrenia. II. Two-year effects of a controlled study on relapse and adjustment. Environmental-Personal Indicators in the Course of Schizophrenia (EPICS) Research Group. *Archives of General Psychiatry*, **48**, 340–7.
Jablensky, A., Sartorius, N., Ernberg, G., Anker, M., Korten, A., Cooper, J.E., Day, R. & Bertelsen, A. (1992). Schizophrenia: manifestation, incidence and course in different cultures. A World Health Organisation ten country study. *Psychological Medicine*, Monograph Supplement, **20**, 1–97.
Jauch, D. A. & Carpenter, W. T. (1988). Reactive psychosis. I: Does the DSM III concept define a third psychosis? *Journal of Nervous and Mental Disease*, **176**, 72–81.
Jones, P. B., Bebbington, P., Foerster, A., Lewis, S. W., Murray, R. M., Russell, A., Sham, P. C., Toone, B. K. & Wilkins, S. (1993). Premorbid social underachievement in schizophrenia. Results from the Camberwell Collaborative Psychosis Study. *British Journal of Psychiatry*, **162**, 65–71.
Kane, J. M., Rifkin, A., Quitkin, F., Nayak, D. & Ramos-Lorenzi, J. (1982). Fluphenazine versus placebo in patients with remitted, acute first-episode schizophrenia. *Archives of General Psychiatry*, **39**, 70–3.
Kissling, W. (1994). Compliance, quality assurance and standards for relapse prevention in schizophrenia. *Acta Psychiatrica Scandinavica*, **89** (Supplement 382), 16–24.
Kosky, R. & Hardy, J. (1992). Mental health: is early intervention the key? *Medical Journal of Australia*, **156**, 147–8.
Larsen, T.K., McGlashan, T. & Moe, L.C. (1996). First episode schizophrenia: I. Early course parameters. *Schizophrenia Bulletin*, **22**, 241–56.
Leff, J., Kuipers, L., Berkowitz, R. & Sturgeon, D. (1985). A controlled trial of social intervention in the families of schizophrenia patients: a two-year follow-up. *British Journal of Psychiatry*, **146**, 594–600.

Lieberman, J. A., Jody, D., Alvir, J. M., Ashtari, M., Levy, D. L., Bogerts, B., Degreef, G., Mayerhoff, D. I. & Cooper, T. (1993). Brain morphology, dopamine, and eye-tracking abnormalities in first-episode schizophrenia: prevalence and clinical correlates. *Archives of General Psychiatry*, **50**, 357–68.

Lincoln, C. V. & McGorry, P. (1995). Who cares? Pathways to psychiatric care for young people experiencing a first episode of psychosis. *Psychiatric Services*, **46**, 1166–71.

Loebel, A. D., Lieberman, A., Alvir, M., Mayerhoff, D. I., Geisler, S. H. & Szymanski, S.R. (1992). Duration of psychosis and outcome in first episode schizophrenia. *American Journal of Psychiatry*, **149**, 1183–8.

Marder, S. R., Wirshing, W. C., Van, P. T., Mintz, J., McKenzie, J., Johnston, C. K., Lebell, M. & Liberman, R. P. (1994). Fluphenazine vs placebo supplementation for prodromal signs of relapse in schizophrenia. *Archives of General Psychiatry*, **51**, 280–7.

McGorry, P. D. (1995). Psychoeducation in first-episode psychosis: a therapeutic process. *Psychiatry*, **58**, 313–28.

McGorry, P. D., Edwards, J., Mihalopoulos, C., Harrigan, S. M. & Jackson, H. J. (1996). EPPIC: An evolving system of early detection and optimal management. *Schizophrenia Bulletin*, **22**, 305–26.

McGuire, P. K., Jones, P., Harvey, I., Bebbington, P., Toone, B., Lewis, S. & Murray, R. M. (1994). Cannabis and acute psychosis. *Schizophrenia Research*, **13**, 161–8.

McNamara, K. & Lewin, T. (1989). General practitioners' recognition and management of psychiatric illness. *Medical Journal of Australia*, **151**, 250–7.

Meares, A. (1959). The diagnosis of prepsychotic schizophrenia. *Lancet*, **i**, 55–9.

Meltzer, D., Hale, S., Malik, S. J., Hogman, G. A. & Wood, S. (1991). Community care for patients with schizophrenia one year after hospital discharge. *British Medical Journal*, **303**, 1023–6.

Merson, S., Tyrer, P., Onyett, S., Lack, S., Birkett, P., Lynch, S. & Johnson, T. (1992). Early intervention in psychiatric emergencies: a controlled clinical trial. *Lancet*, **339**, 1311–4.

Millar, T. & Goldberg, D. P. (1991). Link between the ability to detect and manage emotional disorders: a study of general practitioner trainees. *British Journal of General Practice*, **41**, 357–9.

Mulaik, J. S. (1992). Noncompliance with medication regimens in severely and persistently mentally ill schizophrenic patients. *Issues in Mental Health Nursing*, **13**, 219–37.

Mundy, P., Robertson, M. & Robertson, J. (1990). The prevalence of psychotic symptoms in homeless adolescents. *Journal of the American Academy of Child and Adolescent Psychiatry*, **29**, 724–31.

O'Callaghan, E., Gibson, T., Colohan, H. A., Buckley, P., Walshe, D. G., Larkin, C. & Waddington, J. L. (1992). Risk of schizophrenia in adults born after obstetric complications and their association with early onset of illness: a controlled study. *British Medical Journal*, **305**, 1256–9.

Orleans, C. T., George, L. K., Houpt, J. L. & Brodie, H. K. H. (1985). How primary care physicians treat psychiatric disorders: a national survey of general practitioners. *American Journal of Psychiatry*, **142**, 52–7.

Overall, J. E. & Gorham, D. R. (1962). The Brief Psychiatric Rating Scale. *Psychological Reports*, **10**, 799–812.

Peterson, C. L. (1986). Changing community attitudes toward the chronic mentally ill through a psychosocial program. *Hospital and Community Psychiatry*, **37**, 180–2.

Power, P., Elkins, K., Adlard, S., Curry, C., McGorry, P. & Harrigan, S. (in press). An analysis of the initial treatment phase in first episode psychosis. *British Journal of Psychiatry*.

Ridgely, M. S., Goldman, H. H. & Willenbring, M. (1990). Barriers to care of persons with dual diagnoses: organizational and financial issues. *Schizophrenia Bulletin*, **16**, 123–32.

Royal College of Psychiatrists (1987). A carer's perspective: consensus on caring for the mentally disordered in our communities. *Bulletin of the Royal College of Psychiatrists*, **11**, 237–9.

Shepherd, M., Cooper, B., Brown, A. C. & Kalton, G. W. (1966). *Psychiatric Illness in General Practice*. London: Oxford University Press.

Steinberg, H., Torem, M. & Saravay, S. M. (1980). An analysis of physician resistance to psychiatric consultations. *Archives of General Psychiatry*, **37**, 1007–12.

Strauss, J. S. (1969). Hallucinations and delusions as points on continual function. *Archives of General Psychiatry*, **21**, 581–6.

Sullivan, H. S. (1927). The onset of schizophrenia. *American Journal of Psychiatry*, **7**, 105–34.

Taube, C. A., Morlock, L., Burns, B. J. & Santos, A. B. (1990). New directions in research on assertive community treatment. *Hospital and Community Psychiatry*, **41**, 642–7.

Tsuang, D. & Coryell, W. (1993). An 8-year follow-up of patients with DSM-III-R psychotic depression, schizoaffective disorder, and schizophrenia. *American Journal of Psychiatry*, **150**, 1182–8.

Vardy, M. M. & Kay, S. R. (1983). LSD psychosis or LSD induced schizophrenia? *Archives of General Psychiatry*, **40**, 877–83.

Vlais, R. S. (1993). Mental health promotion: the Western Australian experience. *Mental Health in Australia*, **5**, 41–4.

Weiner, I. B. (1992). *Psychological Disturbance in Adolescence*, 2nd edn. New York: Wiley Interscience.

Weissman, M. M., Myers, J. K. & Harding, P. S. (1978). Rates and risks of depression symptoms in a US urban community. *Acta Psychiatrica Scandinavica*, **57**, 219–31.

Yung, A. R. & McGorry, P. D. (1996a). The prodromal phase of first episode psychosis: past and current conceptualisations. *Schizophrenia Bulletin*, **22**, 353–70.

Yung, A. R. & McGorry, P. D. (1996b). The initial prodrome in psychosis: descriptive and qualitative aspects. *Australian and New Zealand Journal of Psychiatry*, **30**, 587–99.

Yung, A. R., McGorry, P. D., McFarlane, C. A., Jackson, H. J., Patton, G. C. &

Rakkar, A. (1996). Monitoring and care of young people at incipient risk of psychosis. *Schizophrenia Bulletin*, **22**, 283–303.

Zubin, J. & Spring, B. (1977). Vulnerability – a new view of schizophrenia. *Journal of Abnormal Psychology*, **86**, 103–26.

5
Studies of biological variables in first-episode schizophrenia: a comprehensive review

ANJAN CHATTERJEE AND JEFFREY A. LIEBERMAN

Introduction

Since Kraepelin, psychiatrists have been observers of the natural history of schizophrenia. The advent of antipsychotic drugs has been both good and bad from the perspective of the study of the illness. On the one hand, psychiatrists now had an effective treatment modality for this illness, whose clinical efficacy and safety needed to be established. On the other, antipsychotic drug treatment interfered with the natural course of the illness and introduced inextricably confounded effects on biological substrates which were targets of investigations.

Several questions which had been examined in the preneuroleptic era now became much more difficult to resolve due to confounding factors such as drug treatment, differing diagnostic systems, and medication side effects. By focusing on the early periods of the illness, however, this would not only provide a longitudinal perspective, but also an informative window through which competing factors, such as chronicity, medication status and side effects, could be seen and integrated into the clinical picture.

Methods

The purpose of this chapter is to review the neurobiology and treatment of first-episode schizophrenia. To ensure the diagnostic validity of samples, we have searched the world medical/psychiatric literature for English language studies published which utilized diagnostic criteria developed subsequent to DSM-II (i.e. Feighner criteria, RDC, CATEGO,

ICD-9 and 10, DSM-III, III-R and IV). Some studies were not specifically of first-episode schizophrenia, but included such patients in sufficient numbers and reported first-episode results in a manner which warranted inclusion.

The studies identified by this method were grouped into a series of major categories based on the predominant study type. Selected types included neuroimaging, neurophysiology and psychophysiology, neuropsychology, neuroendocrinology and neurochemistry, immunology and treatment (acute and maintenance). Many studies involved combinations of the above strategies. In these instances they were classified by the predominant feature of the study based on our judgement. Categories such as phenomenology, outcome and psychosocial aspects were omitted since they have been covered elsewhere in the book (see Chapters 7 and 9).

Neuroimaging studies

Neuroimaging studies include computed axial tomography (CT scan), magnetic resonance imaging (MRI scan), positron emission tomography (PET scan), single photon emission tomography (SPECT scan), and nuclear magnetic resonance spectroscopy (MRS). The studies are grouped and discussed below by the imaging technique used.

CT studies

A variety of studies involving CT scans support the idea that enlargement of cerebral ventricles may be part of the early pathophysiological process, predating treatment. Weinberger et al. (1982) found that both the schizophreniform and the chronic schizophrenic patients had significantly larger cerebral ventricles than did the other psychiatric or control subjects. Ventricular size in the affective disorder patients was not significantly different than in any of the other groups. The authors concluded that their results suggested that in some schizophrenic patients, ventricular enlargement and, less frequently, cortical atrophy, predated the onset of psychosis and was unrelated to treatment.

Nyback et al. (1982) found that the lateral and third ventricles were significantly wider in 46 schizophrenic patients than in the corresponding 46 healthy volunteers. Also, while there was a significant correlation between age and the size of the lateral ventricles in the volunteers, in the patients with schizophrenia no such correlation was observed. These results indicated that schizophrenia may be associated with pathophysiological processes which interfere with the normal age-related enlargement of the ventricles. Signs of cortical atrophy, CSF circulation disturbances, and reversed asymmetry of the occipital lobes, were also more frequent in the patient group than among the controls.

Schulz et al. (1983) found that on CT scan, the ventricular brain ratios of teenage patients with schizophrenia spectrum disorders ($n=15$) were significantly larger than those of borderline patients ($n=8$), and those of control subjects ($n=18$). This supports the hypothesis that ventricular enlargement was present early in the course of schizophrenia.

Likewise, Turner, Toone & Brett-Jones (1986) found that the schizophrenia patient group of 30 had significantly greater ventricular–brain ratios (VBR) when compared with the 26 individuals comprising the control group. The VBR values were positively correlated both with average alcohol intake and with early physical trauma, and negatively correlated with a family history of schizophrenia.

First-episode schizophrenic patients described by Iacono et al. (1988) had larger third ventricles but not larger lateral ventricles or cortical sulci than the normal subjects. Although other psychosis patients were also examined, they did not differ from the normal control group on these measures.

In Andreasen et al. (1990), significant differences in ventricular–brain ratio were noted in a sample of 108 schizophrenic individuals versus 75 normal volunteers. However, male schizophrenic patients accounted for the bulk of this, with 19% of their ventricular–brain ratios being greater than two standard deviations from the control mean and 43% greater by at least one SD. In this study, first admission schizophrenic patients also had significant ventricular enlargement when compared to their age-equivalent normal controls. From their examination of ventricular size in schizophrenic patients and normal subjects covering a broad age range, the authors suggested that ventricular enlargement does not progress over time at a greater rate in patients than in normal subjects.

Holsenbeck et al. (1992), in comparing ventricular–brain ratios from 33 very recent onset schizophrenic patients with those from 45 neurology patients who served as controls, initially found no significant differences between the two groups in terms of VBRs. However, when control subjects with a neurological diagnosis of vertigo, who had significantly higher VBRs than the remainder of the control group or the psychotic patients, were removed, this changed. With these patients excluded, the schizophrenic patients had significantly greater VBRs. The authors also found an association between positive symptoms in the schizophreniform group and smaller VBRs, but no relationship was found with negative symptoms.

CT scans in Rubin et al. (1993) showed that newly diagnosed schizophreniform disorder ($n = 22$) and schizophrenia patients ($n = 27$), who had at most only briefly been treated with neuroleptics, had significantly reduced brain volume and length than the controls ($n = 24$). The patients had greater widths of the sylvian and intrahemispheric fissures and surface sulci in the frontal and parietal regions, with sulcal enlargement more pronounced in the male patients and on the left hemisphere. Also, a trend towards the enlargement of the third ventricle in the patients was revealed. However, there was no enlargement of the lateral ventricles, causing the authors to speculate that such enlargement may occur during the course of the illness and may not always be present at the outset.

MRI studies

Using magnetic resonance imaging (MRI), researchers have detected everything from increased lateral ventricular size in first-episode patients to less asymmetry in the superior and temporal lobes when patients are compared with control individuals.

DeLisi et al. (1991), who examined brain morphology in 30 first-episode patients, 15 chronic schizophrenics, and 20 neurological controls, found that lateral ventricular size was increased in both first-episode and chronic schizophrenics, with greater significance on the left than the right side. Only the chronic patients had reduced temporal lobe size also on the left side. The authors concluded that enlarged ventricular size was present at the outset in schizophrenia, and was not related to chronicity.

When Lieberman et al. (1992, 1993a) examined brain morphology in MRIs from 62 first-episode patients, 24 chronic schizophrenic patients, and 42 healthy volunteers, they found schizophrenic patients had significantly higher rates of definite abnormalities (using a three-point scale of definite, questionable and no structural abnormality) than healthy volunteers; specifically, 31%, 42% and 5%, of first-episode, chronic schizophrenic, and control patients, respectively, had definite abnormalities. The highest regional rates of abnormalities (control, lateral and third ventricular and mesiotemporal) were seen in the lateral ventricles (first-episode patients 18%, chronic patients 33%, healthy subjects 2%).

Qualitative assessments were significantly correlated with quantitative ones performed on the same sample (Bogerts et al., 1990; Degreef et al., 1992a). The authors here concluded that, whilst some evidence of structural neuropathology is present in patients at the onset of their illness, it is less prevalent and severe than in chronic patients.

In the same series of first-episode patients, Degreef et al. (1992a) also measured volumes of the ventricular system and its subdivisions using MRI on 40 first-episode patients and 25 normal controls. The schizophrenia patients had a significantly larger total ventricular volume (the sum of all lateral ventricular segments plus third and fourth ventricles) than the control subjects, with the left side volumes being larger for all the ventricular segments except the temporal horn.

Positive symptom measures correlated significantly only with left temporal horn volumes, and negative symptom measures correlated with temporal horn volumes. Measures of affective flattening reached significance in correlating with the third ventricle volumes. The authors concluded that lateral ventricle enlargement is present early in the course of the schizophrenic disease process, and the enlargement of specific regions is directly related to the core symptoms of the disorder. Disturbance of the limbic and paralimbic regions of the brain that lie next to the temporal horn may be affected by the pathology and may mediate some of the symptoms of schizophrenia.

More recently, Nopoulos et al. (1995), in examining brain morphology in first-episode schizophrenia using MRI scanning, found that, since structural abnormalities are present early in the course of the illness, this may be the result of a neurodevelopmental mechanism. MRI scanning showed that the 24 first-episode patients had significantly more intersulcal and ventricular CSF than the 24 comparison subjects. There were no differences in terms of the total volume of brain tissue between the two groups. However, the patient group had a regionally specific decrement in frontal lobe tissue significantly different from that of the normal subjects.

There has been discussion in the literature concerning the possibility that non-communicating septum pellucidum defects in the brain may be associated with psychosis. Degreef et al. (1992b) examined this hypothesis, finding that a cavum septum pellucidum was found in 23% of the schizophrenic patients ($n=62$) as compared with 2% of the control groups ($n=46$). Also, pronounced enlargement of the cavum septum and cavum vergae were noted in two of the schizophrenic patients, while agenesis (partial) of the corpus callosum was seen in one of the patients, this leading the authors to conclude that anomalous brain development is an important aspect of the pathogenesis of schizophrenia.

DeLisi et al. (1994) examined asymmetries in the superior temporal lobe in the brains of male and female first-episode schizophrenic patients. The authors hypothesized that since disordered language is a hallmark of schizophrenia there may be abnormalities present in the planum temporale and related superior temporal gyrus in schizophrenic patients. Eighty-five first-episode schizophrenic patients and 40 control subjects (normal healthy subjects) had measurements of the sylvian fissure taken from coronal slices. Researchers found that the pattern of asymmetry in control subjects was longer for the right than the left, in the anterior slices, and that the reverse was true in the posterior slices (corresponding to the planum temporale). As a group, schizophrenic patients demonstrated less asymmetry (R > L) in anterior slices, and female patients showed a trend for less (L > R) asymmetry in posterior slices. The authors concluded that their data lent support to the theory that at least some schizophrenia could be associated with a lack of development of normal cerebral asymmetries.

Likewise, Kleinschmidt et al. (1994) examined planum temporale structural asymmetry in 24 first-episode schizophrenic patients and 26 healthy volunteers. Asymmetry coefficients obtained for the planum temporale did not differ significantly between patients and the control group and were not correlated with standard psychopathological measures. The authors felt that disease heterogeneity and/or technical and methodological issues may explain their failure to find any difference in asymmetry measures.

Bilder et al. (1994) also examined MRI scans of first-episode schizophrenic patients for regional cerebral hemispheric volumes or asymmetries, finding an absence of normal hemispheric asymmetries. Researchers felt this suggested an anomaly in the development of laterally-specialized cerebral systems in schizophrenia, and might be associated with an initial presentation of a non-paranoid psychosis.

Absence of the normal asymmetry was more common among patients initially diagnosed with the undifferentiated, rather than with the paranoid, subtype of schizophrenia, and was associated with more severe negative symptoms among men. Asymmetries were related to sex and handedness regardless of diagnosis. Specifically, dextral men showed more asymmetry than non-dextral men or women, and women (both patients and controls) had less asymmetry.

In another study, Bilder et al. (1995) examined the relationship of mesiotemporal lobe tissue volumes with neuropsychological functions in first-episode schizophrenia. The authors found that morphological abnormalities in the mesiotemporal lobe were associated with impairment of 'frontal lobe' functions, which they believe implicates a defect in an integrated functional system which includes both frontal and mesiotemporal components. The findings are consistent with the hypothesis that neurodevelopmental defects affecting the morphology of the anterior hippocampal formation may be manifested later in life as impairments in frontolimbic regulation.

Examining the caudate nucleus with MRI in a subsample of first-

5 BIOLOGICAL VARIABLES IN FIRST-EPISODE SCHIZOPHRENIA

episode schizophrenics with minimal previous antipsychotic exposure, Chakos et al. (1994) found that volumes increased 5.7% in patients over an 18-month period, while decreasing by 1.6% in the control group. Greater amounts of antipsychotic medication received by patients at the time of the first scan, and younger age, were both associated with larger increases in caudate volume, leading researchers to conclude that early caudate volume increases may be the result of the effects of antipsychotic treatment on dopaminergic neuronal systems.

PET studies

Positron emission tomography (PET) is an in vivo tracer kinetic method which uses a radioactively labelled molecule as an indirect tool for exploring a functional system and its localization within the brain. Although PET has a unique power and sensitivity for examining physiological events, it has the drawback of fairly low spatial resolution. Different tracers have to be used for different biochemical and physiological systems.

Two major areas of brain function studied in first-episode schizophrenia using this method include regional brain energy metabolism and analysis of neuroreceptor function.

Regional brain energy metabolism

Using PET scanning oxygen-15, Sheppard et al. (1983) examined regional cerebral blood flow and the regional cerebral metabolic rate of oxygen in a group of predominantly 'never-medicated' schizophrenics ($n = 12$), and matched normal controls ($n = 12$). The results of the procedure did not reveal the hypofrontality previously described in chronic patients. None of the differences between the schizophrenic group and control group came close to the significance level.

The authors determined, however, that there was reduced metabolic activity in the basal ganglia in the schizophrenia population. Also, whilst there were no differences in the laterality of central structures measured, there were significant differences regarding the peripheral structures. The authors concluded that the abnormal laterality may be due to the illness or, alternatively, is a part of the deeper underlying schizophrenic process.

Volkow et al. (1986) used PET scanning with 11–C-deoxyglucose (11–C-2–deoxyglucose or 11–DG) to compare regional brain metabolism in 12 normal controls and 4 patients with chronic schizophrenia (mean duration of illness = eight years) who had never been treated with antipsychotic drugs. Patients underwent a second PET scan after an injection of thiothixene to evaluate the effects of acute neuroleptics on glucose metabolism. The authors found that the patients showed higher glucose metabolism than the controls and did not demonstrate the metabolic hypofrontality earlier reported in chronic medicated schizophrenic populations. Administration of the antipsychotic drug, in this never-medicated population, did not have a significant effect on the metabolic pattern of the patients. The authors concluded that their findings gave support to the hypothesis that it was prolonged medication use that may contribute to the metabolic hypofrontal pattern seen in chronic schizophrenia.

When Cleghorn et al. (1989) used a tracer of 18–fluorodeoxyglucose (18–F) to measure frontal and parietal lobe metabolism in eight never-medicated, acutely ill schizophrenic patients and ten control subjects, they found that the frontal lobe metabolism of glucose was significantly greater in the schizophrenic patients. The authors noted that this finding differed from earlier reports of the hypofrontality found in scans of chronic medicated patients.

Relative glucose metabolism in the interior parietal lobe, however, was significantly lower in schizophrenic patients than in controls. Likewise, frontal–parietal lobe metabolism ratios were increased in schizophrenic patients. The authors hypothesized that a resting or 'basal' level of metabolism in the parietal lobe may be lower in schizophrenic individuals than in controls.

Buchsbaum et al. (1992) evaluated glucose metabolism in a group of never-medicated schizophrenics ($n = 18$), and 20 age- and sex-matched control subjects, using 18–F-fluorodeoxyglucose as a radioligand. The authors reported that the patients with schizophrenia had relative hypofrontality as compared with the controls, which was in accordance with previous reports in medicated patients, suggesting that this finding was not an artifact of medication status. Significantly reduced ratios of inferior and medial frontal regions to occipital cortex were found which, together with the finding of diminished metabolism in the basal ganglia, led the authors to conclude that a combined fronto-striatal dysfunction in schizophrenia might exist.

Gur et al. (1995) examined resting glucose metabolism in 22 first-episode and 20 previously treated schizophrenic patients, and compared the results with data obtained from 42 control subjects. Fluorodeoxyglucose was used as a radioligand and patients were also scanned by a 1.5 Tesla GE medical MR scanner for anatomical localization. There were no differences between groups, regarding either whole brain metabolism, regional ratios, or in anterior–posterior gradients, but left midtemporal metabolism was relatively higher in patients. This was pronounced in the negative and Schneiderian subtypes of schizophrenia and absent in the paranoid subtypes.

Higher metabolism and lower relative left hemispheric values were associated with better premorbid adjustment and outcome. A higher subcortical–cortical gradient was noted in first-episode patients. The authors concluded that, although no resting metabolic abnormalities were found in patients, abnormal gradients were evident varying according to subtype. In addition, they found that laterality was associated with functioning. These results support the idea of a temporolimbic dysfunction in schizophrenia, which is already present at the onset of illness.

Neuroreceptor studies in first-episode psychosis

The three most commonly used ligands in PET studies of neuroreceptors include 11–C-N-methylspiperone, 76–Br-bromo-spiperone, and 11–C-raclopride. Of these ligands, C-11 raclopride has the highest selectivity with regard to specific binding to D-2 dopamine receptors. However, 11–C-N-methylspiperone and 76–Br-bromo-spiperone have higher affinities to D-2 dopamine receptors. These ligands, however, also have significant affinities for serotonin 5HT-2 receptors as well as other binding sites.

Wong et al. (1986) used 11–C-N-methylspiperone as a radioligand to measure D-2 dopamine receptor densities in the caudate nucleus of 10 never-medicated patients, 5 previously treated schizophrenic individuals, and 11 normal volunteers. The first of two scans was taken while patients were drug-free and receptors were not blocked. The second scan was preceded by the administration of the unlabelled D-2 dopamine receptor antagonist haloperidol, which produced a partially blocked state. Using these measurements to calculate the D-2 receptor density, the authors found that the density of the D-2 dopamine receptors was substantially higher in both drug-naïve and drug-treated schizophrenic patients as compared with normal controls.

The finding that D-2 dopamine receptors are substantially increased in schizophrenic patients, even in those never treated, raises the possibility that abnormalities in dopamine receptors are involved in the disease process and are not solely a treatment artifact. Alternatively, the authors concluded that the increased D-2 receptor number may reflect presynaptic factors such as decreased endogenous dopamine levels. Without conducting similar experiments in non-schizophrenic psychotic populations, they argued it would be premature to conclude that this increase is specific to schizophrenia itself.

Using 11–C-raclopride as a radioligand, Farde et al. (1990) examined D-2 dopamine receptors in 18 neuroleptic-naïve schizophrenic patients and 20 healthy controls. In the first of two PET experiments performed, raclopride with high-specific activity was infused and, in the second, raclopride with low-specific activity was used. In contrast to the Wong et al. (1986) study, researchers here found no increase in the density of dopamine D-2 receptors. Their findings also failed to support the hypothesis that schizophrenia is related to a generalized increase in dopamine-2 receptor densities.

This discrepancy between the two studies has created considerable controversy and raised questions regarding the validity of PET methods for examining brain function.

State-dependent variables could partly account for D-2 receptor density variability, according to Martinot et al. (1990), who also looked at this question. In their study, the radioligand 76–Br-bromospiperone was used to evaluate striatal D-2 dopaminergic receptors in 12 male schizophrenic patients, 9 of whom were neuroleptically naïve and 3 others had minimal drug exposure. Twelve healthy normal subjects were also scanned as a control group. As in the Farde et al. (1990) study, researchers here did not find an increase in dopamine receptor density in schizophrenic patients.

Hietala et al. (1994), using C-11 raclopride as a radioligand, also looked at striatal D-2 dopamine receptor density. In a method similar to that employed by Farde et al. (1990), this group scanned both patients (13 neuroleptic-naïve schizophrenic individuals) and control subjects (10 healthy volunteers) twice in the same day. The quantification of striatal D-2 dopamine receptor density and affinity was accomplished using an equilibrium model, as described for raclopride, labelled with carbon-11. Raclopride with high-specific activity was used the first time and with low-specific activity on the second occasion. No statistically significant alterations were found in D-2 receptor densities between the patient and control groups. However, a subgroup of four patients with relatively high striatal D-2 density was identified. The authors concluded that there were no general changes in D-2 dopamine receptor density in neuroleptic-naïve schizophrenic individuals, but there may be a subgroup of patients with aberrant striatal D-2 dopamine receptor characteristics in vivo.

SPECT studies

Single proton emission computed tomography (SPECT), using technetium Tc99m-d,l,hexamethyl propyleneamine oxime (HMPAO), was employed by Rubin et al. (1991), to measure prefrontal and subcortical activity of the brain during a cognitive task in schizophrenic patients. The patient sample was drug-naïve or treated over a short period of time (maximum 18 days), and consisted of 19 patients admitted for the first time. Seven healthy volunteers served as controls. Using two

SPECT studies for each subject, one at rest and the second upon activation with the Wisconsin Card Sorting Test (WCST) – a problem-solving, abstract-reasoning test related to frontal functioning – researchers measured prefrontal and subcortical activity of the brain.

At rest, the regional cerebral blood flow was not significantly different between the patient (drug-naïve and briefly treated) and control groups. During the WCST, however, the healthy volunteers activated the inferior, as well as the superior, prefrontal cortex, while the patients did not. Also, the volunteers were able to suppress the relative activity of the striatum (specifically the left striatum) upon activation, but the relative flow in the left striatum was nearly unchanged. The ratio of activation to rest again indicated a difference between the groups in the prefrontal cortex and striatum. The differences were most pronounced in the left hemisphere and in the left inferior prefrontal region. Also, the patient group performed significantly poorer than the control group on the WCST.

The authors concluded that the patients' inability to activate the left prefrontal cortex, considered together with their poor performance on the WCST, indicates that they had an altered function of the left prefrontal region. This defect was detectable at initial presentation of the illness and was not confounded by chronicity or medication status, and therefore may reflect pathology intrinsic to schizophrenia. The inability of the patient group to suppress striatal activity may have been due to a lack of corticostriatal feedback during prefrontal activation.

Andreasen et al. (1992) examined the issue of hypofrontality in schizophrenic patients by employing SPECT scans using xenon-133 (Xe-133) as a tracer. Two scans were conducted using three groups which included 13 neuroleptic-naïve schizophrenic patients, 23 non-naïve patients who were off medications for at least three weeks, and 15 normal volunteers. The control condition consisted of looking at undulating coloured shapes on a video monitor, while the experimental task involved the Tower of London, a cognitive task that assesses prefrontal function.

The authors observed the Tower of London to be a relatively specific stimulant of the left mesial frontal cortex (probably including parts of the cingulate gyrus) in normal healthy volunteers. The patient groups (drug-naïve and previously treated) lacked activation of this area, as well as a related one in the right parietal cortex (representing circuitry specifically activated by the Tower of London). Decreased activation occurred only in patients with high scores for negative symptoms. The authors concluded that their results suggested that hypofrontality is related to negative symptoms and is not a long-term effect of medication or chronicity of illness.

Pilowsky et al. (1994) used SPECT with 123–I-IBZM as a tracer to evaluate striatal D-2 dopamine receptor binding in 20 antipsychotic-free schizophrenic patients (including both never-medicated and previously treated, patients) and 20 age- and sex-matched normal control subjects.

The authors did not find any overall elevation of D-2 receptor binding in the patient group as compared with the controls. However, a specific lateralized asymmetry of striatal D-2 receptor binding was found in the male patients. Moreover, an age-dependent decline of striatal D-2 receptors was present in controls, but not in patients. These results suggested that alterations in striatal D-2 receptor distribution and density do occur in schizophrenia, and possibly reflect wider disruptions in prefrontal–striatal–limbic circuits.

Magnetic resonance spectroscopy

Pettegrew et al. (1991) studied membrane phospholipid and high-energy phosphate metabolism (using in vivo phosphorus-31 nuclear magnetic resonance spectroscopy: MRS) in the dorsal prefrontal cortex of 11 drug-naïve first-episode schizophrenic patients, and compared them with 10 healthy control volunteers.

Phosphorus-31 has a nuclear magnetic moment and is present in natural abundance, so no isotope had to be given to the patients. Phosphorus-31 NMR spectroscopy provides direct in vivo assessment of brain membrane phospholipid and high-energy phosphate metabolism.

Schizophrenia patients enrolled in the study had significantly reduced levels of phosphomonoesters and inorganic orthophosphate and significantly increased levels of phosphodiesters and adenosine triphosphate, when compared with the control subjects. Also, adenosine triphosphate and inorganic orthophosphate findings suggested functional hypoactivity of the dorsal prefrontal cortex. Phosphomonoester and phosphodiester results were compatible with either premature ageing, or an exaggeration of normal programmed regressive events occurring in the neural systems sampled.

In Renshaw et al. (1995) researchers evaluated temporal lobe abnormalities in the brains of schizophrenic patients by using 1–H nuclear MRS, which is present in relatively high concentrations in neurons and absent in most glial cell lines. Temporal lobe 1–H MRS was performed bilaterally on 13 patients with first-episode psychosis and 15 comparison subjects. The N-acetyl aspartate–creatine-phosphocreatine and choline–creatine-phosphocreatine ratios of the psychotic patients were significantly lower than that of the comparison subjects, with the authors concluding that their data suggested that abnormalities in temporal lobe N-acetyl aspartate concentrations are present early in the course of psychotic illness.

Summary

While it is difficult to extract a clear picture from this range of neuroimaging studies, it is clear that this area of research will continue to expand and has the potential to illuminate greatly the pathophysiology of the onset of psychosis. One of the most important questions to resolve is the relative contribution of neurodevelopmental (i.e. pre-psychotic) pathological processes on the one hand, and neurodegenerative processes on the other. The evidence to date concerning the issue is by no means conclusive, since whilst it is likely that structural changes predate the onset of psychosis in many cases, it is also becoming apparent that structural change can continue post-onset in a number of ways. Functional MRI, MRS and PET are likely to play an increasing role in future studies; however, a number of important methodological weaknesses will need to be seriously addressed. In addition to technical considerations, the weaknesses include problems with the representativeness of samples and statistical power. Some authors seem to have overinterpreted their data due to a failure to acknowledge fully the impact of these problems.

Neurophysiology

EEG and sleep

The electroencephalographic (EEG) sleep findings in schizophrenia which have most often been reported include: (1) fragmentation of sleep and decrease in total sleep time; (2) decreased percentage of slow-wave sleep; (3) decreased, as well as increased, amounts of rapid eye movement (REM) sleep; and (4) reduced REM compensation following REM deprivation. Some studies have also reported finding a shortened REM latency for the first REM period. Two studies examined sleep EEGs in well defined samples of neuroleptic-naïve first-episode patients.

When Ganguli, Reynolds & Kupfer (1987) compared sleep in eight neuroleptic-naïve first-episode patients, eight patients with delusional depression, 16 patients with non-delusional depression, and 16 healthy control subjects, they found that the schizophrenic patients showed diminished sleep efficiency and early morning awakening, comparable to the older delusional depressives. Patients also had greater wakefulness after sleep onset and diminished sleep maintenance when compared with the non-delusional depressives and healthy subjects.

Both schizophrenic patients and healthy subjects showed comparable percentages of slow-wave sleep and had similar REM latency means compared with both groups of depressives who had significantly lower means. The duration of the first REM period was nearly identical in both the schizophrenic patients and the healthy subjects. A significant inverse correlation was found between the natural log of slow-wave sleep minutes in schizophrenic individuals and the severity of negative symptoms. The authors concluded that there may not be any *pathognomonic* changes in sleep in schizophrenia and that the principal sleep abnormality appears to be in diminished sleep continuity (at least in the sample of young neuroleptic-naïve first-episode patients). The amount of slow-wave sleep appears to be inversely correlated with the presence of negative symptoms, with less slow-wave sleep being seen in patients with more severe negative symptoms.

Tandon et al. (1992) also examined sleep EEG changes in both drug-naïve and chronic schizophrenic patients. Using 20 drug-naïve patients, 20 previously treated patients, and 15 healthy control subjects, they also found that the schizophrenic sample (both drug-naïve and treated) had significant impairment of sleep continuity. The previously treated schizophrenic group had significantly more REM and less stage 2 sleep than the healthy subjects and the drug-naïve patients. Drug-naïve and previously-treated schizophrenics had a shorter REM latency than the controls. REM latency in the drug-naïve sample was inversely correlated with global severity and severity of positive symptoms. In the previously treated sample, it was also inversely correlated with the severity of negative symptoms.

No differences in sleep architecture were seen in either schizophrenic groups as compared with the controls, with no correlation being obtained between measures of REM latency and depressive symptom scores. Tandon et al. (1992) attempted to resolve the discrepancy between their study's REM results and those of Ganguli, Rabin & Belle (1989) by noting that an expanded sample from the latter study demonstrated a significant decreased REM latency, thereby replicating the findings of Tandon and colleagues. Researchers here also noted an inverse relationship between REM latency and positive symptoms, negative symptoms and global severity.

In summary, there appears to be impaired sleep continuity in schizophrenia as well as reduced REM latency. Slow-wave sleep appears to be unaffected, and the REM latency appears to be inversely correlated with positive, negative and global symptom scores in schizophrenia.

Event-related potential studies

Lindstrom et al. (1990) studied the relationship between brain stem auditory-evoked potentials (ERPs) and the cerebrospinal fluid (CSF) levels of HVA and 5–HIAA in first-episode schizophrenic patients ($n = 24$ out of a total of 39 drug-free patients). Clear-cut abnormal ERPs, identified as a lack of one or more peaks or abnormal peak latencies, were found in 15 patients. In 47 controls and patients who had normal ERPs, there was a significant positive correlation between the CSF levels of HVA and 5–HIAA. Schizophrenic individuals with abnormal ERPs had significantly lower levels of HVA, but not of 5–HIAA, in the CSF when compared with controls. Those with normal ERPs ($n = 24$), did not differ from the controls with regard to amine metabolites in the CSF.

A comparison of the CSF levels of HVA and 5–HIAA yielded no significant differences between patients with normal, and those with abnormal, ERPs. In contrast, when only first-episode schizophrenic patients were considered, patients with abnormal ERPs ($n = 10$) had significantly lower levels of both HVA and 5–HIAA as compared with patients with normal ERPs ($n = 14$). The results indicated an association between brain stem dysfunction and reduced CNS dopaminergic, and possibly also serotonergic, activity in schizophrenia.

Mintz et al. (1995) examined late positive components of visual event-related potentials (vERPs) in the first month of neuroleptic treatment, recorded vERPs in drug-naïve schizophrenics during passive attention and active attention tasks. Patients, compared with normal controls, had much lower late positive components (LPC) in both sessions, but nearly normal LPC increase from passive to active tasks.

Neuroleptic treatment during this period produced amelioration of symptoms evidenced by a reduction in BPRS scores. Schizophrenic patients showed a session-related increase in LPC amplitude, when compared with controls, but this process of LPC recovery was too minor to normalize fully the low LPC amplitude in patients. Furthermore, the treatment either did not improve, or even reduced, the LPC reaction to the active attention task. The findings indicated that normalization of low LPC in schizophrenia might require a long period of treatment, and that the patients' reduced LPC may be contributed to by the neuroleptics.

Electrodermal studies in first-episode schizophrenia

Ohman and Ohlund (1989) examined electrodermal non-response and premorbid adjustment as predictors of long-term social functioning in schizophrenic individuals, which was tested over a two-year period in

37 patients. Electrodermal non-responding, poor premorbid adjustment, and negative symptomatology, predicted poor social functioning during the second follow-up year, but the relationship to non-responding pertained exclusively to a group of 15 first-episode patients. Discriminant analysis showed that electrodermal non-responding and symptoms were the only independent predictors of outcome.

Dawson, Neuchterlein & Schell (1992) also examined the relationship between electrodermal anomalies and symptoms and progress in recent-onset schizophrenia, measuring this in 98 recent-onset schizophrenic patients and 40 matched normal controls. Heightened electrodermal activity, as measured at the inpatient phase of treatment, was associated with a number of symptoms in the male patients and with poor recovery from the acute schizophrenic episode. Follow-up tests, conducted both when the patients were in states of remission and suffering a psychotic relapse, revealed that tonic electrodermal arousal measures qualify as state-sensitive episode indicators, whereas phasic non-responding may qualify as an atypical vulnerability indicator. Preliminary data from three patients suggested that an increase in tonic electrodermal arousal may temporally precede psychotic relapses. The authors concluded that their findings were consistent with a vulnerability–stress model which posits that electrodermal hyperarousal is part of a transient intermediate state that may lead to a psychotic episode in a vulnerable individual.

Summary

Electrophysiological studies of first-episode patients have used diverse methodologies. The results are not conclusive with any of the techniques used. The most promising of these would seem to be measures of eye movement function and event-related potentials which appear to be assessing trait-dependent features of the illness.

Neuropsychology

While investigations of neuropsychological function in schizophrenia have consistently indicated deficits, the developmental and neuropathological processes leading to these deficits are poorly understood and also are the subject of some controversy. Studies have shown that chronic schizophrenic patients demonstrate a diffuse pattern of cognitive impairment frequently indistinguishable from brain-damaged patients (Goldstein, 1978; Heaton, Baade & Johnson, 1978). Major dimensions of impairment include attention vigilance, abstraction flexibility, verbal intelligence and language function skills and memory and learning (Andreasen, 1979; Goldberg et al., 1987; Mirsky, 1988; Weinberger, Berman & Zec, 1986). Other studies have suggested a focal pattern of deficit, such as left hemisphere dysfunction (e.g. Gur, 1978), frontal lobe impairment or dysfunction of the temporal–limbic cortex (Goldberg et al.,1987; Kolb & Whisman, 1983).

Because of limitations resulting from medication and chronicity in these studies, it is unclear what degree of cognitive dysfunction is present at the onset of schizophrenic illness. To address these concerns there has been recent interest in characterizing neuropsychological performance in patients experiencing their first episode of illness.

Studying the effects of neuroleptics on attention in adolescent schizophrenic patients, Erickson et al. (1984) compared the performance of these patients with that of healthy subjects, patients with conduct disorder, attention deficit disorder, and a mixed group of patients with anxiety and eating disorders. Response time was not found to be significantly different among the test subjects and the healthy controls; the addition of antipsychotic medication did nothing to improve the performance of affected adolescents. Thus, attentional disorders in schizophrenic adolescents may not be significantly different from those of other non-psychotic psychiatric adolescents.

Likewise, psychotropic medication had no effect on the intellectual performance of 39 psychotic adolescent subjects in Goldberg et al. (1988). At the onset of the illness, performance IQ was significantly lower in the psychotic group and was similar to the pattern displayed by adult schizophrenic patients. Interestingly, their academic achievement was similar to the control subjects, despite the marked difference in the performance IQs. Goldberg et al. concluded that deficits in the processing of novel material seemed to be present at the outset of the illness and may be non-progressive thereafter.

In evaluating the stability of neuropsychological functioning in a one-year follow-up study of first-episode patients, Sweeney et al. (1991) found that considerable improvement in neuropsychological performance can occur following symptomatic recovery from acute psychosis. Analyses of a battery of tests done on 39 ready-to-be-discharged patients, of whom 15 were first-episode patients, indicated significant improvement in neuropsychological functioning from the first to the second testing on several tasks including trails A and B, digit symbol, Wisconsin Card Sorting Test (WCST), finger tapping test, recognition memory on the Rey auditory verbal learning test, and judgement of line orientation. These improvements were unrelated to treatment history and were similar in both chronic and first-episode samples.

When Bilder et al. (1992) compared intellectual functioning in three groups, namely, healthy volunteers, first-episode schizophrenic patients, and chronic schizophrenic patients, they found that schizophrenic patients may suffer both early developmental *and* deteriorative effects on intellectual functioning over the course of their illness. Wechsler Adult Intelligence Scale – revised (WAIS – R) testing undertaken by Bilder et al. (1992) indicated that the normal controls were superior to both patient groups. The first-episode schizophrenia group had significantly higher performance IQ than the chronic sample, but differences in full scale IQ (FSIQ) and verbal IQ (VIQ) was not statistically significant. The first-episode sample was superior to the chronic group on digit span, arithmetic, picture arrangement, and digit symbol subtests, but the two groups did not differ significantly on other subtest scores.

Sweeney, Haas & Li (1992) found that 33 chronic schizophrenic patients showed more severe pursuit eye movement dysfunction than the 27 first-episode patients. They also had more severe disturbances of neuropsychological performance on tests sensitive to prefrontal and left temporal cortical function, implying that deterioration had taken place. First-episode patients were superior on psychomotor testing, emphasizing visual search and flexibility (trails B), verbal fluency, verbal learning and memory, complex problem-solving, and the ability to shift cognitive set (WCST).

When Hoff et al. (1992a) conducted neuropsychological testing in a group of 56 consecutively-admitted schizophreniform patients upon first admission and stabilization, and again two years into the illness, they found a diffuse pattern of neuropsychological impairment which appeared to improve over time. An atypical pattern of anatomical lateral symmetry was found in female schizophreniform patients, with females appearing to have a reduction in the normally occurring 'left-greater-than-right' length of the lateral sulcus. Such atypical asymmetry was associated with better cognitive function, and thus language disturbance may have an impact in cognitive functioning in schizophrenic illness.

In another study, Hoff et al. (1992b) compared 32 first-episode patients with healthy volunteers and 26 patients with chronic schizophrenia. Both groups of patients did worse than the healthy controls and the first-episode patients were no different from the chronic sample in terms of cognitive impairment. Also, both patient groups showed greater left than right hemisphere dysfunction. Researchers concluded that substantial cognitive deficits in first-episode patients, and comparable to those in chronic patients, are present early on in the course of psychotic illness. It is important to note that both groups of patients were on medication at the time of their testing.

5 BIOLOGICAL VARIABLES IN FIRST-EPISODE SCHIZOPHRENIA

Saykin et al. (1994) found the presence of verbal memory and learning deficits when comparing 37 patients with first-episode psychosis, 65 unmedicated previously treated schizophrenics (off medication for at least two weeks), and 131 healthy control subjects. Spatial cognition, fine motor speed and visual memory, were more impaired in the previously treated group than in the first-episode group. Saykin et al. concluded that the results implicate the left temporal–hippocampal system in schizophrenia.

Summary

It seems that substantial neuropsychological impairments are present at the time of the first episode of schizophrenia. It is also likely that these are not of equal severity to those seen in patients with chronic schizophrenia, so that progression is possible, although sampling issues could create an artifactual impression of that in cross-sectional studies. More attention needs to be directed to the phase of illness and of episode, to study design, and to utilizing more appropriate and sophisticated methods and tools for assessing the domain of cognitive psychology in future research.

Neuroendocrinology and neurochemistry

Several different neurochemical and neuroendocrine studies have been undertaken in first-episode psychosis. In addition to characterizing the neurobiology of this population, some were intended to elucidate diagnosis, others to predict outcome.

After having performed dexamethasone suppression tests (DSTs) and the thyrotropin releasing hormone (TRH) stimulation test on 21 newly admitted acute patients with schizophreniform disorder, Targum (1983) found that neuroendocrine challenges may be useful in the early assessment of first-episode psychosis. Nine patients showed dysregulation on one or the other test. When 17 patients were divided into two groups – those with persistent dysfunction and/or psychotic symptoms, and those in full remission – and followed up for six months, 14% of patients with symptoms, in contrast to 70% of patients with full remission, showed evidence of dysregulation. Targum concluded that dysregulation may be an indicator of episodic illness with a better prognosis, possibly reflecting a diagnosis of affective disorder.

Banki, Arato & Rihmer (1984) investigated neuroendocrine differences among different subtypes of schizophrenic disorder using the DST in 45 recently hospitalized female patients with schizophrenia and schizophreniform disorder. Nineteen patients showed non-suppression, most being of the catatonic subtype (9 of 10) and none of the paranoid subtype. The authors concluded that limbic pathology in schizophrenia is heterogeneous and the finding of non-suppression in the catatonic subtype may indicate shared biology with affective disorders.

Demisch et al. (1987) studied the incorporation of 14–C labelled arachidonic acid (14–C-AA) into membrane phospholipids (into platelets) in a group of 33 untreated patients with schizophrenia (12 of whom were first-episode schizophrenic patients). Platelets from patients with schizophreniform or schizoaffective disorder incorporated > 50% less 14–C-AA than those from a healthy control group. The incorporation rates from schizophrenic patients were slightly, but not significantly, reduced from controls. The authors concluded that the difference in platelet uptake between schizophreniform and schizophrenic patients may be useful in the search for biological variables associated with recurrent episodes and recovery.

Markianos, Botsis & Arvanitis (1992) estimated the main metabolites of dopamine, noradrenaline, and serotonin (homovanillic acid (HVA), methoxyhydroxyphenyl glycol (MHPG), and 5–hydroxyindoleacetic acid (5–HIAA)) in the plasma of drug-naïve young male schizophrenic patients and compared it with healthy control subjects. No significant differences were found between the two groups. However, strong associations were found between the patients' 5–HIAA levels and their scores on the Brief Psychiatric Rating Scale (BPRS), with 5–HIAA correlating positively with hostility and negatively with somatic concerns, and MHPG plasma levels associated positively with disorientation and negatively with emotional withdrawal and unco-operativeness. The authors suggest that levels of neurotransmitter metabolites may be related to specific psychological dysfunctions rather than to the disease process *per se*.

As part of a comprehensive study of first-episode psychosis, Lieberman et al. (1993a) studied growth hormone secretion (GH), and behavioural response to methylphenidate (MPH) infusion, as indices of dopamine neural functioning. Patients, but not control subjects, demonstrated an increase in psychotic symptoms, such as delusions, distrustfulness, impaired understandability, and bizarre behaviour, upon the MPH infusion. This change occurred in 59% of the first-episode patients, which was higher than the psychotogenic response rate to psychostimulants (40%) in all types of schizophrenic patients found in the literature (Lieberman, Kane & Alvir, 1987).

The authors suggested that the difference was due to generally increased pharmacological sensitivity in young first-episode subjects in the early stages of their illness. Behavioural response to methylphenidate is believed to reflect a functional increase in the activity of the mesolimbic or mesocortical DA neural systems. If the schizophrenic pathophysiological condition involves deafferentation of limbic and cortical dopamine (DA) neurons (Weinberger, 1987) and is progressive, then the proportion of patients exhibiting symptom activation to psychostimulants should diminish as the illness progresses and patients become chronically ill. Non-activator patients may have already progressed to that stage of illness, or this population may represent a distinct subgroup with a different pathophysiological condition.

Elevated GH levels are believed to reflect a regulatory defect in DA input to the hypothalamus. Male schizophrenic subjects, to whom the study was limited, obtained significantly higher basal GH levels than the controls. Although male patients had a broader response to apomorphine administration, neither the post-administration GH response, mean or maximum response, was significantly different between patients and controls.

The GH findings of this study are consistent with previous reports (Meltzer, 1987) in patients with chronic multi-episode schizophrenia and in patients with first-episode schizophrenia. The increase in basal GH secretion may reflect a regulatory disturbance mediated by DA afferents to the arcuate nucleus of the hypothalamus or hypothalamic dysfunction involving peptidergic factors (Brown et al., 1978). The fact that anterior pituitary GH response to GH-releasing factor has been reported to be unimpaired, suggests that the dysfunction is at the hypothalamic or the suprahypothalamic level (Mayerhoff et al., 1990).

The authors found a positive correlation between methylphenidate activation and basal GH levels. GH response to apomorphine stimulation was associated with third ventricle enlargement on MRI and suggested a selective disturbance in DA neural function. Patients with abnormal ratings on the MRI had lower GH responses to apomorphine. The hypothalamus, which regulates GH secretion by the anterior pituitary, forms the lateral boundary of the third ventricle. Thus, this anatomical region would be the most likely to be associated with neuroendocrine abnormalities. This finding is consistent with the previously suggested hypothesis of an inverse relationship between the dual pathological processes, structural and biochemical (Crow, 1980), in which decreased measures of neurochemical function would be associated with increased levels of structural neuropathology.

Levy et al. (1993) reported that, unlike methylphenidate which increases thought disorder in first-episode schizophrenic individuals, apomorphine does not. This is interesting in light of the fact that both drugs are either directly or indirectly dopamine agonists (DA). The difference in the effects of these two drugs on thought disorder could be referable to relatively specific actions of MPH on mesolimbic–mesocortical DA systems, to low-dose APO being a less potent potentiator of DA in mesolimbic and mesocortical DA systems than MPH, or to MPH's effects on non-dopaminergic systems.

As a part of the previous comprehensive study, Koreen et al. (1994a) measured plasma HVA (pHVA) levels in a first-episode patient sample, compared them with healthy volunteers, and assessed their association to psychopathology and treatment response. Previous studies which examined pHVA levels in patients with chronic schizophrenia found that pHVA levels increase with short-term treatment, decrease with long-term treatment, and are correlated with psychopathology (Amin, Davidson & Davis, 1991). Basal and neuroleptic-induced changes in pHVA levels have been shown in some studies to have prognostic significance, with responders having higher pretreatment levels of pHVA and greater decreases in pHVA levels with continuous antipsychotic treatment.

Koreen et al. (1994a) found that there were no differences in baseline pHVA between first-episode patients and healthy control subjects, but suggested that pHVA levels have prognostic significance for response and time to reach remission. Baseline and week-1 pHVA levels were higher in responders than in non-responders. The pattern of pHVA response was similar in all the patients with a short-term rise followed by a decrease toward baseline values. There was also a significant gender effect with both patients and control females having higher pHVA levels than the males.

Koreen et al. (1994b) also examined the relationship that plasma fluphenazine levels have to treatment response and to EPS. Examining data from 36 first-episode patients, the authors found that plasma levels of fluphenazine for weeks 1 to 4 of the one-month study, were significantly correlated with each other, but were not correlated with age, gender, diagnosis or race. Mean neuroleptic levels (weeks 3 and 4) did not differ between responders and non-responders and were not correlated with measures of psychopathology or extrapyramidal symptoms. The authors concluded that the differences between their results and those of previous studies may be due to methodological or biologically-based differences between first-episode and chronic patients.

Szymanski et al. (1995) examined gender differences in onset of illness, response to treatment, course and biological measures in first-episode schizophrenia. Fifty-four neuroleptic-naïve schizophrenic patients, 29 of whom were males, were studied at baseline and during standardized treatment. The female schizophrenic patients had a later onset and better treatment response than the men. Plasma homovanillic acid (pHVA) levels at baseline and week 1, and changes in prolactin levels from baseline to weeks 1 to 6, were greater among the women.

The authors concluded that gender differences in first-episode schizophrenia appear to mirror those of more chronic schizophrenia and are present at the onset of the illness. The greater pharmacological responsivity of the female patients, as indicated by the neuroendocrine results, is consistent with the gender difference in degree of symptom improvement with medication.

Summary

In general, these studies of neuroendocrine functioning and neurochemistry in first-episode psychosis are relatively preliminary. They reveal some interesting differences between patients at this stage of illness and those later in the course, and may prove to have some value as prognostic markers or predictors of treatment response.

Studies of movement disorders and neurological abnormalities

Studies of movement disorders and neurological abnormalities in first-episode schizophrenia have been of three different types: abnormal movements and spontaneous dyskinesias, neurological 'soft' signs, and extrapyramidal signs of parkinsonism in never-medicated first-episode schizophrenic patients.

Extrapyramidal signs

Extrapyramidal signs (EPS) in schizophrenic populations are generally associated with antipsychotic drug effects and are thought to be the consequence of dopamine receptor antagonism. EPS was observed in patients long before the introduction of neuroleptic treatment (Mettler & Crandell, 1959; Reiter, 1926) and may be directly involved in the pathophysiology of schizophrenia. Since the introduction of neuroleptics in the 1950s and the nearly universal use of these agents for schizophrenia, it has become extremely difficult to assess the contribution of the disease process itself to the motor abnormalities observed.

In one of two studies of unmedicated patients reported in the literature, Caligiuri, Lohr & Jeste (1993) found that 21% of the schizophrenic patients had rigidity and 12% had bradykinesia (on clinical examination). In contrast, none of the normal controls were affected. The authors concluded that the presence of the EPS was not correlated with total BPRS score, positive or negative symptom factor scores, and that the EPS observed was asymmetric (right > left).

These findings, when coupled with the fact that there is a relative absence of other studies in this area, underscore the need for investigation into the role of the basal ganglia structures and extrapyramidal pathways in the pathophysiology of schizophrenia.

Chatterjee et al. (1995) examined the prevalence of EPS and spontaneous dyskinesias in 89 neuroleptic-naïve first-episode patients. Fifteen patients (16%) in the sample had scores of mild or more on the Simpson Angus Extrapyramidal Sign Scale (SAEPS). The subsample with baseline (pretreatment) EPS had more negative symptoms, took longer to remit from their acute episode, and had a poorer level of remission than the sample without EPS. In addition, the patients with EPS at baseline developed parkinsonism secondary to antipsychotic medication more readily than the non-EPS group. However, there was no increased tendency on their part to develop tardive dyskinesia as compared with the non-EPS group.

The fact that 'hypodopaminergic' EPS could co-exist with 'hyperdopaminergic' schizophrenic symptoms might seem paradoxical. However, the results of post-mortem and cerebrospinal fluid studies of DA metabolites do not make a convincing case for a homogenous dopamine excess in schizophrenia.

Several recent studies (e.g. Pickar et al., 1990) indicate that hypodopaminergic activity may be important in the negative symptoms of schizophrenia. Neuroimaging studies of cortical and subcortical regions in patients with schizophrenia have revealed abnormalities suggestive of both hypo- and hyper-functional dopaminergic states (Weinberger et al., 1986). Thus, the conception of uniformly increased dopamine activity in all brain regions in schizophrenia is probably simplistic and inaccurate, with present theories suggesting the possibility of a co-existence of both states in different areas of the brain.

Chakos et al. (1992) were the first to examine the incidence and correlates of acute EPS in the first-episode schizophrenic patient, and found that patients with acute parkinsonism (34%) had higher baseline psychopathology, and higher positive and negative symptom scores. Those with acute dystonia (36%) also had higher baseline psychopathology, higher positive symptom scores, and a trend toward higher negative symptom scores. There was no significant correlation between the forms of EPS and time to remission. The authors speculated that the patients who are vulnerable to developing acute EPS have greater levels of dopaminergic activity and this may give rise to more florid psychopathology.

Sanders, Keshavan & Schooler (1994) performed neurological examinations in first-episode patients who were neuroleptic-naïve, and compared them with healthy control subjects. The neurological performance of the patients was significantly more impaired than that of the comparison subjects overall, and on each of the subscales of motor sequencing, motor co-ordination, and sensory integration. These findings considered along with the previously described EPS in treatment-naïve patients, indicate that neurological abnormalities exist as a part of the pathology of schizophrenia independent of medication effects.

Assessing the prevalence of neurological soft signs, Gupta et al. (1995) compared never-medicated schizophrenic patients with patients treated with antipsychotics and normal controls. While soft signs were present in 23% of the never-medicated and 46% of the treated schizophrenics, developmental reflexes were seen in 19% of the neuroleptic-naïve patients and 12% of the medicated patients; neither soft sign was found in controls.

The presence of soft signs in both never-medicated and treated schizophrenic patients reflects dysfunction primarily in the areas of motor co-ordination, integrative sensory function, and execution of complex motor tasks. Several neural substrates may be involved, but this remains unclear.

Circling behaviours

Circling behaviours exhibited by never-medicated patients appear to have a dopaminergic connection, according to Bracha (1987). This behaviour in animals is related to asymmetry in dopaminergic activity between the left and right basal ganglia, or left and right frontal cortex. As a rule, animals rotate toward the hemisphere with lower striatal dopaminergic activity. In a human model, left-prone circling behaviour (neglect of right-sided turning) was found in 10 unmedicated schizophrenic patients, whereas 85 normal controls demonstrated almost equal right and left turning. The authors suggested the presence of a dopaminergic asymmetry in some unmedicated schizophrenic patients, with right anterior subcortical or cortical areas of the brain possibly manifesting a relative dopaminergic overactivity compared to left anterior structures.

Spontaneous dyskinesia

Spontaneous dyskinesias (SD: dyskinetic movements present in schizophrenic patients before the initiation of antipsychotic treatment and unrelated to medication) have been described since the pre-neuroleptic era. Rates appear to vary widely (0% to 100% in some populations –

McCreadie & Ohaeri, 1994; Waddington & Youssef, 1990) registering an increase over time, a fact not entirely explained by the increased vigilance for these disorders (Kane et al., 1982). Casey & Hansen (1984), described an overall prevalence rate of 4.2%. Despite the wide divergence of rates some general patterns have emerged, with SD appearing to increase with age and occurring more often in females (Casey & Hansen, 1984).

Finding only one patient with SD out of 89 first-episode never-medicated cases, Chatterjee et al. (1995) concluded that, in this young population, prevalence of SD may be quite limited. However, more sensitive testing may increase these numbers.

Some clinical correlates have also recently been described for SD (Fenton, Wyatt & McGlashan, 1994). These include an association with a more malignant course – originally described by Kleist as parakinetic catatonia (Fish, 1958) – the presence of more negative symptoms, and the fact that these patients had lower IQs than the non-dyskinetic schizophrenic patients.

Summary

The existence of these neurological abnormalities in a subgroup of never-medicated patients provides further support for the neurodevelopmental origins of at least some cases of schizophrenia, and also indicates the involvement of the basal ganglia in some forms of the illness. These features also have potential as markers to assist with early intervention in prepsychotic phases of illness and in prediction of outcome.

Immunological studies in first-episode schizophrenia

It has long been hypothesized that there might be an autoimmune component to schizophrenia. Several clinical features, namely onset in adolescence, excess of winter births, a remitting and relapsing course, triggering by infections, drug abuse and physical injury, all suggest a possible place for autoimmune factors in the schizophrenic pathophysiology (Ganguli et al., 1993). Furthermore, an association between schizophrenia and other autoimmune illnesses is well known, e.g. Graves disease and systemic lupus erythromatosus (Ganguli et al., 1993; Knight, 1982). Abnormalities in autoimmune function in laboratory tests have also been reported in schizophrenia (Ganguli et al., 1993; Kirch, 1993).

Of all the reported immunological findings in the area, the linkage

5 BIOLOGICAL VARIABLES IN FIRST-EPISODE SCHIZOPHRENIA

with abnormal lymphokine physiology has been the most replicable. This includes decreased interleukin-2 (IL-2) production following mitogenic stimulation reported by four studies (Ganguli, Rabin & Belle, 1989; Kolyaskina et al., 1988; Sirota et al., 1990; Villemain et al., 1989).

Looking at mitogen-stimulated IL-2 production in neuroleptic-naïve first-episode patients and controls, Ganguli et al. (1995) found that the production of IL-2 was significantly reduced in the patients. There was also a significant positive correlation between IL-2 production and age at onset, and a negative correlation between IL-2 production and negative symptom scores. No correlations were found between IL-2 levels and positive symptoms and depressive symptoms. These findings confirm that IL-2 production is lower in schizophrenic patients and is not a confound of medication status. Also, the relationship between the levels and age at onset and negative symptoms argues that IL-2 may be a marker for a subtype of illness or severity.

Summary

The evidence for an autoimmune hypothesis, however, has met with some scepticism due to the fact that there has been inconsistent replication of results. Only a small portion of patients has been found to have these abnormalities, and no antigen-specific antibody has been shown to be exclusively associated with schizophrenia. Finally, methodological shortcomings and the potentially confounding effects of medication status of these samples have clouded interpretation of results.

Treatment studies

To date, five treatment studies have been described in first-episode schizophrenia. Drugs such as fluphenazine, lithium, pimozide and flupenthixol have all been assessed, as has ECT and psychotherapy.

The aim of May et al. (1976, 1981) was to compare the outcomes of five different modalities of treatment for schizophrenia. A patient group consisting of 228 first-admission male and female schizophrenic patients received either psychotherapy alone, antipsychotic drug therapy alone, psychotherapy plus drug therapy, ECT, or milieu therapy. Over a period of 2–5 years after first admission and first 'release', researchers found that patients who were originally treated with psychotherapy alone, on the whole stayed significantly longer in hospital over the entire follow-up period, when compared with those who received ECT, drug alone or drug plus psychotherapy. The milieu group did not differ significantly regarding outcome from the psychotherapy group.

The positive advantage from drug treatment began to dissipate after three years post-admission, with the authors concluding that, in in-patient settings, drug therapy and/or ECT was superior to milieu therapy or psychotherapy as a form of treatment for acute first-admission schizophrenia. However, they were unsure of the long-term advantage of drug treatment in this population.

In other studies, drug treatments have likewise fared well. Kane et al. (1982), who compared fluphenazine with placebo in 28 remitted acute first-episode patients, found that those receiving the drug were much less likely to relapse. In this double blind trial 41% of patients on placebo relapsed as against none receiving fluphenazine.

In Garver et al. (1984) lithium, which had been associated with remission of psychosis in other instances, such as with schizophreniform disorder, likewise resulted in significant improvement for first-episode schizophrenic patients. Essentially, full and sustained remission of psychosis began during periods of lithium treatment in 4 of 15 of the study patients. When these same patients failed to show sustained improvement while on placebo, researchers concluded that continued response to lithium occurred at a rate at least four times greater than that which could be attributed to spontaneous remission.

First-episode patients in Crow et al. (1986) relapsed less frequently on medication than those on placebo (46% versus 62%). A correlation was also found between duration of illness and poor prognosis. This led the authors to speculate that either susceptibility of illness is reduced by early institution of treatment, or that those who experience an extended duration of symptoms before admission for treatment are intrinsically more likely to do poorly.

In McCreadie et al. (1987a, b, c, d) two drug treatments, flupenthixol and pimozide, studied for five weeks in 46 first-episode schizophrenic patients, proved to be equally effective. There was no significant difference between patients receiving a mean daily dose of 18.8 mg of pimozide and those who received 20 mg/day of flupenthixol. Poor response was associated with 'organicity'. Just 54% of patients with successful outcome, who switched to a maintenance treatment after five weeks, achieved satisfactory results; this may be attributed to poor drug compliance and also possibly a short acute treatment phase. Intermittent oral pimozide was as effective as intramuscular flupenthixol.

Lieberman et al. (1989, 1993a, b) conducted a comprehensive prospective study which examined the neurobiology, treatment and outcome of first-episode psychosis. Seventy first-episode patients underwent four biological assessment procedures (brain magnetic resonance imaging, behavioural response to methylphenidate infusion, measurement of plasma growth hormone (GH) levels and smooth pursuit eye movements) and were treated with a standardized antipsychotic drug protocol until recovery.

Response was measured in terms of psychopathology by time to, and degree of, remission. Using survival analysis, the proportion of patients remitting by one year was estimated at 83%. Mean and median times to remission were 35.7 weeks and 11 weeks, respectively. While no baseline demographic or psychopathological measure significantly predicted time or level of remission, some other factors were indicative. Males tended to respond to treatment less frequently than females and to have diagnoses of schizophrenia rather than schizoaffective disorder. Also, brain pathomorphology and abnormal basal growth hormone levels did significantly predict time to remission. Specifically, abnormalities of the lateral and third ventricle predicted a longer time to remission, whereas cortical and medial temporal lobe abnormalities played no role in this. The GH analysis was limited to the male patients and indicated that patients with high basal levels had a significantly longer time to remission and that the degree of remission was poorer.

Antipsychotic treatment response of first-episode schizophrenia patients was better than that of chronic multi-episode patients, the authors concluded. This suggested that specific pathobiological markers reflect pathophysiological processes which mediate antipsychotic treatment response or are associated with more severe (i.e. less responsive) forms of illness.

In another arm of the Lieberman study, Loebel et al. (1992) assessed the effect of duration of untreated illness on outcome in the same group of 70 first-episode patients. The mean duration of psychotic symptoms before initial treatment was 52 weeks, preceded by a substantial prodromal or prepsychotic period. By survival analysis, duration of illness before treatment was found to be significantly associated with time to, as well as level of, remission. The effect of duration of illness on outcome remained significant when diagnosis and gender variables, themselves associated with outcome, were controlled in a regression analysis. Duration of illness was not correlated with age at onset, mode of onset, premorbid adjustment, or severity of illness at entry into the study. The authors determined that acute psychotic symptoms may reflect an active morbid process which, if not ameliorated by antipsychotic drug treatment, may result in lasting morbidity.

Summary

Clearly, a great deal more research is required in relation to the treatment of first-episode psychosis. The key decision points need data to allow informed choices to be made regarding the dose, route and sequence of medications, and the optimal use of adjunctive and combination therapies. Studies of combined drug and psychological interventions are urgently required and the role of the new antipsychotic medications and clozapine needs clarification. The treatment requirements of special subgroups need attention, especially women, young people, and a variety of different ethnic populations.

Conclusions

To summarize such a large body of literature is a formidable task. The findings encompass diverse areas involving changes in brain structure and function (physiological as well as biochemical) and link to aspects covered in other chapters, such as the impact of the illness on social function and its long-term prognosis. In some respects, the findings in this population of patients are similar to those found in more chronic schizophrenia. There are, however, many and important differences.

The importance, then, of this literature is the information it provides us regarding the early years of these illnesses, the pathology present at the outset, the changes which occur over time, and the potential effects of treatment on the measures of interest.

References

Amin, F., Davidson, M. & Davis, K. L. (1991). Homovanillac acid measurement in clinical research: a review of methodology. *Schizophrenia Bulletin*, **18**, 123–48.

Andreasen, N. C. (1979). Thought, language, and communication disorders. *Archives of General Psychiatry*, **36**, 1315–30.

Andreasen, N. C., Rezai, K., Alliger, R., Swayze, V. W., Flaum, M., Kirchner, P., Cohen, G. & O' Leary, D. S. (1992). Hypofrontality in neuroleptic naïve patients and in patients with chronic schizophrenia. Assessment with Xenon133 single-photon emission computed tomography and the Tower of London. *Archives of General Psychiatry*, **49**, 943–58.

Andreasen, N. C., Swayze, V. W., Flaum, M., Yates, W. R., Arndt, S. & McChesney, C. (1990). Ventricular enlargement in schizophrenia evaluated with computed tomographic scanning. *Archives of General Psychiatry*, **47**, 1008–15.

Banki, C. M., Arato, M. & Rihmer, Z. (1984). Neuroendocrine differences among subtypes of schizophrenic disorder. *Neuropsychobiology*, **11**, 174–7.

Bilder, R. M., Bogerts, B., Ashtari, M., Wu, H., Alvir, J. M., Jody, D., Reiter, G., Bell, L. & Lieberman, J. A. (1995). Anterior hippocampal volume reductions predict frontal lobe dysfunction in first-episode schizophrenia. *Schizophrenia Research* **17**, 47–58.

Bilder, R. M., Lipschutz-Broch, L., Reiter, G., Geisler, S. H., Mayerhoff, D. I. & Lieberman, J. A. (1992). Intellectual deficits in first episode schizophrenia: evidence for progressive deterioration. *Schizophrenia Bulletin*, **18**, 437–48.

Bilder, R. M., Wu, H., Bogerts, B., Degreef, G., Ashtari, M., Alvir, J. M. J., Snyder, P. J. & Lieberman, J. A. (1994). Absence of regional hemispheric volume asymmetries in first episode schizophrenia. *American Journal of Psychiatry*, **151**, 1437–47.

Bogerts, B., Ashtari, M., Degreef, G., Alvir, J. M., Bilder, R. M. & Lieberman, J. A. (1990). Reduced temporal limbic structure volumes on magnetic resonance images in first episode schizophrenia. *Psychiatry Research*, **35**, 1–13.

Bracha, H. S. (1987). Asymmetric rotational behavior, a dopamine-related asymmetry: preliminary findings in unmedicated and never medicated schizophrenic patients. *Biological Psychiatry*, **22**, 995–1003.

Brown, G. M., Seggie, J. A., Chambers, J.W. & Ettigi, P.G.(1978). Psychoendocrinology and growth hormone: a review. *Psychoendocrinology*, **3**, 131–53.

Buchsbaum, M. S., Haier, R. J., Potkin, S. G., Neuchterlein, K., Bracha, H. S., Katz, M., Lohr, J., Wu, J., Lottenberg, S., Jerabek, P. A., Trenary, M., Tafalla, R., Reynolds, C. & Bunney, W.E., Jr. (1992). Frontostriatal disorder of cerebral metabolism in never medicated schizophrenics. *Archives of General Psychiatry*, **49**, 935–42.

Caligiuri, M. P., Lohr, J. B. & Jeste, D. V. (1993). Parkinsonism in neuroleptic naïve schizophrenic patients. *American Journal of Psychiatry*, **150**, 1343–8.

Casey, D. E. & Hansen, T. E. (1984). Spontaneous dyskinesias. In *Neuropsychiatric Movement Disorders*, ed. D. V. Jeste & R. J. Wyatt, pp. 68–95. Washington DC: American Psychiatric Press.

Chakos, M. H., Lieberman, J. A., Bilder, R. M., Borenstein, M., Lerner, G., Bogerts, B., Wu, H., Kinon, B. & Ashtari, M. (1994). Increase in caudate nuclei volumes of first episode schizophrenic patients taking antipsychotic drugs. *American Journal of Psychiatry*, **151**, 1430–6.

Chakos, M. H., Mayerhoff, D. I., Loebel, A. D., Alvir, J. M. J. & Lieberman, J. A. (1992). Incidence and correlates of acute extrapyramidal symptoms in first episode schizophrenia. *Psychopharmacology Bulletin*, **28**, 81–6.

Chatterjee, A., Chakos, M., Koreen, A., Geisler, S., Sheitman, B., Woerner, M., Kane, J. M., Alvir, J. & Lieberman, J. A. (1995). Prevalence and clinical correlates of extrapyramidal signs and spontaneous dyskinesia in never medicated schizophrenic patients. *American Journal of Psychiatry*, **152**, 1724–9.

Cleghorn, J. M., Garnett, E. S., Nahmias, C., Firnau, G., Brown, G. M., Kaplan, R., Szechtman, H. & Szechtman, B. (1989). Increased frontal and reduced parietal glucose metabolism in acute untreated schizophrenics. *Psychiatry Research*, **28**, 119–33.

Crow, T.J. (1980). Molecular pathology of schizophrenia. More than one dimension of pathology? *British Medical Journal*, **280**, 66–8.

Crow, T. J., Macmillan, J. F., Johnson, A. L. & Johnstone, E.C. (1986). A randomised controlled trial of prophylactic neuroleptic treatment. *British Journal of Psychiatry*, **158**, 120–7.

Dawson, M. E., Neuchterlein, K. H. & Schell, A. M. (1992). Electrodermal anomalies in recent onset schizophrenia: relationship to symptoms and prognosis. *Schizophrenia Bulletin*, **18**, 295–311.

Degreef, G., Ashtari, M., Bogerts, B., Bilder, R. M., Jody, D. N., Alvir, J. M. J. & Lieberman, J. A. (1992a). Volumes of ventricular system subdivisions measured from magnetic resonance images in first episode schizophrenic patients. *Archives of General Psychiatry*, **49**, 531–7.

Degreef, G., Lantos, G., Bogerts, B., Ashtari, M. & Lieberman, J. A. (1992b). Abnormalities of the septum pellucidum on MR scans in first episode schizophrenic patients. *American Journal of Neuroradiology*, **13**, 835–40.

DeLisi, L. E., Hoff, A. L., Neale, C. & Kushner, M. (1994). Asymmetries in the superior temporal lobe in male and female first episode schizophrenic patients: measures of the planum temporale and superior temporal gyrus by MRI. *Schizophrenia Research*, **12**, 19–28.

DeLisi, L. E., Hoff, A. L., Schwartz, J. E., Shields, G. W., Halthore, S. L., Gupta, S. M., Henn, F. A. & Anand, A. K. (1991). Brain morphology in first episode schizophrenic-like psychotic patients: a quantitative magnetic resonance imaging study. *Biological Psychiatry*, **29**, 159–75.

Demisch, L., Gerbaldo, H., Gebhart, P., Georgi, K. & Bochnik, H. J. (1987). Incorporation of 14-C arachidonic acid into platelet phospholipids of untreated patients with schizophreniform or schizophrenic disorders. *Psychiatry Research*, **22**, 275–82.

Erickson, W. D., Yellin, A. M., Hopwood, J. H., Realmuto, G. M. & Greenberg, L. M. (1984). The effects of neuroleptics on attention in adolescent schizophrenics. *Biological Psychiatry*, **19**, 745–53.

Farde, L., Wiesel, F.-A., Elander, S. S., Haldin, C., Nordstrom, A. L., Hall, H. & Sedvall, G. (1990). D-2 dopamine receptors in neuroleptic naïve schizophrenic patients. *Archives of General Psychiatry*, **47**, 213–19.

Fenton, W. S., Wyatt, R. J. & McGlashan, T. H. (1994). Risk factors for spontaneous dyskinesias in schizophrenia. *Archives of General Psychiatry*, **51**, 643–50.

Fish, F. (1958). Leonhard's classification of schizophrenia. *Journal of Mental Science*, **104**, 943–71.

Ganguli, R., Brar, J. S., Chengappa, K. N. R., DeLeo, M., Yang, Z. W., Shurin, G. & Rabin, B. S. (1995). Mitogen stimulated interleukin-2 production in never medicated first episode schizophrenic patients: the influence of age at onset and negative symptoms. *Archives of General Psychiatry*, **52**, 668–72.

Ganguli, R., Brar, J. S., Chengappa, K. N. R., Yang, Z. W., Nimgaonkar, V. L. & Rabin, B. S. (1993). Autoimmunity in schizophrenia. *Annals of Medicine*, **25**, 489–96.

Ganguli, R., Reynolds, C. F. 3rd & Kupfer, D. J. (1987). Electroencephalographic sleep in young, never-medicated schizophrenics. A comparison with delusional and nondelusional depressives and with healthy controls. *Archives of General Psychiatry*, **44**, 36–44.

Ganguli, R., Rabin, B. S. & Belle, S. H. (1989). Decreased interleukin-2 production in schizophrenic patients. *Biological Psychiatry*, **26**, 427–30.

Garver, D. L., Hirschowitz, J., Fleishmann, R. & Djuric, P. E. (1984). Lithium response and psychosis: a double blind placebo controlled study. *Psychiatry Research*, **12**, 57–68.

Goldberg, T. E., Weinberger, D. R., Berman, K. F., Pliskin, N. H. & Podd, M. H. (1987). Further evidence for dementia of the prefrontal type in schizophrenia? *Archives of General Psychiatry*, **44**, 1008–14.

Goldberg, T. E., Carson, C. N., Leleszi, J. P. & Weinberger, D. R. (1988). Intellectual impairment in adolescent psychosis. *Schizophrenia Research*, **1**, 261–6.

Goldstein, G. (1978). Cognitive and perceptual differences between schizophrenics and organics. *Schizophrenia Bulletin*, **4**, 160–85.

Gupta, S., Andreasen, N. C., Arndt, S., Flaum, M., Schultz, S. K., Hubbard, W. C. & Smith, M. (1995). Neurological soft signs in neuroleptic naïve and neuroleptic treated schizophrenic patients and in normal comparison subjects. *American Journal of Psychiatry*, **152**, 191–6.

Gur, R.E. (1978). Left hemisphere dysfunction overactivation in schizophrenia. *Journal of Abnormal Psychology*, **87**, 226–38.

Gur, R. E., Mozley, P. D., Resnick, S. M., Mozley, L. H., Shtasel, D. L., Gallacher, F., Arnold, S. E., Karp, J. S., Alavi, A., Reivich, M. & Gur, R. C. (1995). Resting cerebral glucose metabolism in first episode and previously treated patients with schizophrenia relates to clinical features. *Archives of General Psychiatry*, **52**, 657–67.

Heaton, R. K., Baade, L. E. & Johnson, K. L. (1978). Neuropsychological test results associated with psychiatric disorders in adults. *Psychological Bulletin*, **85**, 141–62.

Hietala, J., Syvalahti, E., Vuorio, K., Nagren, K., Lehikoinen, P., Ruotsalainen, U., Rakkolainen, V., Lehtinen, V. & Wegelius, U. (1994). Striatal D-2 dopamine receptor characteristics in neuroleptic naïve schizophrenic patients studied with positron emission tomography. *Archives of General Psychiatry*, **51**, 116–23.

Hoff, A. L., Riordan, H., O'Donnell, D., Stritzke, P., Neale, C., Boccio, A., Anand, A. K. & DeLisi, L. E. (1992a). Anomalous lateral sulcus asymmetry and cognitive function in first episode schizophrenia. *Schizophrenia Bulletin*, **18**, 257–70.

Hoff, A. L., Riordan, H., O'Donnell, D. W., Morris, L. & DeLisi, L. E. (1992b). Neuropsychological functioning of first episode schizophreniform patients. *American Journal of Psychiatry*, **149**, 898–903.

Holsenbeck, L. S. 3rd, Davidson, L. M., Hostetter, R. E., Casanova, M. F., Taylor, D. O., Kelley, C. T., Perrotta, C. Jr., Borison, R. L. & Diamond, B. (1992). Ventricle-to-brain ratio and symptoms at the onset of first-break schizophrenia. *Schizophrenia Bulletin*, **18**, 427–35.

Iacono, W. G., Smith, G. N., Moreau, M., Beiser, M., Fleming, J. A. E., Lin, T.-Y. & Flak, B. (1988). Ventricular and sulcal size at the onset of psychosis. *American Journal of Psychiatry*, **145**, 820–4.

Kane, J. M., Rifkin, A., Quitkin, F., Nayak, D. & Ramos-Lorenzi, J. R. (1982). Fluphenazine vs placebo in patients with remitted acute first episode schizophrenia. *Archives of General Psychiatry*, **39**, 70–3.

Kirch, D. G. (1993). Infection and autoimmunity as etiologic factors in schizophrenia. *Schizophrenia Bulletin*, **19**, 355–70.

Kleinschmidt, A., Falkai, P., Huang, Y., Schneider, T., Furst, G. & Steinmetz, H. (1994). In vivo morphometry of planum temporale asymmetry in first episode schizophrenia. *Schizophrenia Research*, **12**, 9–18.

Knight, J. G. (1982). Dopamine receptor stimulating autoantibody: a possible cause of schizophrenia. *Lancet*, **2**, 1073–5.

Kolb, B. & Whisman, I.Q. (1983). Performance of schizophrenic patients on tests sensitive to left or right frontal temporal parietal function in neurological patients. *Journal of Nervous and Mental Disease*, **171**, 435–43.

Kolyaskina, G. I., Morozov, T. P., Sekirina, T. P. & Burbeyeya, G. S. (1988). *Immunological and Virological Studies in Schizophrenia*. Paper presented at the Second World Congress on Viruses, Immunity and Mental Health, Quebec, Canada, 6th October 1988.

Koreen, A. R., Lieberman, J. A., Alvir, J., Mayerhoff, D., Loebel, A., Chakos, M., Amin, F. & Cooper, T. (1994a). Plasma homovanillic acid levels in first episode schizophrenia. *Archives of General Psychiatry*, **51**, 132–8.

Koreen, A. R., Lieberman, J. A., Alvir, J., Chakos, M., Loebel, A., Cooper, T. & Kane, J. M. (1994b). Relation of plasma fluphenazine levels to treatment response and extrapyramidal side effects in first episode schizophrenic patients. *American Journal of Psychiatry*, **151**, 35–9.

Koreen, A. R., Siris, S. G., Chakos, M., Alvir, J., Mayerhoff, D. & Lieberman, J. (1993). Depression in first episode schizophrenia. *American Journal of Psychiatry*, **150**, 1643–8.

Levy, D. L., Valentino, C., Smith, M., Robinson, D., Jody, D., Lerner, G., Alvir, J., Geisler, S. H., Szymanski, S. R., Gonzalez, A., Mayerhoff, D. I., Woerner, M. G., Lieberman, J. A. & Mendell, N. R. (1993). Methylphenidate increases thought disorder in recent onset schizophrenics but not in normal controls. *Biological Psychiatry*, **34**, 507–14.

Lieberman, J. A. (1993). Prediction of outcome in first episode schizophrenia. *Journal of Clinical Psychiatry*, **54** (Supplement 3), 13–17.

Lieberman, J. A., Kane, J. M. & Alvir, J. (1987). Provocative tests with psychostimulant drugs in schizophrenia. *Psychopharmacology*, **91**, 415–33.

Lieberman, J. A., Alvir, J., Woerner, M., Degreef, G., Bilder, R. M., Ashtari, M., Bogerts, B., Mayerhoff, D. I., Geisler, S. H., Loebel, A., Levy, D. L., Hinrichsen, G., Szymanski, S., Chakos, M., Koreen, A., Borenstein, M. & Kane, J. M. (1992). Prospective study of psychobiology in first episode schizophrenia at Hillside Hospital. *Schizophrenia Bulletin*, **18**, 351–71.

Lieberman, J. A., Jody, D., Alvir, J., Ashtari, M., Levy, D. L., Bogerts, B., Degreef, G., Mayerhoff, D. I. & Cooper, T. (1993a). Brain morphology, dopamine, and eye tracking abnormalities in first episode schizophrenia. *Archives of General Psychiatry*, **50**, 357–67.

Lieberman, J. A., Jody, D., Geisler, S., Alvir, J., Loebel, A., Szymanski, S., Woerner, M. & Borenstein, M. (1993b). Time course and biologic correlates of treatment response in first episode schizophrenia. *Archives of General Psychiatry*, **50**, 369–76.

Lieberman, J. A., Jody, D., Geisler, S., Vital-Herne, J., Alvir, J. M. J., Walsleben, J. & Woerner, M. G. (1989). Treatment outcome of first episode schizophrenia. *Psychopharmacology Bulletin*, **25**, 92–5.

Lindstrom, L. H., Wieselgren, I.-M., Klockhoff, I. & Svedberg, A. (1990). Relationship between abnormal brainstem auditory evoked potentials and subnormal CSF levels of HVA and 5–HIAA in first episode schizophrenic patients. *Biological Psychiatry*, **28**, 435–42.

Loebel, A. D., Lieberman, J. A., Alvir, J. M. J., Mayerhoff, D. I., Geisler, S. H. & Szymanski, S. R. (1992). Duration of psychosis and outcome in first episode schizophrenia. *American Journal of Psychiatry*, **149**, 1183–8.

Markianos, M., Botsis, A. & Arvanitis, Y. (1992). Biogenic amine metabolites in plasma of drug naïve schizophrenic patients: associations with symptomatology. *Biological Psychiatry*, **32**, 288–92.

Martinot, J.-L., Peron-Magnan, P., Huret, J.-D., Mazoyer, B., Baron, J.-C., Boulenger, J.-P., Loc'h, C., Maziere, B., Caillard, V., Loo, H. & Syrota, A. (1990). Striatal D-2 dopaminergic receptors assessed with positron emission tomography and [76–Br] bromospiperone in untreated schizophrenic patients. *American Journal of Psychiatry*, **147**, 44–50.

May, P. R., Tuma, A. H., Dixon, W.J., Yale, C., Thiele, D. A. & Kraude, W. H. (1981). Schizophrenia: a follow up study of the results of five forms of treatment. *Archives of General Psychiatry*, **38**, 776–84.

May, P. R. A., Tuma, A. H., Yale, C., Potepan, P. & Dixon, W. J. (1976). Schizophrenia – a followup study of results of treatment. *Archives of General Psychiatry*, **33**, 481–86.

Mayerhoff, D. I., Lieberman, J. A., Lemus, C. Z., Pollack, S. & Schneider, B.S. (1990). Growth hormone response to growth hormone-releasing hormone in schizophrenic patients. *American Journal of Psychiatry*, **147**, 1072–4.

McCreadie, R. G. & Ohaeri, J. W. (1994). Movement in never and minimally treated Nigerian schizophrenic patients. *British Journal of Psychiatry*, **164**, 184–9.

McCreadie, R. G., Crocket, G. T., Livingston, M. G., Todd, N. A., Loudon, J., Batchelor, D. & Menzies, C. W. (1987a). The Scottish first episode schizophrenia study. I. Patient identification and categorisation. *British Journal of Psychiatry*, **150**, 331–3.

McCreadie, R. G., Crocket, G. T., Livingston, M. G., Todd, N. A., Loudon, J., Batchelor, D. & Menzies, C. W. (1987b). The Scottish first episode schizophrenia study. II. Treatment. Pimozide versus flupenthixol. *British Journal of Psychiatry*, **150**, 334–8.

McCreadie, R. G., Crocket, G. T., Livingston, M. G., Todd, N. A., Loudon, J., Batchelor, D. & Menzies, C. W. (1987c). The Scottish first episode schizophrenia study. III. Cognitive performance. *British Journal of Psychiatry*, **150**, 338–40.

McCreadie, R. G., Crocket, G. T., Livingston, M. G., Todd, N. A., Loudon, J., Batchelor, D. & Menzies, C. W. (1987d). The Scottish first episode schizophrenia study. IV. Psychiatric and social impact on relatives. *British Journal of Psychiatry*, **150**, 340–4.

Meltzer, H. Y. (1987). Biological studies in schizophrenia. *Schizophrenia Bulletin,* **13,** 77–111.

Mettler, F. A. & Crandell, A. (1959). Relation between parkinsonism and psychiatric disorder. *Journal of Nervous and Mental Disease,* **129,** 551–7.

Mintz, M., Hermesh, H., Glicksohn, J., Munitz, H. & Radwan, M. (1995). First month of neuroleptic treatment in schizophrenia: only partial normalization of the late positive components of visual ERP. *Biological Psychiatry,* **37,** 402–9.

Mirsky, A. F. (1988). Research on schizophrenia in the NIMH Laboratory of psychology and psychopathology, 1954–1987. *Schizophrenia Bulletin,* **14,** 151–6.

Nopoulos, P., Torres, I., Flaum, M., Andreasen, N. C., Ehrhardt, J. C. & Yuh, W. T. C. (1995). Brain morphology in first episode schizophrenia. *American Journal of Psychiatry,* **152,** 1721–3.

Nyback, H., Wiesel, F.-A., Bergren, B. M. & Hindmarsh, T. (1982). Computed tomography of the brain in patients with acute psychosis and in healthy volunteers. *Acta Psychiatrica Scandinavica,* **65,** 403–14.

Ohman, A. & Ohlund, L. S. (1989). Electrodermal nonresponding, premorbid adjustment, and symptomatology as predictors of long term social functioning in schizophrenics. *Journal of Abnormal Psychology,* **98,** 426–35.

Owens, D. G. C., Johnstone, E. C. & Frith, C. D. (1982). Spontaneous involuntary disorders of movement. *Archives of General Psychiatry,* **39,** 452–61.

Pettegrew, J. W., Keshavan, M. S., Panchalingam, K., Strychor, S., Kaplan, D. B.,Tretta, M. G. & Allen, M. (1991). Alterations in brain high energy phosphate and membrane phospholipid metabolism in first episode, drug naïve schizophrenics. *Archives of General Psychiatry,* **48,** 563–8.

Pickar, D., Litman, R. E., Konicki, P.E., Wolkowitz, O.M. & Breier, A. (1990). Neurochemical and neural mechanisms of positive and negative symptoms in schizophrenia. *Modern Problems of Pharmacopsychiatry,* **24,** 124–51.

Pilowsky, L. S., Costa, D. C., Ell, P. J., Verhoeff, N. P. L. G., Murray, R. M. & Kerwin, R. W. (1994). D-2 dopamine receptor binding in the basal ganglia of antipsychotic free schizophrenic patients. *British Journal of Psychiatry,* **164,** 16–26.

Rabiner, C. J., Wegner, J. T. & Kane, J. M. (1986). Outcome study of first episode psychosis. Relapse rates after 1 year. *American Journal of Psychiatry,* **143,** 1155–8.

Reiter, P. J. (1926). Extrapyramidal motor disturbances in dementia praecox. *Acta Psychiatrica Neurologia,* **1,** 287–310.

Renshaw, P. F., Yurgelun-Todd, D. A., Tohen, M., Gruber, S. & Cohen, B. M. (1995). Temporal lobe proton magnetic resonance spectroscopy of patients with first episode psychosis. *American Journal of Psychiatry,* **152,** 444–6.

Rubin, P., Holm, S., Friberg, L., Videbech, P., Anderson, H. S., Bendsen, B. B., Stromso, N., Larsen, J. K., Lassen, N. A. & Hemmingsen, R. (1991). Altered modulation of prefrontal and subcortical brain activity in newly diagnosed schizophrenia and schizophreniform disorder. *Archives of General Psychiatry,* **48,** 987–95.

Rubin, P., Karle, A., Moller-Madsen, S., Hertel, C., Povlsen, U. J., Noring, U. &

Hemmingsen, R. (1993). Computerised tomography in newly diagnosed schizophrenia and schizophreniform disorder. *British Journal of Psychiatry*, **163**, 604–12.

Sanders, R. D., Keshavan, M. S. & Schooler, N. R. (1994). Neurological examination abnormalities in neuroleptic naïve patients with first break schizophrenia: preliminary results. *American Journal of Psychiatry*, **151**, 1231–3.

Saykin, A. J., Shtasel, D. L., Gur, R. E., Kester, D. B., Mozley, L. H., Stafiniak, P. & Gur, R. C. (1994). Neuropsychological deficits in neuroleptic naïve patients with first episode schizophrenia. *Archives of General Psychiatry*, **51**, 124–31.

Schulz, S. C., Koller, M. M., Kishore, P. R., Hamer, R. M., Gehl, J. J. & Friedel, R. O. (1983). Ventricular enlargement in teenage patients with schizophrenia spectrum disorder. *American Journal of Psychiatry*, **140**, 1592–5.

Sedvall, G. (1992). The current status of PET scanning with respect to schizophrenia. *Neuropsychopharmacology*, **7**, 41–54.

Sheppard, G., Gruzelier, J., Manchanda, R., Hirsch, S. R., Wise, R., Frackowiak, R. & Jones, T. (1983). 15-O positron emission tomographic scanning in predominantly never treated acute schizophrenic patients. *The Lancet*, Dec 24/31, 1448–52.

Sirota, P., Fishman, P., Elizur, A. & Djaldetty, M. (1990). Lymphokine production in schizophrenic patients (Abstract). *Biological Psychiatry*, **27**, 173A.

Sweeney, J. A., Haas, G. L., Keilp, J. G. & Long, M. (1991). Evaluation of the stability of neuropsychological functioning after acute episodes of schizophrenia: one year follow up study. *Psychiatry Research*, **38**, 63–76.

Sweeney, J. A., Haas, G. L. & Li, S. (1992). Neuropsychological and eye movement abnormalities in first episode and chronic schizophrenia. *Schizophrenia Bulletin*, **18**, 283–93.

Szymanski, S., Lieberman, J. A., Alvir, J., Mayerhoff, D., Loebel, A., Geisler, S., Chakos, M., Koreen, A., Jody, D., Kane, J., Woerner, M. & Cooper, T. (1995). Gender differences in onset of illness, treatment response, course, and biological indexes in first episode schizophrenic patients. *American Journal of Psychiatry*, **152**, 698–703.

Tandon, R., Shipley, J. E., Taylor, S., Greden, J. F., Eiser, A., DeQuardo, J. & Goodson, J. (1992). Electroencephalographic sleep abnormalities in schizophrenia. *Archives of General Psychiatry*, **49**, 185–94.

Tardive Dyskinesia. A Task Force Report of the American Psychiatric Association. Washington, DC: American Psychiatric Press.

Targum, S. (1983). Neuroendocrine dysfunction in schizophreniform disorder: correlation with six month clinical outcome. *American Journal of Psychiatry*, **140**, 309–13.

Turner, S. W., Toone, B. K. & Brett-Jones, J. R. (1986). Computerised tomographic scan changes in early schizophrenia – preliminary findings. *Psychological Medicine*, **16**, 219–25.

Villemain, F., Chatenoud, L., Galinowski, A., Delarche, F. H.-G., Ginistet, D., Loo, H., Zarifian, E. & Bach, J. F. (1989). Aberrant T-cell mediated immunity in untreated schizophrenic patients: deficient interleukin-2 production. *American Journal of Psychiatry*, **146**, 609–16.

Volkow, N. D., Brodie, J. D., Wolf, A. P., Angrist, B., Russell, J. & Cancro, R. (1986). Brain metabolism in patients with schizophrenia before and after acute neuroleptic administration. *Journal of Neurology, Neurosurgery and Psychiatry*, **49**, 1199–202.

Waddington, J. L. & Youssef, H. A. (1990). The lifetime outcome and involuntary movements of schizophrenia never treated with neuroleptic drugs. *British Journal of Psychiatry*, **156**, 106–8.

Weinberger, D. R. (1987). Implications of normal brain development for the pathogenesis of schizophrenia. *Archives of General Psychiatry*, **44**, 660–9.

Weinberger, D. R., Berman, K. F. & Zec, R. F. (1986). Physiologic dysfunction of dorsolateral prefrontal cortex in schizophenia. I. Regional blood flow evidence. *Archives of General Psychiatry*, **43**, 114–24.

Weinberger, D. R., DeLisi, L. E., Perman, G. P., Targum, S. & Wyatt, R. J. (1982). Computed tomography in schizophreniform disorder and other acute psychiatric disorders. *Archives of General Psychiatry*, **39**, 778–83.

Wong, D. F., Wagner, H.N. Jr, Tune, L. E., Dannals, R. F., Pearlson, G. D., Links, J. M., Tamminga, C. A., Broussolle, E. P., Ravert, H. T., Wilson, A. A., Toung, J. K. T., Malat, J., Williams, J. A., O'Tuama, L. A., Snyder, S. H., Kuhar, M. J. & Gjedde, A. (1986). Positron emission tomography reveals elevated D-2 dopamine receptors in drug naive schizophrenics. *Science*, **234**, 1558–63.

Part III

Assessment and clinical management of early psychosis

6

Initial assessment of first-episode psychosis

PADDY POWER AND PATRICK D. MCGORRY

Introduction

The comprehensive clinical assessment of first-episode psychosis is fundamental to developing an initial formulation of a person's condition, and provides the foundation for later management. Earlier chapters of this book emphasize the importance of early detection of the emerging symptoms of first-episode psychosis (see Chapters 1, 2, 3, and 4). It seems probable, although not yet proven, that early detection has the potential to reduce morbidity and mortality (Loebel et al., 1992; McGorry et al., 1996) through enhancing treatment responsiveness (Loebel et al., 1992; Wyatt, 1991), and even attenuating the deficit processes of schizophrenia (McGlashan & Johannessen, 1996). A key feature of early detection is the provision of service delivery models which aim to ensure prompt access to clinicians skilled in the clinical assessment of early psychosis. The focus of this chapter is on outlining the essential components of this clinical assessment.

The entry phase – an avoidable crisis?

One of the fundamental principles in the assessment of first-episode psychosis is that it represents a 'crisis'. Indeed, it may represent a potential 'personal disaster' (Raphael, 1986), with both patient and family typically experiencing considerable trauma and multiple losses. Assessment should therefore occur within the broad framework of 'crisis intervention'. Yet despite these factors, there are a number of obstacles to accessing timely and appropriate assessment and treatment. The annual incidence of first-episode psychosis is relatively low, making it difficult for primary care clinicians to maintain a high level of vigilance and clinical expertise in its detection (Jablensky et al., 1992; WHO, 1973). In one year, for a population of 100,000, one would expect between one and six new cases of schizophrenia (Jablensky et al., 1992; WHO, 1973) and one to eight new cases of mania (including non-psychotic forms) to present (Daly, Webb & Kaliszer, 1996). Even when detected, patients are generally more fearful of the consequences of referring themselves on to psychiatric services and frequently become reluctant or unwilling participants in referrals mediated by concerned family or carers. Once the patient is referred, the clinician is often faced with the dilemma of when, and how assertively, to intervene. This is particularly so for those suspected to be in the prodromal phase of psychosis for whom treatments have yet to be shown to be of proven benefit, notwithstanding the significant dysphoria and disability they experience (see Chapters 2 and 4). Once psychosis has clearly developed, this dilemma poses less of an issue, as the risks tend to be more immediate and, in principle at least, services generally have a mandate to intervene promptly in order to prevent further deterioration. Yet, even then, delays are very common, particularly when services are reactive rather than proactive, promote a narrow definition of 'serious mental illness' based on established disability and immediate risk, and limit access in order to minimize case loads. Emerging first-episode psychosis patients may be regarded as not 'serious' enough, or too difficult to engage, or as not requiring monitoring and follow-up if no signs of psychosis are evident on first assessment. This scenario generally means that a more severe crisis must develop in addition to the presence of psychotic symptoms before entry to services is assured. This confers additional risk and trauma to an already serious situation. These problems may be overcome if services were to adopt a greater emphasis on prevention, as well as broader criteria for maintaining continuity of follow-up after first contact.

The clinical landscape of onset

In addition to the above obstacles in accessing services, the assessment of first-episode psychosis presents a number of particular clinical problems. The onset of early psychosis is often complicated by slowly evolving and fluctuating symptoms which are intimately entwined with psychosocial stressors or developmental issues. Symptoms may mimic non-psychotic disorders commonly seen in adolescence, e.g. adjustment disorders and emergent personality and mood disorders. Confirmation of psychosis itself may be difficult, particularly in the early stages of non-bizarre delusional disorders, manic psychosis and paranoid schizophreniform disorder, as patients may conceal subjective changes. Differential diagnosis within the global domain of psychotic disorders, particularly distinguishing between affective and non-affective psychosis, may be hampered by difficulties in eliciting affective symptoms, which may manifest as behavioural or personality disturbances, mimic prodromal symptoms of a schizophrenic disorder, or fluctuate during the early course, thereby causing significant diagnostic flux and instability.

There is a common belief that a stable categorization within the DSM or ICD system is necessary for initiation of treatment, e.g. waiting until it is clear that the patient meets the criteria for schizophrenia. This view, which can hold up appropriate treatment, fails to acknowledge that these categorizations remain syndromal and arbitrary, have only a partial connection with treatment strategies, and are essentially subtypes of psychotic disorder (McGorry, 1995). Thus, recognition of psychosis is the key step, followed by a consideration of associated or comorbid syndromes with treatment implications, e.g. mania. Substance abuse further complicates diagnostic confusion in many cases, and has the potential to delay definitive treatment of persistent psychotic vulnerability because a less stigmatizing explanation for the symptoms has been chosen instead (see also Chapter 13).

It is useful to be aware of the epidemiological landscape of the onset phases in approaching the assessment process. Psychosis (excluding delusional disorders and paraphrenia) usually first presents in adolescents or young adults (Häfner et al., 1995). Males tend to have an earlier age of onset of psychosis than in females (Häfner et al., 1995). By virtue of this, males are more likely to be single, living with parents, and their presentations are frequently complicated by adolescent issues, e.g. separation/individuation factors, antisocial behaviours, drug abuse, adjustment disorders, and family disruption. In contrast, females are often at the next developmental stage, have an established partner, and not infrequently have young children. Their presentations are commonly complicated by tensions with partners and parenting issues. The potential pervasive and rapidly disruptive effect of psychosis at these critical developmental phases demands that engagement and assessment strategies be crisis-orientated and developmentally informed, as well as broad and flexible in approach, catering for both the individual's and the family's needs. Particular care needs to be taken to avoid interventions that might further threaten an increasingly fragile support system so that further losses can be prevented.

The following section delineates principles which may aid in the initial engagement and assessment of patients presenting with first-episode psychosis.

Guidelines for engagement and initial clinical assessment

Style and context

The first contact of the patient and family with the service is a critical one. Every effort should be made to begin 'on the right foot' with an emphasis on establishing continuity of care. While, in theory, the assessment task is distinct from that of engagement and treatment, in practice they merge inextricably. Strategies which facilitate this blend are to be encouraged, so that engagement, assessment and early treatment occur as parallel processes during the initial phase, and indeed beyond. This can be achieved by enabling the initial clinician to continue with the care of the patient, or from the onset allowing for the introduction of key players in ongoing management, e.g. case managers. Unfortunately, in many services, the response in this early phase of management is fragmented, with patients and families undergoing several independent assessments by different clinicians working in different components of services, e.g. 24-hour community assessment teams with rostered staff, after-hours inpatient admission staff, and case managers. Such dislocation during the assessment phase may threaten engagement, may cause patients to reframe their symptoms in response to clinicians' reactions, and may risk key information being lost or misinterpreted between clinicians. From a service point of view, the process is unwieldy and inefficient.

Regrettably, by the time many first-episode patients present, their condition has reached crisis point. Frequently, concerned families and/or carers will have already made several unsuccessful attempts to encourage the patient to attend for psychiatric assessment. By this stage, the risks of violence or self-harm may have substantially increased with the potential for aversive experiences with police involvement. Consequently, patients frequently experience considerable posttraumatic stress symptoms (McGorry et al., 1991) following such initial experiences. The traumatizing effects of these aversive experiences can obstruct the best efforts of clinicians to promote a therapeutic alliance or protect the patient's fragile social milieu.

In our experience, engagement is usually more successful if the contact occurs as early as possible prior to a major crisis, with prompt outreach assessments being conducted in a non-threatening and collaborative manner in the patient's own familiar environment with primarily one or two identifiable clinicians and, if necessary, over several visits. In these early stages, the person often maintains an awareness that something is not quite right and, due to the subjectively distressing nature of the symptoms, may be more amenable to assistance and treatment.

6 INITIAL ASSESSMENT OF FIRST-EPISODE PSYCHOSIS

Engaging and understanding the first-episode patient

Planning the initial engagement with a patient is essential. As much information as possible should be gathered from referring sources about the patient before arranging a formal assessment. This will assist in determining the most appropriate setting for interviewing the patient, who and how many should be involved, whether the presence of family members or friends will be of assistance, and whether safety issues need to be addressed by drawing upon the support of other services.

While the general principles of developing a therapeutic alliance, such as warmth, empathy, and respect are essential, there are several additional factors to be considered for first-episode psychosis patients. Dispelling the patient's fears and establishing trust is a particularly difficult task. A balance needs to be struck between respecting the patient's interpretation of their psychotic experiences while conveying to the patient one's own clinical judgment and advice regarding treatment. Clearly, as the risks increase, the potential for confrontation increases. Initial contacts may be of a highly emotionally charged nature and severely disturbed or agitated patients may provoke unwary clinicians to resort to criticism, implied threats, or be seen to ally themselves excessively with carers in an attempt to control the situation.

A calm, reassuring professional friendly manner, and a commitment to flexibly negotiating the best initial outcome for each person is required. In our experience, spending more time initially to engage the patient and family, develop rapport, and encourage the patient to help work out a range of options to deal with the concerns identified, has a much greater potential for co-operation in the long run. The first step is to very deliberately and consciously attempt to understand the personal context in which the person's psychosis has developed.

Understanding the personal context of the patient's psychosis

Traditional views have emphasized that psychosis, specifically schizophrenia, was difficult or impossible to understand (Jaspers, 1923). More recently, however, a more comprehensive understanding has been emerging of the experience and the personal struggle of young people coping with psychosis, in particular, their first episode (Jackson et al., 1996; McGorry, 1995). Psychotic illness can create havoc across virtually all aspects of the person's life, threatening personal safety, impairing physical health, disrupting the sense of self and fundamentally changing the person's relationships with, and perspectives of, family, friends, and their environment. The adaptive tasks involved are enormous and are beyond most people in the short term without skilled help. An understanding of these factors is assisted by asking oneself the following questions.

(1) How rapidly did the psychosis and prodrome evolve?

A more slowly evolving course may allow the person to acclimatize to the deleterious effects of psychosis, yet carrying with it the potential for a more insidious effect on the person's self-identity and awareness of change. In this way the psychotic experience becomes more ego-syntonic with less dysphoria, reduced awareness of change or of the possibility of 'illness'. This all reduces motivation to seek or accept help. Family perceptions may be similarly biased with negative expectations of recovery and mislabelling of symptoms as part of the person's usual self and character, particularly in adolescence, when personality has yet to fully develop.

(2) What kind of person is being affected by the psychosis and what are their reactions?

A full assessment of the person's premorbid personality structure, self-concept, phase of development, defence style, coping skills, current conflicts, social strengths and resources as well as accommodation, occupation, financial, cultural and family issues will aid in understanding the interaction between the individual patient's psychological and social framework and their psychosis.

The personal meaning of a particular psychotic experience may vary greatly between patients, potentially affecting their emotional responses, behaviour and likely compliance with treatment. The experience of psychosis may disturb the patient's perspective of previously protective or secure relationships, creating intense and often labile feelings of persecution, violation, despair or impending doom.

(3) In what kind of environment or culture has the patient's psychosis arisen?

The sociocultural milieu in which a patient lives may profoundly influence detection, pathway to services, and compliance with interventions offered. Birchwood et al. (1992) noted considerable variations in the mode and timing of presentation between different cultures. These factors may influence the person's reaction to admission and treatment methods. For example, refugees with first-episode psychosis who have previously been incarcerated and maltreated or tortured in their country of origin, may be severely distressed and react in an extreme fashion in the context of an involuntary inpatient admission. Additional factors which appear to be associated with delays in presentation and compulsory admissions of first-episode psychotic patients via the police, include being single, having no GP involvement, and the absence of help-seeking relatives or friends (Cole et al., 1995).

While an intimate knowledge of cultural factors in all cultures is not feasible, an openness on the part of the clinician to new understanding and the capacity to draw on the skills of bicultural workers and interpreters is essential.

(4) What kind of family supports exist and what are their reactions to the illness?

Families are an invaluable source of collateral information and no assessment should be concluded without trying to involve the family. Moreover, this process should always include the provision of immediate support and information for family members. However, information should be gathered while fostering a therapeutic alliance with the patient and, if possible, families should be interviewed with the patient's consent. Families are often the first to detect subtle changes in their relative's mental state or functioning and are an invaluable guide in determining the rate and severity of deterioration. Many parents already suspect a diagnosis of schizophrenia or a related disorder and the family's explanatory model should be explored and enhanced with timely and relevant information. An honest, frank, concerned, supportive and optimistic approach is advised from the outset. Finally, a careful assessment of the current coping resources of the family is critical in determining the location of initial treatment.

Interview technique

Establishing rapport should begin with putting the patient at ease by spending time with introductions and explanations of one's role, acknowledging, listening carefully, respecting the patient's viewpoint, and trying to identify common ground. At the same time, one should make note of signs of the patient's appearance, responsiveness, attention span, affect, level of anxiety, agitation, hostility and unpredictability, in addition to the patient's movements, communication, responses and willingness to engage. One should pay attention to the interview setting and one's own body language in order to minimize confrontation, particularly with paranoid, anxious or manic patients, while at the same time ensuring that one is safe and assistance is easily available. It is wise to position oneself sideways to the patient, avoiding direct face-to-face eye contact, and allowing for adequate personal space for an agitated patient to move around. This strategy aims to reduce the risk of projection of internal distress, and has been termed counter projective (Havens, 1986). With patients who are highly aroused or hostile, one should ensure that one is accompanied by other staff, maintain oneself between the patient and the door, retreat back from the situation should it escalate, and avoid stating a position if one has not the resources at hand to support it, e.g. suggesting hospitalization when the patient is likely to react in a hostile manner.

Once the interview process has been established, one should begin to explore the patient's view of recent experiences with open-ended questions which allow the patient to provide his or her own account while, at the same time, allowing for an initial assessment of thought form, stream and content, evidence of responses to perceptual disturbances, and level of insight. In finding common ground and enhancing or building rapport, it is useful to identify the focus of distress or suffering and empathize with this. It is also important to isolate and deal with the patient's immediate fears regarding treatment.

Particular interview techniques include adopting the 'Colombo technique' in which the interviewer adopts an excessively ingenuous stance which facilitates greater disclosure from otherwise cautious or guarded patients, 'curbing techniques' with thought-disordered or pressured patients, aggrandisement with manic patients, and distraction techniques with hostile confrontational patients. For adolescent patients, even greater skill may be required in using these techniques.

Towards the end of the interview one should go through a brief checklist of symptoms not yet covered, e.g. suicidal ideation. One should then attempt to provide initial feedback to the patient of one's impressions, together with the options for the 'next step'. It is best to link these options to problem areas agreed by the patient to warrant attention and, maybe, special support. This is a more secure foundation on which to build in additional treatment initiatives.

Comprehensive clinical assessment

Clinical history

Over as brief a period as possible, one should accumulate from different sources a detailed and systematic history of evolving prodromal symptoms and primary or secondary symptoms of psychosis: their onset, course, duration, aggravating or relieving factors, patient's responses, indications of risk of violence or suicide or at risk behaviours, any attempts to access health services and the effect of any treatment interventions already tried. The factors influencing the transition from prodrome to psychosis should be determined, e.g. stressors or drugs of abuse. Included in the above should be a careful screening in the history for any potentially associated or aetiologically significant physical conditions (see below). A history of previous episodes of psychiatric disorder should be investigated, e.g. depressive episodes, drug abuse, and undetected low grade symptoms of psychosis. The aim is to build up a careful and complete reconstruction of the evolution of the psychotic disorder in the context of the life story of this particular individual.

Family history, perinatal history, developmental history and premorbid personality and functioning may reveal risk factors for psychosis, clarify the context within which the patient's psychosis has developed, how it might impact on the life of the patient and carers, and what reactions might be expected. Especially invaluable sources of collateral information come from families and every effort should be made to interview families as soon as possible. This can be further explored by contacting professionals who may have had prior contact with the patient, e.g. the family doctor, teachers, and community support agencies. In particular, it is important to elicit a family history of mood or psychotic disorder, substance abuse, suicide, and any relevant neurological conditions, e.g. Huntington's disease, Wilson's disease, and porphyria, or mental retardation. An understanding of the patient's best level of premorbid functioning will reveal any co-existing personality, emotional or developmental problems, may give clues as to when prodromal symptoms first began to emerge, and will set a ceiling for the recovery process.

Mental state examination
A patient's mental state may vary considerably in response to different settings and to different staff members. In addition to this dynamic fluctuation in presentation, one should not underestimate patients' ability to maintain control over their symptoms. Patients quickly learn not to reveal information about psychotic phenomena to hospital staff if they sense it will prolong an unwanted stay in hospital or prompt treatment which they wish to avoid. Patients with paranoid psychosis are frequently more willing to reveal elaborate information about their psychotic experiences to visiting research staff than to their treating clinicians. For these various reasons serial clinical assessments, undertaken by different clinicians, should be blended in a single comprehensive clinical assessment summary (McGorry, Copolov & Singh, 1989, 1990a,b), and regular formal reviews of the progress of the assessment process should be undertaken by the treating team or clinician. These reviews then give rise to a systematic individual service plan.

Clinical signs may vary significantly depending on diurnal influences, with signs of depression being more prominent in the morning and signs of mania escalating in the late evening. In our experience, the potential for interpersonal conflicts appears to peak in the late afternoon or early evening when most homes and inpatient units are at their most socially interactive. In patients who are socially phobic, or have prominent deficit symptoms, social withdrawal may be most obvious in the mornings with many of the young people remaining in bed until early afternoon. Bizarre behaviours may be more obvious in quieter isolated settings or late at night when patients might believe they are less likely to be observed.

Much of the remainder of the mental state examination follows standard guidelines; however, the phenomena are usually less well formed and the patients less 'schooled' in their descriptions. The quality of such descriptions is variable and depends upon a number of factors.

Consideration should be given to determining the phase of the psychotic episode. In the early phase of a rapidly developing florid psychosis, patients are often perplexed and frightened, with fleeting poorly systematized delusions. In the early phases of less precipitous presentations, confirmation of psychosis may prove difficult as the features may be brief, mild or fleeting, with the potential to be interpreted as dissociative phenomena or experiences which might be culturally sanctioned. Patients presenting with more prolonged episodes of untreated psychosis often have developed more systematized or bizarre delusions, or interpretations of psychotic phenomena. As stated previously, complicating affective features may vary considerably during the evolution of a psychosis and it is important to remember that there is substantial syndromal flux and complexity generally in first-episode psychosis (Fennig et al., 1996; McGorry, 1994).

The patient's level and quality of insight should be explored. Insight is a complex construct and involves several elements, including awareness of change in mental functioning, that the change phenomena are due to symptoms of an illness, and that the illness requires treatment (Kemp & David, 1996). Insight varies dramatically between patients and appears to have little association with severity or phase of psychosis. Even in the same patient, insight may vary markedly during an interview depending on the patient's level of arousal or mood state. A suspicious guardedness may imply a degree of insight, while a frank denial of symptoms may be a manifestation of complete unawareness of change.

Negative symptoms in first-episode psychosis appear to be more responsive to treatment than in subsequent episodes and many of these features prove to be secondary in nature (McGorry et al., 1996). The assessment of deficit states in first-episode psychosis may prove to be important for the prediction of prognosis, with studies reporting deficit features in 23% of first-episode schizophrenia patients, of whom 17%

met all the criteria for a deficit syndrome, i.e. 4% of the total sample (Mayerhoff et al., 1994). An emerging area requiring careful serial assessment, both acutely and during the recovery phase, is that of cognitive functioning, which is more highly predictive of functional outcome in later phases of illness than is symptom severity. Consequently, it is a dimension which should be periodically assessed along with psychopathology during clinical reviews.

Assessment of comorbid disorders in first-episode psychosis

Comorbid psychiatric and medical disorders are commonly seen in first-episode patients and may be associated with poorer outcome (Strakowski, Shelton & Kolbrener, 1993; Strakowski et al., 1993). Alcohol and drug abuse appear to be the most frequent complicating disorders in 32–70% of first-episode psychosis patients (Strakowski et al., 1993; Power et al., 1998).

Assessment of substance abuse disorders has been described by Linszen and Lenoir in Chapter 13. In summary, it is important to take a detailed history of the type, amount, frequency, method, reasons for and effects of substance used, particularly during the phase of emerging psychosis. The patient's attitude towards substance use and his or her motivation to cease its use should be explored. It is a common clinical experience that these patients frequently deny substance use initially but later give quite accurate accounts of previous drug use as they recover from the acute psychosis, although marijuana use tends to be more accurately reported than psychostimulant usage (Hillier et al., 1996). Not infrequently, one observes that patients and families focus on the substance abuse as a less stigmatizing reason for the psychotic episode.

Less frequently associated disorders include obsessive compulsive disorder, affective and anxiety disorders, eating disorders, and medical conditions (Strakowski et al., 1993). It is particularly important to assess the onset, course and relationship of these disorders with a patient's emerging prodrome and psychosis. Frequently, it is virtually impossible to separate the features of these conditions from the emerging psychotic process. Personality deterioration is a common complication of the prodrome phase (Jones et al., 1993). Confirmation of these features through collateral sources is advised, as patients' recall is often unreliable, at least during the acute phase of illness, due to the pervasive effects of the illness upon cognition and memory.

Risk assessment

Clinicians should always remain mindful of the serious risks associated with psychosis and ensure that prompt and regular risk assessments (both short-term and long-term) are formally made and communicated to other staff and carers involved in the patient's management and supervision. New patients are 'unknown quantities' for clinicians and the first priority is to ensure that the patient and his or her environment is safe.

(1) Suicide risk assessment
Suicide risk assessment is described in detail in Chapter 12. The importance of assessing suicide risk at the first interview cannot be overstated, given the high risk of suicide in this early phase of illness. Up to 23% of first-episode psychosis patients experience suicide thoughts, with around 15% of first-episode patients reporting a previous suicide attempt (Bromet et al., 1996; McGorry, Henry & Power, 1998). Despite this, patients are infrequently asked about suicide. An exploration of suicide ideation and intent should be undertaken near the end of the interview once some rapport has been established. A useful introduction is to explore how distressing the patient's experiences have been and then to inquire whether the patient has ever considered life unbearable. One should always conclude the inquiry with a discussion on the nature of suicidality in psychosis and negotiate help-seeking mechanisms should the patient later become suicidal. It is important to note that suicidality is often a transient and variable state which requires regular monitoring, particularly in those identified to be at high risk. Suicide risk assessment relies heavily on a comprehensive clinical evaluation of predisposing and precipitating factors along with counterbalancing protective factors. Current clinical measures of suicide risk have limited predictive value in chronic schizophrenia (Roy, Schreiber & Mazonson, 1988); however, the early phases of disorder are a time of especially high risk and the chances of prediction and prevention may prove to be better (McGorry, Henry & Power, 1998).

(2) Assessment of risk of neglect and death
There are other sources of excess mortality and morbidity in young people with psychosis apart from suicide. These include exposure to high risk lifestyles, such as homelessness, with greater risk of accidental death, assault or murder, exposure to HIV infection, gambling, excess cigarette smoking (Elkins et al., 1997), and substance abuse (Hambrecht & Häfner, 1996; Strakowski et al., 1993). Death from the physical complications of psychosis is now very rare. However, in patients with catatonia, signs of physical status, and for example hydration and electrolyte balance, should be monitored closely.

(3) Violence risk assessment

It is useful in clinical practice to conceptualize violence associated with psychosis as reactive, either to the patient's own symptoms, to the responses of others, or to the patient's perceived threats in their environment. Certain subgroups appear more prone to violent reactions. Research with community samples suggests that demographic variables, such as younger age and male sex, are more important long-term predictors of violence than clinical variables (Swanson et al., 1990). However, studies of acutely ill patients, evaluated shortly before or in hospital, suggest that clinical variables are better short-term predictors than demographic factors (McNeil, Binder & Greenfield, 1988). These include hostility, suspiciousness, agitation, and cognitive disorganization, while the diagnoses associated with assaultive behaviour include schizophrenia, acute mania, and organic psychosis (McNeil & Binder, 1994). Our own audits of inpatient violence reveal a peak in the number of incidents occurring in, and among, the most recently admitted male patients.

As inpatient units become more acute in their focus, a number of studies have reported a recent increase in the levels of interpersonal conflicts and assaults in psychiatric hospitals (Aquilina, 1991; James et al., 1990), especially for first-admission patients. Limited staffing levels and poor building design may exacerbate these problems. A volatile mix can quickly develop in these busy noisy units with groups of young and unfamiliar people (mainly male) confined in locked areas by the distressing process of involuntary hospitalization and agitated by their psychotic experiences or mood disturbances. Vicious cycles can rapidly be established within the ward milieu, as new arrivals find their worst fears about psychiatry realized, become insecure and threatened, and actively reject the patient role and identification with co-patients. As the potential for fostering a therapeutic alliance breaks down, staff or carers may attempt to manage the problems by limit setting and escalating confrontation, further increasing the risk of violence.

It may be possible to minimize incidents of violence through careful attention to both staff morale and the quality of the inpatient milieu, as well as conducting specific staff training in aggression management, especially preventive strategies. Such training should be routine for all clinicians working in these services, and at least the preventive elements of this training should be provided to relatives and friends, especially where home-based acute management is undertaken. However, it must be remembered that despite the best efforts and such training, violence can be difficult to predict. Useful violence-prevention guidelines for policies and designs in acute inpatient units are outlined by Atakan (1995).

(4) Assessment of risk of victimization by others

Violence risk assessments have traditionally concentrated on the perpetrators of violence, but with the increasing trend towards highly acute inpatient units, the potential impact of violence within these units on the more vulnerable residents, and the staff, must also be considered. A recent study by Thomas, Bartlett & Mezey (1995) reported that 75% of inpatients surveyed reported unwanted physical and sexual experiences mainly from other patients, with 39% of the sample being physically assaulted at least once during the admission, and female patients reporting a high incidence of sexual harassment and even two cases of alleged rape. More subtle forms of harassment and intimidation are often unrecognized, not reported to, or not recorded by, staff. This is especially common in younger patients. Highly vulnerable patients should be identified from the outset and precautions put in place for their protection, e.g. one-to-one patient care. A discussion of risks with carers and relatives often avoids unrealistic expectations by relatives of the level of patient monitoring, and assists in negotiating better options, e.g. intensive home management with relatives on a 24–hour roster or 'rooming in'. Mechanisms should be found to improve the quality and safety of inpatient environments for young people. Prevention of victimization outside the 'safety' of hospital is also important to ensure, e.g. avoidance of entrapment in the criminal justice system, homelessness, and contact with police services.

(5) Assessment of risk of non-adherence to treatment

Normal responses to treatment recommendations and levels of treatment adherence have not been well studied in first-episode psychosis. Non-adherence is likely to be substantially greater than in established illness, and can probably be seen as a normative response in these young people, one which is inevitably going to be difficult to change. This leads into a consideration of strategies to promote adherence, for example, avoiding side effects at all costs through a very low dose neuroleptic strategy. Even a brief assessment of patients' attitudes towards proposed intervention or treatment may prove invaluable in identifying fears and misconceptions which can be effectively addressed, with the potential to enhance treatment adherence (McGorry & Kulkarni, 1994). Management of treatment adherence is discussed in Chapter 7.

(6) Assessment of risk of absconding from hospital
Rates of premature discharges of patients, either discharging themselves against medical advice or being absent without leave, have been reported in the literature to be between 6 and 35% of psychiatric hospital admissions (Chanderasena, 1987). Absconded patients are a cause of considerable anxiety for relatives and staff, and suicide risk is commonly identified in this group (Tomison, 1989).

In the EPPIC inpatient unit which is an open ward, the rates of absconding average 10% of admissions, with over 90% of patients being returned by family or staff within 24 hours. Absconder characteristics tend to concur with the above reports, and it is of note that, over a two-year period with 600 admissions, one absconding patient was found dead at his home with no explicable cause found at autopsy, while another was shot dead by police within hours of absconding. No suicides occurred in this post-absconding time period. Patients most at risk of absconding appear to be younger males with frequent readmissions, with prominent manic or paranoid features, and frequent complicating substance abuse or antisocial personality traits (Tomison, 1989). A key inpatient policy issue is how to balance the competing needs so as to maintain an open and flexible therapeutic milieu for young people, while addressing the seriousness of the risks of absconding. Very individualized strategies are likely to be most helpful.

'Neuroleptic-free' assessment phase
A 'neuroleptic-free' assessment period of at least 48 hours is recommended, whether the patient is managed in the home or in hospital. This allows clinicians adequate time to make a more detailed formulation of a patient's presentation through repeated reassessment of the evolving mental state and the gathering of further clinical information and review of biological investigations. This is intended to reduce the potential for premature and inappropriate diagnostic and treatment interventions. It also allows for preparation and psychoeducation for the patient, so as to engage in the pharmacological treatment, and avoids the perception of a 'knee-jerk' response, instead conveying the impression of a thoughtful and considered treatment response.

This 'neuroleptic-free' period of several days of assessment is essential when presentations are complicated by drug abuse, or where symptoms of psychosis are vague, transient and possibly dissociative in nature, and where they are denied by the patient or where probable non-bizarre delusional ideas have not been substantiated as such, e.g.

hypochondriacal or paranoid delusions. In such situations, premature prescription of neuroleptics may mask the correct diagnosis. It is important to note that 'neuroleptic-free' does not necessarily mean 'drug-free', as benzodiazepines can be used to restore the patient's sleep cycle and to reduce anxiety or agitation. It certainly does not mean 'treatment-free' since the patient and family are receiving intensive support and evaluation. It should be remembered that neuroleptics will take weeks to impact significantly on core psychotic symptoms in first-episode psychosis, while the features, such as agitation, insomnia and anxiety, which need to be addressed in the initial phase, will respond best and most rapidly to benzodiazepines, support and nursing interventions.

Hospitalization: when and how?

Despite the best efforts of all concerned, it must be recognized that a significant proportion of newly presenting first-episode patients will be unable or unwilling to engage in assessment, or will require the immediate provision of intensive care in hospital in order to minimize serious risks of selfharm or violence. Involuntary recommendation should not be viewed as a failure, but merely as an aid in ensuring access to appropriate levels of care and treatment. Criteria for admission will depend on the complexion of the rest of the service. With the availability of an integrated intensive mobile outreach team it is possible to reserve inpatient care primarily for risk management. In EPPIC where such a team exists, over a third of first-episode psychosis patients avoid hospitalization during the first three months of treatment, and when hospitalization does occur, it is generally brief in duration (average 18 days) (Power et al., 1998).

It is essential to recognize the potentially traumatizing nature of hospitalization or involuntary recommendation, in which the patient is likely to feel disempowered and threatened. Frequent concerns expressed by first-episode patients admitted to hospital at EPPIC are: that they will forfeit basic legal rights, be incarcerated indefinitely, injected with chemically restraining medications, or assaulted. Sometimes, patients believe that a mistake has been made, and they are not unwell like the other patients. These concerns can be countered by providing patients with clear choices regarding their options, and by ensuring that they have access to second opinions, legal assistance and rights of appeal against their involuntary status. Of particular benefit is when the assessing clinician accompanies the patient and family to hospital, provides a sympathetic description of the hospital process, introduces them to hospital staff and ensures a full orientation to the inpatient unit and its policies. Transport via ambulance or police services should be avoided if possible. Our own experience with police admissions is that, while often uneventful and well managed, they can be extremely traumatizing for the patient, and in some cases even physically dangerous, especially where close liaison processes do not exist between police and mental health systems. Consumer input into these policies and procedures can be invaluable.

Providing debriefing for both the patient and the family is an essential component of hospitalization, particularly when it occurs involuntarily. This form of counselling should follow immediately after the event and be followed up regularly, particularly at the time of discharge from hospital. It is important to remember that, although a minority of patients maintain negative attitudes about their recommendation to hospital, most are subsequently able to develop a more positive perspective on the inpatient experience (Edelsohn & Hiday, 1990).

Biomedical evaluation of first-episode psychosis

Only about 3% of first-episode psychosis patients have a defined organic aetiology for their illness (Johnstone et al., 1986). This percentage is higher (5–8%) if late-onset presentations are included (Lewis & Flint, 1994). Often, this can be detected from a clinical examination and some have suggested that current laboratory or radiological investigations in otherwise healthy young patients may be of little benefit (Remington, 1996). Nevertheless, if an organic screen is not undertaken at this stage of illness, it is our experience that it is unlikely to be carried out subsequently. Our recommendation is that such a serious disturbance of brain function deserves an initial routine comprehensive organic investigation (Kulkarni, Copolov & Keks, 1991).

A number of physical conditions are associated with a higher risk of psychosis. These include: Cushing's syndrome; thyroid and parathyroid disorders; cerebral sarcoidosis; systemic lupus erythematosus; HIV-AIDS; sex chromosome abnormalities; demyelinating diseases such as multiple sclerosis and Schilder's disease, particularly if they involve the temporal lobes; encephalitic diseases such as cerebral syphilis and herpes simplex encephalitis; Wilson's disease; Huntington's disease; Friedreich's ataxia; vitamin B_{12} deficiency; subarachnoid haemorrhage; and cerebral tumours. Head injury and, in particular, temporal lobe epilepsy, have also been associated (Lishman, 1987). During this initial assessment phase, young people with little or no previous experience of medical procedures are not infrequently very anxious and suspicious of physical examinations and investigations. Reassurance and careful explanations of the procedures or results are therefore essential.

Physical examination

Physical examination may not only usefully provide clues as to an organic cause for psychosis but may also be useful in assessing the impact of the psychosis on the patient's physical health, e.g. state of physical neglect. Ideally, the first community-based assessment should include a brief physical examination of a patient's vital signs, including temperature, pulse, blood pressure, respiratory rate, and a brief neurological examination, particularly in patients with catatonic features or signs suggestive of movement disorder. A more complete physical examination is generally more appropriately undertaken later in the setting of a clinic or hospital, when laboratory investigations are being carried out. The former should include examination for soft neurological signs and minor physical abnormalities. Rates of minor congenital physical abnormalities (Green, Satz & Christenson, 1994) and soft neurological signs (Walker, Savoie & Davis, 1994) are significantly higher in populations of patients with schizophrenia, although as yet the significance, i.e. predictive power and sensitivity, of these findings remains unclear. Some studies suggest a correlation between these findings and aetiological–neurodevelopmental factors in psychosis. It is possible that they may signify poorer prognosis (Lieberman, 1993).

Laboratory investigations

Recommended and optimal physical investigations are reported in Tables 6.1 and 6.2, respectively. By far the most useful laboratory investigation is the simple urine drug screen. Illicit substance abuse is a common problem in this group of patients and regular laboratory investigation is important to establish the role of drug abuse in the presentation or perpetuation of psychosis. Seventy per cent of patients presenting to the EPPIC programme with first-episode psychosis have a complicating history of marijuana use (Power et al., 1998) in the last 12 months.

Lumbar puncture Being quite an invasive and painful procedure, lumbar puncture for CSF assays is generally only recommended if meningitis or encephalitis is suspected. Its use outside these areas remains limited to research investigations.

Neuro-imaging studies Weinberger (1984) recommends a CT brain scan in all first-episode psychosis patients. It is preferable to wait until the patient's psychosis has settled sufficiently so that they can tolerate and co-operate with the procedure, as patients report finding the noise and restrictions of the machinery to be particularly distressing. They may also be fearful of what could happen to them; fears which are enhanced by the fact that this is their first experience of psychiatric

Table 6.1. *Recommended routine physical investigations*

Before commencing antipsychotic medication	As early as possible
Urine tests Drug screen General urine microscopy *Blood tests* Full blood examination ESR Renal function tests (urea, creatinine) Electrolytes Serum calcium and phosphate Liver function tests Thyroid function tests	CT brain scan or, ideally, MRI scan EEG

Table 6.2. *Optional investigations depending on clinical indications*

Urine tests
Pregnancy test
Urinary porphyrins

Blood tests
Pregnancy test
Fasting blood glucose
Nutritional indices (B_{12}, folate, iron studies)
Autoantibody screens
Hepatitis screens
HIV and syphilis screens
Copper studies

Imaging
Chest x-ray

Electrocardiogram

treatment, and by persecutory ideation. Urgent CT and MRI scans are recommended only when there is a strong indication of an organic cause for the patient's presentation. Any abnormalities detected on a CT scan should be followed up by an MRI scan. The clinical significance of abnormalities found on CT brain scans or MRI in first-episode psychosis patients remains unclear. This is a rapidly developing field covered more extensively in Chapter 5.

Electroencephalograms   In our experience with the current level of EEG interpretation, the cost effectiveness of routine EEG in early psychosis is questionable, given the low yield of reports of clinically significant findings. However, EEGs should be undertaken if there is a history of epilepsy, birth trauma, head injury, mental handicap, and significant findings on neuro-imaging. With improved levels of sophistication in EEG interpretation, e.g. EEG coherence measures (Norman et al., 1997), it is possible that in the future the EEG may become a useful routine investigation in psychosis.

Neuropsychological assessments
There is considerable evidence (mainly from studies of patients with chronic schizophrenia) suggesting an association between psychosis and a range of neuropsychological deficits, in particular attentional or information processing and verbal memory or learning impairments. These deficits are apparent even in first-episode psychosis patients (Brewer et al., 1996; Hoff et al., 1992; Rubin et al., 1995; Saykin et al., 1994) with similar levels to those of patients with chronic schizophrenia, thereby suggesting that the deficits may not be progressive (Hoff et al., 1992, Saykin et al., 1994), or may even develop during the prodrome (Brewer et al., 1996). The deficits point towards prefrontal and temporohippocampal dysfunction and correlate with abnormal CT scan findings (Rubin et al., 1995). Deficits in verbal memory function may be useful as additional markers of vulnerability to psychosis in high-risk groups (Brewer et al., 1996). Given the extent to which these neuropsychological findings may prove useful in determining prognosis and treatment response, routine mapping of the course of these seems increasingly important. The recovery of neurocognitive functioning will probably become a key goal in treatment.

Accurate IQ and personality testing is generally invalidated while patients continue to experience acute psychotic symptoms, although both elements may contribute to a heightened risk for psychotic disorder. Differentiating primary (premorbid) personality traits from traits induced by, or complicating, acute psychosis is a highly complex endeavour, especially in younger populations (Hulbert, Jackson & McGorry, 1996).

Social and educational assessment
Assessment of a patient's premorbid level of psychosocial functioning is essential in determining the duration of prodrome, level of premorbid limitations in functioning, degree of current impairment, and the expected level of functional recovery. This information can be con-

firmed by the patient's educational reports, work references, and collateral information from relatives.

Assessment of the home environment, family dynamics and their adaptive responses provides invaluable information for determining not only the nature and degree of stressors for both patient and family, but also the cultural factors which require consideration when making decisions about psychosocial interventions. Judgements about the level of expressed emotion (EE) within a family should be cautiously assessed in the context of the duration and severity of the relative's illness, competing family stressors, and available family support (see also Chapter 14). It is useful to try to distinguish state-related from trait-related high EE phenomena (Schreiber, Breier & Pickar, 1995).

Diagnosis and formulation

An adequate diagnosis and formulation becomes the foundation stone upon which a management plan and critical decisions about appropriate engagement and treatment strategies can be made. It is essential to allow sufficient time to gather information from a number of sources in order to develop a comprehensive working formulation of the patient's condition based on a multidisciplinary approach using an integrated biopsychosocial model.

Is there sufficient evidence to confirm that the patient suffers from a psychosis?

Confirmation of psychosis is notoriously difficult in these early stages of illness. Chapter 2 provides a more detailed discussion of these problems. To qualify for a diagnosis of psychotic disorder, one can set an arbitrary threshold where the intensity and duration of psychotic symptoms indicate that neuroleptics would generally be indicated. We have operationalized this as the presence of clearcut delusions, hallucinations or severely disorganized speech sustained for at least one week.

What form of psychosis exists?

Once the presence of psychosis has been confirmed, the common forms of psychoses are schizophrenia spectrum disorders, affective psychosis, and drug-induced psychosis. Brief reactive psychosis is relatively uncommon. Organic psychoses and delusional disorders generally present later in life. It is rare for factitious disorders and dissociative conditions to present with features suggestive of psychosis, and the majority of such presentations are later confirmed as psychotic in nature.

In simple terms, the major distinguishing factor between a schizophrenic spectrum disorder and affective psychosis is the presence of prominent affective features during the acute phase of psychosis (APA, 1992). However, mood disturbance, in particular depression, is a common complication during the prodrome and recovery phases of a schizophreniform psychosis. Catatonia is commonly underestimated as a consequence of bipolar disorder (Fein & McGrath, 1990). The consequence of failing to recognize the potential affective features may deny the patient access to adequate treatment using combined pharmacotherapies, e.g. antidepressant or mood stabilizer added to neuroleptic treatment.

With first-episode psychosis complicated by substance use, assessment is, in our experience, commonly complicated by either premature prescribing of neuroleptic medication or continued drug abuse. The distinction between the functional psychoses and drug-induced psychosis remains controversial (Poole & Brabbins, 1996) and often blurred in clinical practice (see Chapter 13). Patients with psychosis may self-medicate in an attempt to either mask positive symptoms, assist with negative symptoms or mitigate side effects of medication (Decker & Ries, 1993). Psychoactive drugs may have a pathoplastic effect in functional psychosis, either modifying the presentation of psychosis or precipitating psychosis itself (Poole & Brabbins, 1996). Failure to recognize this may result in the underlying functional psychosis being untreated and mistaken for a drug-induced psychosis.

Problems with diagnosis in early psychosis

It is important to be mindful that premature decisions about diagnosis may condemn patients to inappropriate expectations and treatments. Distinctions between diagnostic categories are frequently difficult to make in emerging early psychosis due to the frequent presence of a complex interplay between premorbid developmental or personality vulnerabilities, stressors, drugs, and affective features. This is further complicated by the changing patterns of symptoms with age or phase of illness (McGorry, 1995). The diagnostic value of key symptoms of acute psychosis is complicated by their lack of specificity, the continuing syndromal basis of psychiatric diagnosis (Kendell, 1975), and by the changing concepts of diagnostic categories (Hegarty et al., 1994). Even with improved diagnostic criteria, considerable variability still exists in clinical practice, with Fennig et al. (1994) reporting poor concordance (one-third agreement for common diagnoses) between research and clinical psychiatrists' decisions about diagnoses in first-admission psychosis patients. Similar slippage in concordance exists even between alternative procedures applying a common diagnostic system (McGorry et al., 1995). Furthermore, within the first six months of treatment, about 25% of first-episode diagnoses were found to be changed (Fennig, Bromet & Jandorf, 1993). It is important to be clear that we are not advocating a non-diagnostic stance here, merely that to aim for subtyping among psychotic disorders at this phase of illness is to seek a precision which often turns out to be spurious. Psychiatric diagnosis is still a syndromal endeavour, and broad syndromes are diagnostically appropriate at this phase of disorder, enhancing rather than inhibiting psychoeducational efforts.

A model for diagnosis in early psychosis is outlined in McGorry (1995). This model is compatible with existing terminology but is more transparent to the assumptions involved in our current approach to diagnosis in early psychosis. Figure 6.1 sets out a template on which to date an individual patient's symptoms and phase of illness.

How best to formulate the patient's condition?

An individual understanding of the person as a unique individual and the relationship of the illness to the course of his or her life is a key element of the formulation which complements the diagnostic 'look'. In formulating the patient's condition, it is useful to identify the patient's duration of prodrome, psychosis, complicating comorbidity, risk factors, and the immediate issues facing both patient and carers. This should be elaborated in the context of the patient's premorbid level of functioning and how the patient's psychosis is influenced by predisposing, precipitating and perpetuating factors. It is helpful to integrate biological, psychological, and social aetiological influences. Zubin's stress vulnerability model (Zubin & Spring, 1977) provides a useful premise from which to start and to explain the nature of the problem to patients and family. At the onset, diagnosis should be provisional in nature, emphasizing what a psychiatric diagnosis means in practical terms and what the potential differential diagnoses might be.

Comorbid disorders

Comorbid disorders such as physical or substance abuse disorders should be considered from the outset. This includes DSM-IV (APA, 1994) axis II disorders, e.g. personality disorders, and non-psychotic axis I disorders such as depression, although the therapeutic signifi-

		Early Psychosis		Critical Period		Prolonged Psychosis	
		Prodrome	First-episode Psychosis	Persistent	Relapse	Persistent	Relapse
IMPAIRMENT (syndromes)	None						
	PS						
	MS						
	DS						
	NS						
	COM						
	PD						
DISABILITY/ HANDICAP	None						
	Intermittent						
	Sustained						

Key:
PS = Positive Symptoms
MS = Manic Symptoms
DS = Depressive Symptoms
NS = Negative Symptoms
COM = Other Axis I Co-morbidity eg. Panic, PTSD, Substance Abuse
PD = Personality Disorder

Figure 6.1. Phase-oriented classification of psychosis: a template on which to rate an individual patient's symptoms and phase of illness.

cance is complex. Earlier age of onset of psychosis is generally associated with greater personality disturbance, which is not infrequently confused by clinicians to be due to borderline personality features, with its potential to attract a pejorative label. In many cases, the features of these other disorders (depression is the classic example) are secondary to the psychotic process and will gradually resolve with effective primary treatment of the psychosis. However, in more severe or persistent comorbid presentations specific interventions for these conditions may provide significant amelioration of symptoms (Hulbert, Jackson & McGorry 1996; Jackson et al., 1996).

Conclusion

A comprehensive and thorough assessment of biological, psychological and social factors in this early phase of management of first-episode psychosis is essential in determining the predisposing, precipitating and perpetuating influences. This then allows for a proper formulation of the patient's condition, treatment options, likely responses, risks, available supports, likelihood of treatment compliance, and prognosis. It provides the essential basis upon which initial management of early psychosis can be structured. It is critically dependent upon a good level of engagement and a stable treatment environment within the initial treatment period.

All too often, particularly where the initial episode is treated in a fragmentary way, key elements of this process are missing. This not only leads to errors in decision-making but contributes to failures in engagement, understanding of the patient and family and their needs, and in continuity of care. Optimal assessment and engagement provides a strong foundation for optimal treatment experiences and more complete recovery.

References

American Psychiatric Association (1992). *Report from the DSM-IV Field Trial for Schizophrenia and Related Psychotic Disorders* (M. Flaum, Field Trial Co-ordinator). Iowa City, Iowa: University of Iowa.

American Psychiatric Association (1994). *Diagnostic and Statistical Manual of Mental Disorders*, 4th edn, DSM-IV. Washington, DC: American Psychiatric Association.

Aquilina, C. (1991). Violence by psychiatric in-patients. *Medicine, Science and the Law*, **31**, 306–12.

Atakan, Z. (1995). Violence on psychiatric in-patient units: What can be done? *Psychiatric Bulletin: The Journal of Trends in Psychiatric Practice*, **19**, 593–6.

Birchwood, M., Cochrane, R., Macmillan, F., Copestake, S., Kucharska, J. & Cariss, M. (1992). The influence of ethnicity and family structure on relapse in first episode schizophrenia. A comparison of Asian, Afro-Caribbean, and white patients. *British Journal of Psychiatry*, **161**, 783–90.

Brewer, W. J., Edwards, J., Anderson, V., Robinson, T. & Pantelis, P. (1996). Neuropsychological, olfactory, and hygiene deficits in men with negative symptom schizophrenia. *Biological Psychiatry*, **40**, 1021–31.

Bromet, E. J., Jandorf, L., Fennig, S., Lavelle, J., Kovasznay, B., Ram, R., Tanenberg-Karant, M. & Craig, T. (1996). The Suffolk County Mental Health Project: demographic, pre-morbid and clinical correlates of 6-month outcome. *Psychological Medicine*, **26**, 953–62.

Chanderasena, R. (1987). Premature discharges: a comparative study. *Canadian Journal of Psychiatry*, **32**, 259–63.

Cole, E., Leavey, G., King, M., Johnson-Sabine, E. & Hoar, A. (1995). Pathways to care for patients with a first episode of psychosis: a comparison of ethnic groups. *British Journal of Psychiatry*, **167**, 770–6.

Daly, I., Webb, M. & Kaliszer, M. (1996). First admission incidence study of mania, 1975–1981. *British Journal of Psychiatry*, **167**, 463–8.

Decker, K. P. & Ries, R. K. (1993). Differential diagnosis and psychopharmacology of dual disorders. *Psychiatric Clinics of North America*, **16**, 703–18.

Edelsohn G. A. & Hiday V. A. (1990). Civil commitment: a range of attitudes. *Bulletin of the American Academy of Psychiatry and the Law*, **18**, 65–77.

Elkins, K., Curry, C. M., Harrigan, S. M. & McGorry, P. D. (1997). *Cigarette Smoking: the First Episode Experience*. Poster Presented at the International Congress on Schizophrenia Research, Colorado, USA, 12–16 April, 1997.

Fein, S. & McGrath, M. G. (1990). Problems in diagnosing bipolar disorder in catatonic patients. *Journal of Clinical Psychiatry*, **51**, 203–5.

Fennig, S., Bromet, E. & Jandorf, L. (1993). Gender differences in clinical characteristics of first-admission psychotic depression. *American Journal of Psychiatry*, **150**, 1734–6.

Fennig, S., Craig, T., Tanenberg-Karant, M. & Bromet, E. (1994). Comparison of facility and research diagnoses in first admission psychotic patients. *American Journal of Psychiatry*, **151**, 1423–9.

Fennig, S., Bromet, E. J., Galambos, N. & Putman, K. (1996). Diagnosis and six-month stability of negative symptoms in psychotic disorders. *European Archives of Psychiatry and Clinical Neuroscience*, **246**, 63–70.

Green, M. F., Satz, P. & Christenson, C. (1994). Minor physical anomalies in schizophrenia patients, bipolar patients, and their siblings. *Schizophrenia Bulletin*, **20**, 433–40.

Häfner, H., Maurer, K., Löffler, W., Bustamante, S., an der Heiden, W., Riecher-Rössler, A. & Notwotny, B. (1995). Onset and early course of schizophrenia. In *Search for the Causes of Schizophrenia*, Vol. III, ed. H. Häfner & W. F. Gattaz, pp. 43–66. New York: Springer-Verlag.

Hambrecht, M. & Häfner, H. (1996). Substance abuse and the onset of schizophrenia. *Biological Psychiatry*, **40**, 1155–63.

Havens, L. (1986). *Making Contact: Uses of Language in Psychotherapy*. Cambridge, Massachusetts: Harvard University Press.

Hegarty, J. D., Baldessarini, R. J., Tohen, M., Waternaux, C. & Oepen, G. (1994). One hundred years of schizophrenia: a meta-analysis of the outcome literature. *American Journal of Psychiatry*, **151**, 1409–16.

Hillier, R., McPhillips, M. A., Puri, B., Joyce, E. & Barnes, T. R. E. (1996). *Prevalence of Substance Misuse Among People with First-episode Schizophrenia: a Study Using Hair Analysis*. Paper Presented at the First Psychotic Episode of Schizophrenia Conference, Amsterdam, The Netherlands, Nov. 28–29, 1996.

Hoff, A. L., Riordan, H., O'Donnell, D. W., Morris, L. & DeLisi, L. E. (1992). Neuropsychological functioning of first-episode schizophreniform patients. *American Journal of Psychiatry*, **149**, 898–903.

Hulbert, C. A., Jackson, H. J. & McGorry, P. D. (1996). The relationship between personality and course and outcome in early psychosis: a review of the literature. *Clinical Psychology Review*, **16**, 707–27.

Jablensky, A., Sartorius, N., Ernberg, G., Anker, M., Kroten, A., Cooper, J. E., Day, R. & Bertelsen, A. (1992). Schizophrenia: manifestations, incidence and course in different cultures. A World Health Organization ten-country study. *Psychological Medicine* (Monograph, Supplement **20**), 1–97.

Jackson, H. J., McGorry, P. D., Edwards, J. & Hulbert, C. (1996). Cognitively orientated psychotherapy for early psychosis (COPE). In *Early Intervention and Prevention in Mental Health*, ed. P. Cotton & H. Jackson, pp. 131–54. Melbourne, Australia: Australian Psychological Society.

James D. G., Fineberg, N. A., Shah, A. K. & Priest, R. G. (1990). An increase in violence on an acute psychiatric ward, a study of associated factors. *British Journal of Psychiatry*, **156**, 846–52.

Jaspers, K. (1923). *General Psychopathology*, 7th edn. Translated by J. Hoenig & M. W. Hamilton (1963). Berlin: Springer-Verlag.

Johnstone, E., Crow, T., Johnson, A. & Macmillan, J. (1986). The Northwick Park Study of first episodes of schizophrenia. I: Presentation of illness and problems relating to admission. *British Journal of Psychiatry*, **148**, 115–20.

Jones, P. B., Bebbington, P., Foerster, A., Lewis, S. W., Murray, R. M., Russell, A., Sham, P. C., Toone, B. K. & Wilkins, S. (1993). Premorbid social underachievement in schizophrenia: Results from the Camberwell Collaborative Psychosis Study. *British Journal of Psychiatry*, **162**, 65–71.

Kemp, R. & David, A. (1996). Psychological predictors of insight and compliance in psychotic patients. *British Journal of Psychiatry*, **169**, 444–50.

Kendell, R. E. (1975). *The Role Of Diagnosis In Psychiatry*. London: Blackwell Scientific Publications.

Kulkarni, J., Copolov, D. & Keks, N. (1991). Laboratory investigations in psychiatry. In *Mental Health and Illness: A Textbook for Health Science Students*, ed. R. Kosky, H. Eskevari & V. Carr, pp. 136–42. London: Butterworths.

Lewis, S. & Flint, J. (1994). The differentiation of organic and functional psychosis. In *The Assessment of Psychosis: A Practical Handbook*, ed. T. Barnes & H. Nelson, pp. 173–90. London: Chapman & Hall.

Lieberman, J. A. (1993). Prediction of outcome in first-episode schizophrenia. *Journal of Clinical Psychiatry*, **54** (Supplement), 13–17.

Lishman, W. A. (1987). *Organic Psychiatry. The Psychological Consequences of Cerebral Disorder*, 2nd edn. Oxford, UK: Blackwell Scientific Publications.

Loebel, A. D., Lieberman, J. A., Alvir, J. M., Mayerhoff, D. I., Geisler, S. H. & Szymanski, S. R. (1992). Duration of psychosis outcome in first episode schizophrenia. *American Journal of Psychiatry*, **149**, 1183–8.

Mayerhoff, D. I., Loebel, A. D., Alvir, J. M., Szymanski, S. R., Geisler, S. H., Borenstein, M. & Lieberman, J. A. (1994). The deficit state in first-episode schizophrenia. *American Journal of Psychiatry*, **151**, 1417–22.

McGlashan, T. H. & Johannessen, J. O. (1996). Early detection and intervention with schizophrenia: rationale. *Schizophrenia Bulletin*, **22**, 201–22.

McGorry, P. D. (1994). The influence of illness duration on syndrome clarity and stability in functional psychosis: does the diagnosis emerge and stabilise with time? *Australian and New Zealand Journal of Psychiatry*, **28**, 607–19.

McGorry, P. D. (1995). A treatment-relevant classification of psychotic disorders. *Australian and New Zealand Journal of Psychiatry*, **29**, 555–8.

McGorry, P., Copolov, D. L. & Singh, B. S. (1989). The validity of the assessment of psychopathology in the psychoses. *Australian and New Zealand Journal of Psychiatry*, **23**, 469–82.

McGorry, P. D., Copolov, D. L. & Singh, B. S. (1990a). The Royal Park Multidiagnostic Instrument for Psychosis. Part 1. Rationale and review. *Schizophrenia Bulletin*, **16**, 501–15.

McGorry, P. D., Copolov, D. L. & Singh, B. S. (1990b). Current concepts in functional psychosis: the case for a loosening of associations. *Schizophrenia Research*, **3**, 221–34.

McGorry, P. D., Chanen, A., McCarthy, E., Van Riel, R., McKenzie. D. & Singh, B. S. (1991). Post-traumatic stress disorder following recent-onset psychosis: an unrecognised post-psychotic syndrome. *Journal of Nervous and Mental Disease*, **179**, 253–8.

McGorry, P. & Kulkarni, J. (1994). Prevention and preventively oriented clinical care in psychotic disorders. *The Australian Journal of Psychopharmacology*, **7**, 62–9.

McGorry, P. D., Mihalopoulos, C., Henry, L., Dakis, J., Jackson, H. J., Flaum, M., Harrigan, S., McKenzie, D., Kulkarni J. & Karoly, R. (1995). Spurious precision: procedural validity of diagnostic assessment in psychotic disorders. *American Journal of Psychiatry*, **152**, 220–3.

McGorry, P. D., Edwards, J., Mihalopoulos, C., Harrigan, S. M. & Jackson, H. J. (1996). EPPIC: an evolving system of early detection and optimal management. *Schizophrenia Bulletin*, **22**, 305–26.

McGorry, P. D., Henry, L. & Power, P. (1998). Suicide in early psychosis: could early intervention work? In *Proceedings of Suicide Prevention. The Global Contact*, ed. R. Kosky, R. Goldney & R. Hassan. New York: Plenum.

McNeil, D., Binder, R. & Greenfield, T. (1988). Predictors of violence in civilly committed acute psychiatric patients. *American Journal of Psychiatry*, **145**, 965–78.

McNeil, D. E. & Binder, R. L. (1994). The relationship between acute psychiatric symptoms, diagnosis, and short-term risk of violence. *Hospital and Community Psychiatry*, **45**, 133–7.

Norman, R. M., Malla, A. K., Williamson, P. C., Morrison-Stewart, S. L., Helmes, E. & Cortese, L. (1997). EEG coherence and syndromes in schizophrenia. *British Journal of Psychiatry*, **170**, 411–15.

Poole, R. & Brabbins, C. (1996). Drug induced psychosis. *British Journal of Psychiatry*, **168**, 135–8.

Power, P., Elkins, K., Adlard, S., Curry, C., McGorry, P. & Harrigan, S. (in press). An analysis of the initial treatment phase in first episode psychosis. *British Journal of Psychiatry* (Supplement) in press.

Raphael, B. (1986). *When Disaster Strikes: How Individuals and Communities Cope With Catastrophe*. New York: Basic Books.

Remington, G. (1996). Topical issues on the diagnosis and drug treatment of first episode schizophrenia. *Journal of Practical Psychiatry and Behavioural Health*, **2** (Supplement), 2–9.

Roy, A., Schreiber, J. & Mazonson, A. (1988). Suicidal behaviour in chronic schizophrenic patients: a follow-up study. *Canadian Journal of Psychiatry*, **31**, 737–40.

Rubin, P., Holm, A., Moller-Madsen, S., Videbech, P., Hertel, C., Povlsen, U. J. & Hemmingsen, R. (1995). Neuropsychological deficit in newly diagnosed patients with schizophrenia or schizophreniform disorder. *Acta Psychiatrica Scandinavica*, **92**, 35–43.

Saykin, A. J., Shtasel, D. L., Gur, R. E., Kester, D. B., Mozley, L. H., Stafiniak, P. & Gur, R. C. (1994). Neuropsychological deficits in neuroleptic naive patients with first-episode schizophrenia. *Archives of General Psychiatry*, **51**, 124–31.

Schreiber, J., Breier, A. & Pickar, D. (1995). Expressed emotion: trait or state? *British Journal of Psychiatry*, **166**, 647–9.

Strakowski, S. M., Shelton, R. C. & Kolbrener, M. L. (1993). The effects of race and comorbidity on clinical diagnosis in patients with psychosis. *Journal of Clinical Psychiatry*, **54**, 96–102.

Strakowski, S. M., Tohen, M., Stoll, A., Faedda, G., Mayer, P., Kolbrener, M. & Goodwin, D. (1993). Comorbidity in psychosis at first hospitalisation. *American Journal of Psychiatry*, **150**, 752–7.

Swanson, J. W., Holzer, C. E., Ganju, V. K. & Jono, R. T. (1990). Violence and psychiatric disorder in the community: evidence from the Epidemiologic Catchment Area surveys. *Hospital and Community Psychiatry*, **41**, 761–70.

Thomas, C., Bartlett, A. & Mezey, G. (1995). The extent and effects of violence among psychiatric in-patients. *Psychiatric Bulletin*, **19**, 600–4.

Tomison, A. R. (1989). Characteristics of psychiatric hospital absconders. *British Journal of Psychiatry*, **154**, 368–71.

Walker, E. F., Savoie, T. & Davis, D. (1994). Neuromotor precursors of schizophrenia. *Schizophrenia Bulletin*, **20**, 441–51.

Weinberger, D. R. (1984). Brain disease and psychiatric illness: when should a psychiatrist order a CAT scan? *American Journal of Psychiatry*, **141**, 1521–7.

World Health Organization. (1973). *The International Pilot Study of Schizophrenia*. Geneva: World Health Organization.

Wyatt, R. J. (1991). Neuroleptics and the natural course of schizophrenia. *Schizophrenia Bulletin*, **17**, 325–51.

Zubin, J. & Spring, B. (1977). Vulnerability – a new view on schizophrenia. *Journal of Abnormal Psychology*, **86**, 103–26.

7
Initial treatment of first-episode psychosis

JAYASHRI KULKARNI AND PADDY POWER

Introduction

Optimizing the initial management of a patient's first-episode of psychosis is not only vital in maximizing the chances of a full recovery, but is critical also in minimizing the potential for future relapses and morbidity.

Previous chapters have outlined the strategies for detection, early intervention, and assessment of the prodromal and acute phases in patients with first-episode psychosis. Initial management can be viewed as an extension of these assessment processes in order to: (*a*) develop a comprehensive formulation of a patient's condition; (*b*) decide on appropriate treatments; and (*c*) engage the patient in initial therapeutic interventions.

The management of first-episode psychosis presents a number of special characteristics. The first-episode of psychosis (excluding delusional disorders and paraphrenia) usually presents in young adults, already at risk due to a range of vulnerability factors. Males develop psychosis earlier than females (Angermeyer & Kuhn, 1988) and in our experience they are usually single, living with, or just recently separated from, their parents by the age of onset of illness. Their presentations are frequently complicated by adolescent issues, e.g. separation and individuation factors, antisocial behaviours, drug abuse, adjustment disorders, and family disruption due to other affected members. Females more often than not already live with established partners (Riecher-Rössler et al., 1992), and not infrequently have children. Presentations are frequently complicated by parenting issues and tensions with their partners.

The potential pervasive disruptive effect of psychosis on this young population, occurring at a critical phase of their development, requires

7 INITIAL TREATMENT OF FIRST-EPISODE PSYCHOSIS

that management strategies be broad in approach, flexible in nature, and able quickly to address the specific individual needs of patients and their family. The patient's career and social supports need particular attention during this early phase to minimize major losses, maintain the patient's potential developmental trajectory, and assist with reintegration during recovery.

Misconceptions about the management of first-episode psychosis

Many 'myths' still abound regarding the management of early psychosis. These are described as follows:

(1) 'Schizophrenia is a chronic, deteriorating illness'
This view (Andreasen, 1984) is not supported by the figures for both short-term and long-term prognosis. Eighty-five per cent of first-episode psychosis patients recover, with most returning to their premorbid level of functioning (Kane, 1993). A 13–year follow-up of 67 people with first-episode schizophrenia (Mason et al., 1995) showed that 55% had good or fair functioning, whilst 52% had no positive or negative symptoms during the last two years of follow-up.
(2) 'All first-episode psychosis patients require hospitalization'
Successful treatment for first-episode psychosis patients can occur in the community, provided that adequate support can be provided for patients and their families or other carers. The home-based treatment of first-episode psychosis is discussed in Chapter 8.
(3) 'Patients with psychosis have no capacity for insight when acutely psychotic'
Bleuler (1950) considered 'lack of insight' as a fundamental and stable phenomenological finding in psychosis. More recent concepts of insight suggest that it is multidimensional (Amador et al., 1993) and fluctuates depending on illness phase (Heinrichs, Cohen & Carpenter, 1985). Many people with a first-episode psychosis maintain an awareness of their dysfunction and, when in remission, are able to recall illness details, external stressors and coping strategies (Breier & Strauss, 1983; McCandless-Glimcher et al., 1986). Acknowledgement that acutely psychotic patients generally retain an awareness of disturbance, and try to explain this,

is important for the involvement of patients in their treatment plans.

(4) 'Low-dose antipsychotic medication is not effective'

Recent studies using low-dose antipsychotic medication in first-episode psychosis confirms good medium-term response rates (Kane, 1993; Lieberman et al., 1993). Emsley, McCreadie & Livingston (1995) reported that 63% of 183 first admission patients responded well to low-dose antipsychotic treatment (average of 6 mg/day haloperidol equivalents). Power et al. (1998) have reported that 63% of 231 patients treated with a mean dose of 4.1 mg/day (haloperidol equivalents) experienced a 50% reduction in their psychotic symptoms, within two months of commencing treatment. McEvoy, Hogarty & Steingard (1991) found that even lower doses of neuroleptics (mean = 2.1 mg haloperidol) were effective for first-episode patients.

(5) 'The only effective treatments for acute psychosis are pharmacological'

Cognitive–behavioural therapy (CBT) has been reported to be effective in patients with medication-resistant psychotic symptoms (Chadwick & Lowe, 1990; Garety et al., 1994). Drury et al. (1996a) demonstrated acceleration of the rate of recovery from acute psychosis with cognitive therapy enhancement, and Jackson et al. (1998) reported on the beneficial effects of adjunctive cognitive therapy in first-episode psychosis patients (see also Chapter 10 and Jackson et al., 1996, 1998).

General early treatment principles

Comprehensive assessment

Optimal treatment of first-episode psychosis begins with a comprehensive biopsychosocial assessment and the development of a good therapeutic alliance between clinicians and patients, as well as the patients' families. A full assessment of current phenomenology, suicide and violence risk, and assessment of the environment and social support, guides decisions about the location of management, and provide basic information for commencing treatment. In addition, it is important to assess the person's premorbid personality, concepts of psychosis, coping skills, current conflicts, sociocultural milieu, social strengths and weaknesses, accommodation, occupation, and financial and family issues. This knowledge helps the clinician to understand the patient's first psychotic episode in the context of the person's whole life situation, and should be used to formulate a working diagnosis so that appropriate treatment can be initiated. More specific details about the comprehensive assessment of the first-episode of psychosis are discussed in Chapter 6.

Identifying phases of illness

Conceptually, separating the first psychotic episode into acute and recovery phases provides a useful framework for clinicians, enabling them to identify and meet the changing needs of patients and families throughout the episode of illness (McGorry, 1992). Thinking about the phases of illness in this way also highlights the prospect of recovery, and conveys a sense of limitation to the acute phase of psychotic symptoms. The illness phases, however, are not independent or identifiable by time constraints. The length and nature of an acute phase differs for each patient and the transition to recovery phase may be marked by episodic relapses.

Consideration of the location of treatment

The location of treatment for people suffering from a first-episode of psychosis remains an area of controversy, with some clinicians adopting rigidly polarized views about hospitalization versus community treatment. Issues of safety, refusal to comply with community assessment or treatment, and lack of appropriate family support, are the three most common reasons for hospitalization in first-episode psychosis. If resources are available and the person's family or carers are coping, treatment can be initiated safely in the community, thus avoiding the anxiety, loss of control, increased stigma and trauma which can accompany hospitalization. The home-based treatment of first-episode psychosis is discussed in Chapter 8. However, even if involuntary hospitalization is required, it is possible to make this difficult situation more acceptable by providing early and ongoing support to the person and their relatives. By permitting flexibility in visiting times, and paying attention to personal comfort, with an emphasis on small but important issues such as diet, personal possessions, access to telephones and accurate information about expected length of stay, the clinician can help to demystify and humanize the experience of hospitalization. An optimal therapeutic milieu needs to promote continuity of care through case-management models located within comprehensive multidisciplinary team structures. Expressed emotion in staff also needs to be addressed in order to ensure that patients receive the best possible care in a genuinely therapeutic environment.

Minimizing the risks and impact of violence in inpatient settings is becoming an increasing challenge for staff in acute inpatient units, given the trend towards admitting only the most acutely disturbed and ill patients for increasingly short stays, with some inner city wards becoming 'untherapeutic' environments, where both staff and patients feel unsafe (Atakan, 1995). Atakan (1995) outlined a number of principles in preventing and managing violence in inpatient settings. These included: the provision of intensive care units or areas; the development of clear policies, ward structures, treatment models and activities for patients; and ensuring that there is good communication between all clinical staff as well as adequate support for the latter. While there are benefits and problems associated with both home-based and hospital treatment, the ultimate decision should best meet the particular needs for each patient and his or her family, and be ideology-free. This is achieved more easily where services are fully integrated and the same clinicians are responsible for the care of the patient in either location.

Addressing precipitants

Psychosocial stressors such as the loss of a significant relationship or other losses, may precede the acute onset of psychosis (Malla & Norman, 1994). Such stressors may lead the patient to abuse substances such as alcohol, cannabis or other drugs, in an attempt to 'self-medicate', thereby potentially exacerbating the psychotic illness. Both the stressors and the patient's method of coping with them need to be addressed early in the treatment of the first episode of psychosis. A relatively under-recognized factor which may aggravate manic psychotic symptoms is sleep deprivation (Wehr et al., 1982). Patients with florid psychotic symptoms may experience sleep deprivation as a reaction to constant and intense hallucinations or delusional beliefs, and an early intervention may include the use of a sedating benzodiazepine medication to prevent future escalation of psychotic symptoms driven by ongoing sleep deprivation.

Using integrated treatment interventions

The importance of an integrated approach cannot be over-stressed. Clinicians need to be able to integrate biological treatments with supportive psychotherapy, cognitive approaches, problem-solving techniques, and educational material, and often advocate on the person's behalf in various community settings such as the workplace, schools, law courts, or even within the family unit. The priorities in treatment vary markedly during the course of the first psychotic episode from the acute phase through to recovery, and clinicians need to be flexible in their approach to accommodate these changing priorities.

Avoidance or minimization of potential harmful effects of treatment

An overarching principle for all treatments used for the management of the first-episode psychosis, is to avoid or minimize any harmful effects of treatment. The type and outcome of treatment offered to patients suffering from a first episode of psychosis serves as a blueprint for their level of recovery and any future psychotic episodes. Therefore, the choice of treatments needs to allow the patient to continue with personal development in relationships, work and leisure, while adequately treating psychotic symptoms.

Since the ultimate object of treatment is to assist patients to return to their normal lives as early as possible, it is obviously counterproductive to employ drug treatments which produce side-effects severe enough to damage the patient's quality of life and future growth. Similarly, psychological treatments and social interventions need to be individualized and tailored to meet the patient's needs and goals, rather than being offered as rigid, standardized processes based on the clinician's own values and perspectives. A truly collaborative approach to treatment forged between patients and clinicians may significantly improve the patient's ultimate outcome, by avoiding or minimizing harmful treatment effects.

Specific treatments for first-episode psychosis

Drug treatments

The efficacy of neuroleptics as a first-line treatment of psychosis has been solidly established (Klein & Davis, 1969). Earlier treatment of acute psychosis with neuroleptic drugs has been shown to be associated with improved prognosis (Loebel et al., 1992; Wyatt, 1991).

Considering the optimal neuroleptic dose required, our clinical experience in treating over 500 first-episode psychosis patients has convinced us that low doses of neuroleptic medication are effective in abolishing or alleviating the psychotic symptoms of hallucinations, delusions, thought disorder and bizarre behaviour, while enabling extra-pyramidal and other side-effects to be minimized. Psychotic symptom response can take at least 10–14 days to begin after drug commencement, and up to six weeks or longer for maximum response to occur even if the initial antipsychotic proves effective (Baldessarini, Cohen & Teicher, 1988), so patience is required. Other authors (Lieberman, 1993; Szymanski et al., 1996) have suggested that the maximum response to neuroleptics in first-episode psychosis may not occur for several months after the commencement of neuroleptics. Impatient prescribing habits do not shorten admission or the length of the acute phase, but merely increase the risk of subsequent poor adherence and relapse.

In a controlled study of neuroleptic threshold in acute schizophrenia, McEvoy, Hogarty & Steingard (1991) described significant responses to neuroleptic threshold doses of haloperidol. A key point made in this McEvoy study, was that a significant number of first-episode psychosis patients had a significant response to a mean dose of 2.1 mg haloperidol. Responses did not improve with higher haloperidol doses. Neuroleptic threshold was defined as the point when individuals developed slight increases in rigidity. This occurred at mean haloperidol doses of 3.7 ± 2.3 mg/day for the whole sample. Response rates did not improve by raising the dose; merely waiting for a longer period produced equal results. Patients receiving a mean dose of 3.7 mg/day of haloperidol did as well as patients receiving three times that dose by the end of the six-week period.

Nordstrom et al. (1993), using positron emission tomography, found that antipsychotic effects occurred when 60–70% of the D2 receptors in the brain were occupied by antagonists, and that even steady doses of 4 mg/day of haloperidol produced 80% blockade. The major clinical goal with conventional or typical neuroleptics, supported by PET studies of this kind, is to produce a clinical response without reaching the threshold for extrapyramidal side-effects (EPS) (Remington, Kapur & Zipursky, 1998). This can be called the 'therapeutic window'.

Even in patients with more established illness, Stone et al. (1995) reported no difference in response rates within the first week of treatment between patients on 4 mg/day, 10 mg/day, or 40 mg/day of haloperidol. By day 4 of treatment, they reported that, overall, patients demonstrated a 25% reduction in their BPRS positive symptom scores, and by day 14 of treatment a 42–45% reduction in scores.

Choice of neuroleptic

Choosing to treat a patient with an antipsychotic drug is a serious decision which should only be made following a comprehensive assessment and subsequent to the diagnosis of psychotic disorder being made.

As discussed in Chapter 6, a neuroleptic-free assessment period is vital. During this time, the patient's agitation and anxieties related to psychosis can be safely managed by prescribing regular benzodiazepines, such as diazepam 10–40 mg/day for up to seven days. Clinicians often feel an urgent need to commence neuroleptic treatment immediately, but should recognize that the prescription of benzodiazepines, in addition to the provision of support, leads to more rapid symptom relief than neuroleptics – the latter take time to exert antipsychotic effects.

Once a carefully considered decision has been made to prescribe neuroleptic drugs, attempts should be made to match the neuroleptic's actions and side-effect profile to the most distressing symptoms, and consideration given to the patient's lifestyle. Clinicians need to be very familiar with neuroleptic side-effects (Keks, Kulkarni & Copolov, 1989).

Patients who are very agitated on account of their symptoms may be best served by neuroleptic treatment, commencing with chlorpromazine or thioridazine, both of which have sedating properties; while the patient experiencing paranoid delusions may feel more secure with a non-sedating neuroleptic such as risperidone or haloperidol. Similarly, lifestyle issues need to be considered. For example, a person whose occupation involves manual dexterity will not benefit from neuroleptics which cause detectable EPS. A major task of the clinician is to minimize side-effects by avoiding the use of more than one neuroleptic at a time, by using small doses below the EPS threshold whenever possible, and by using adjuncts such as benztropine or benzodiazepines to diminish side-effects. A few general rules can be applied to guide the prescription of neuroleptics for patients with first-episode psychosis:

(1) The optimal dosage of drug should aim at maximizing therapeutic benefit while minimizing unwanted side-effects.
(2) Starting doses should be extremely low, particularly in first-episode patients who are drug-naïve.
(3) Dosage adjustments should occur in small increments and at appropriately spaced intervals – in our experience 3–4 weeks.
(4) Polypharmacy should be avoided where possible, but the clinician should remain mindful of the frequent need to use antidepressant or mood stabilizer drugs in conjunction with neuroleptics.

Atypical antipsychotic drugs
The chief advantage of the recently developed serotonin–dopamine antagonist drugs (including risperidone, sertindole, and olanzapine) is the effect on serotonin (5HT2) and cholinergic pathways which provide intrinsic protection against the EPS caused by the dopamine blockage

(D2) also produced by these drugs. Risperidone was shown to be equally, if not slightly more, efficacious when compared to dose equivalents of haloperidol in a multicentre double-blind controlled trial ($n = 183$) of previously untreated first-episode psychosis patients, with significantly higher side-effects being reported in the haloperidol group (Emsley, McCreadie & Livingston, 1995). There is evidence suggesting that risperidone is more effective than traditional neuroleptics for relieving negative symptoms (Hoyberg et al., 1993), but no proper comparison has yet been reported with clozapine (Carpenter & Buchanan, 1994). In treating first-episode psychosis patients, our clinical experience is that low doses of risperidone, i.e. between 2 and 4 mg/day, are effective for most patients.

The use of clozapine in first-episode psychosis has not been well researched, but Szymanski et al. (1994) reported moderate responses with clozapine in a small group ($n = 10$) of treatment-refractory first-episode schizophreniform patients. Meltzer & Okayli (1995) recommended that clozapine should be prescribed early in patients with high risk factors such as suicide. With first-episode psychosis patients, we have found that clozapine is a useful neuroleptic to use in clinical situations where two other neuroleptics have been used but have failed to achieve significant symptom remission. The place of clozapine in treating first-episode psychosis patients requires further research, but clearly it is important to treat refractory psychotic symptoms as vigorously as possible, in order to decrease the duration of illness and prevent deterioration in the quality of life or constraint on the level of recovery.

Mood stabilizers
In schizophreniform disorders, lithium has been shown to be of benefit as an adjunct to neuroleptic treatment in patients, particularly with complicating affective features, its effect typically being evident by the end of the first week of treatment (Zemlan et al., 1984). Lithium potentiates neuroleptic effects (Christison, Kirsch & Wyatt, 1991) and therefore can be a useful addition to, or mainstay of, treatment, enabling neuroleptics to be spared; however, a higher incidence of neurotoxicity has been reported with the combination of lithium and some neuroleptics under certain conditions (Christison, Kirsch & Wyatt, 1991).

In view of the high incidence of affective symptoms found in first-episode psychosis (McGorry, 1992), we recommend the use of adjunctive lithium carbonate as an effective strategy – particularly for those patients who meet the diagnostic criteria for schizoaffective disorders. Lithium remains the recommended first-line treatment for manic psychosis in combination with a neuroleptic, although Bowden et al. (1995)

has reported that mild mania may respond to lithium as a monotherapy. Other mood stabilizers, such as carbamazepine and sodium valproate, have been consistently reported as effective in treating non-responders to lithium (McElroy et al., 1992) and atypical forms of mania.

Antidepressants
Patients who suffer from prominent depressive symptoms as part of their psychotic illness, may require both antidepressant drugs and neuroleptics. Spiker et al. (1985), in a general study, found that four-fifths of patients with delusional depression responded to a combination of antidepressants and antipsychotics. Selective serotonin reuptake inhibitors (SSRIs), prescribed in combination with neuroleptics, have been reported to be as effective as a tricyclic antidepressant combination, but to have lower levels of side-effects (Rothschild et al., 1993). The role of ECT in treating first-episode psychosis is not well studied, but patients who demonstrate depressive symptoms which are resistant to antidepressant medications, may benefit from a course of unilateral ECT. Kellner (1995) discussed a role for ECT in treatment-resistant first-episode psychosis. This therapeutic strategy can be feasible; however, the reasonable and familiar fear of patients and relatives must be carefully explored and responded to. Although used in 5% of cases of first-episode psychosis, and usually with good results, ECT can arouse strong images which resonate with people's worst stereotypes of psychiatric treatment.

Medication decision tree
Some general principles for deciding about the types of medication to be used in treating first-episode psychosis are depicted in Figure 7.1. Time scales are not incorporated in the decision tree because of the considerable variation in medication response times.

Issues related to the administration of medication in first-episode psychosis
A patient's initial experience with medication, and the information provided by others, clearly can play a major role in later adherence to treatment. Weiden, Manewitz & Dixon (1989), in a study of medication compliance among patients with schizophrenia in the first two years of their treatment, reported that 48% of patients were non-compliant in the first year and 74% of patients were non-compliant with medication by the end of two years. In the context of the age of the first-episode psychosis patient group and the preceding data, non-compliance is actually the norm, rather than the exception, under standard conditions.

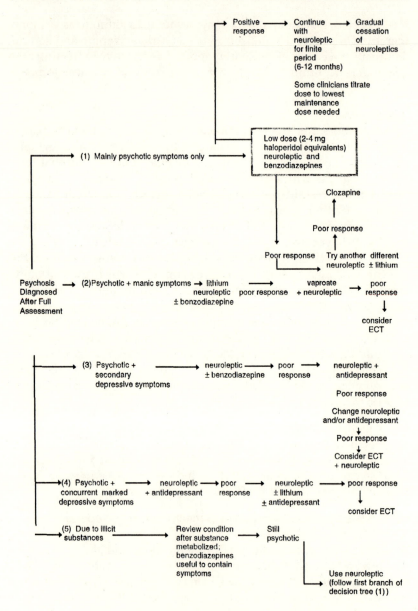

Figure 7.1. Framework for drug treatment of first-episode psychosis.

7 INITIAL TREATMENT OF FIRST-EPISODE PSYCHOSIS

Although adherence to treatment is a more general issue than that of medication, it is medication which usually becomes the particular focus of concern in treatment compliance. Clearly, attitudes towards illness, and insight and concerns about medication effects, are important influences on adherence rates (McEvoy et al., 1989). Even providing a relatively brief commitment to addressing these issues initially may reap considerable benefits in the long term by minimizing later non-compliance, relapses and utilization of acute services.

Administering medication to the patient should be considered as a negotiation between clinician and patient (and his/her family). Identifying, and dealing with, the patient's anxieties about medication empowers the patient which, in turn, leads to greater adherence. Several common fears are expressed by first-episode patients regarding medication and some suggested methods of dealing with them are presented in Table 7.1.

Clinicians managing medication, or aspects of the same, for patients with first-episode psychosis, need to be flexible in their approach and prepared to listen and act on problems experienced by the patient. The premature use of depot medication in these patients usually represents an admission of failure to address the complexity of the issues discussed above, and follows the soft option of blaming the patient for 'non-compliance'. It is justified only in a small minority of patients for specific reasons, such as where denial is extreme and where the risks associated with relapse are severe.

Psychosocial interventions

Cognitive strategies

A detailed description of cognitive behaviour therapy (CBT) interventions in first-episode psychosis is given in Chapter 10.

Briefly, our experience with individual CBT-like interventions suggests that CBT hastens and consolidates the resolution of psychotic symptoms. This may occur through assisting patients to recognize their symptoms, label them appropriately, deal with secondary affective features, and via the use of various distraction or desensitization techniques. More specific targeting of delusional beliefs and hallucinations may also be effective in attempting to attenuate these features before they become too deeply entrenched.

An extended period of engagement is recommended in the initial week of inpatient treatment, during which time the context and evolution of the patient's psychotic experiences are explored collaboratively. In our experience, the second to fourth week of pharmacological

Table 7.1. *Common fears regarding drug therapy in first-episode psychosis*

	Common fears		Suggested strategies
1.	Loss of control for patient by taking mind drugs. Fear of medicine changing personality.	1.	Engage patient as a participant in medication management. Explore the person's explanatory model for his/her current problems or predicament. Find a rationale for drug therapy the person can accept. Education about drug effects and mode of action is very important. Avoid enforced medication (such as intramuscular injections, depot drugs).
2.	Fear of side-effects of drugs. Fear of effects of drugs in all areas of functioning such as work, social, sexual, planning for future. Fears of addiction to medication.	2.	Use lowest possible dose of drug and, if side-effects occur, treat quickly. Avoid pressure to increase dose prematurely. Clear explanations about medications and their side-effects are needed. Explanation should be repeated during different illness phases. Different educational media are usually helpful. Educate family.
3.	Concern about stigma is attached to taking neuroleptics.	3.	Minimize obvious side-effects that may draw undue attention to patient, e.g. rigid posture, salivation, blunt affect, etc. Supportive psychotherapy to enable the patient to deal with stigma. Explore person's own attitudes to psychiatric illness and encourage a review if denial permits.
4.	Fear of altered lifestyle due to medication.	4.	Prescribe doses at times that can be adhered to by the patient. Avoid polypharmacy. Discuss medication interactions with other drugs and alcohol. Be prepared to change medication if side-effects unacceptable to the patient.

Table 7.1. (continued)

	Common fears		Suggested strategies
5.	Fear of emptiness – if symptoms such as long-standing hallucinations are cured by medication then this may create a vacuum in the patient's life.	5.	Institute broad management strategies that assist person to develop or regain skills in occupation and leisure.
6.	Where there is a family history of psychosis, there can be several issues for the patient being prescribed the same medication as a patient or sibling.	6.	Explore the person's feelings about the other family member/s, their attitudes and response to medications. The patient's positive or negative identification with a sick relative has a strong bearing on whether he/she wants to be prescribed the same drug as the relative.
7.	Fears of life-long medication	7.	Give a clear outline of the plan of drug management and a realistic time course (one the particular patient may be able to tolerate). Suggest titration of dose with incremental decrease related to symptom response between 6 and 9 months after illness improves (Baldessarini et al., 1988).
8.	Fears that medication will not work	8.	Ongoing explanation about mode of action. Reinforce and highlight signs of improvement. Utilize family/other staff observations of improvement. Discuss reasons and plans if a change in medication is needed. Outline expected time course and response to medication.

treatment is a crucial phase for introducing CBT techniques which 'challenge' the patient's delusional beliefs and hallucinatory experiences. It is at this stage that most patients will begin to develop insight and their psychotic experiences will begin to resolve along a continuum with normal experiences. During the recovery phase many patients are quite amenable to reframing these psychotic experiences. This is assisted by the immediate nature of those experiences and by the provision of appropriate alternative explanations through psychoeducation. Then the patient is assisted in attempting to validate or invalidate their 'faulty assumptions' by an examination of the evidence and generation of alternative explanations, e.g. stress vulnerability model.

In the early recovery phase, it is essential to follow up these interventions after discharge from hospital in order to provide debriefing and counselling for the patients who may have experienced the psychotic episode as traumatic. Furthermore, CBT may assist with rebuilding the person's self-esteem through addressing negative self-constructs and self-stigmatization. Secondary morbidity such as depression and social anxiety which are commonly experienced in the recovery phase may be usefully addressed by CBT. Skills training, stress management, the teaching of problem-solving techniques and cognitive strategies, help the person to return to previously important activities which will, in turn, further reinforce hope in recovery and self-esteem. Psychoeducation regarding treatment options and relapse prevention strategies promote a sense of mastery over the illness and help instill a realistic appraisal of the risk of relapse. However, this is often a complex and idiosyncratic process in a young person with no prior experience of the health care system.

Nursing interventions
The role of well trained nursing staff is crucial to: risk management, aggression control, collaborative engagement in activities, non-confrontational negotiation of limits to behaviour with presentation of choices, and empowerment of patients in decisions concerning management. By virtue of their more frequent face-to-face contact with patients than other professional staff, inpatient nursing staff may be more aware of the daily experiences of patients and have higher levels of concern about their safety (Thomas, Bartlett & Mezey, 1995).

Special nursing aspects related to the home-based management of first-episode psychosis patients, are considered in Chapter 8. When one focusses on the hospital management of these patients, there are several essential nursing skills. These lead to better care and include: avoidance of excessive use of sedation and PRN medication, avoidance of seclusion and restraint, use of 'specialling' or one-to-one nursing, rather than

7 INITIAL TREATMENT OF FIRST-EPISODE PSYCHOSIS

reliance on physical containment, high dependency units and locked wards. Patients admitted for the first time may be particularly traumatized by these interventions which confirm their worst fears of psychiatric institutions. In a study by Wadeson & Carpenter (1976) of the experiences and feelings of patients about their illness and treatment, one-third of patients recalled their negative feelings about past experiences of seclusion.

Nursing training in CBT and supportive psychotherapy, and careful management of the quality of the inpatient environment, atmosphere and morale, has the considerable potential to enhance the overall acute care provided for the first-episode psychosis patient.

Family interventions

It is vital to provide prompt attention to the needs of carers, adopting a crisis intervention model with psychoeducation aiming at minimizing carers' stress, confusion, and maximizing their support for the patient. Chapter 14 specifically deals with family issues related to the first episode of psychosis.

Families of first-episode patients have several areas of special need. Often, a considerable amount of blame and guilt is experienced by family members as they search for a reason for the illness. In some ways, traditional illness models can ease the burden of guilt on families and patients by initially deflecting aetiology of psychosis onto 'neutral' objects such as neurotransmitter aberrations. Later, when the initial shock has subsided, careful exploration of precipitating and perpetuating stresses in the patient's life may be useful. While some families may not have been functioning optimally, the acute phase is not the time to explore the basis for this and managing the immediate crisis is the first task. Families may need explanation of the patient's behaviour, to understand that paranoid delusions about them or bizarre behaviour in general and negative symptoms spring from illness rather than 'bad' behaviour. Considerable reassurance is needed and engagement of the family as a management ally is an important asset. People suffering a first episode of psychosis are often young and living with parents, so the normal developmental tasks of adolescence can be severely hampered by illness. Often, families may have been experiencing difficulties with 'normal' adolescent behaviour, but this may be exaggerated in the psychotic patient. A major dilemma for families is about 'over-' or 'under-limit-setting' on the patient's activities when recovering from psychosis. Family issues and interventions are further detailed in Chapter 14.

Women generally tend to present with first psychotic episodes between 5 and 10 years later than men (Häfner et al., 1989). This often means that they have left their family of origin, and may have their own children. Family work here involves similar supportive psychotherapy for the spouse and children. A major issue to deal with sensitively and quickly is the question of child care when the single mother is ill. Clinicians have a responsibility to both the woman and her children. Unfortunately, there is often little understanding of the nature of good recovery from psychosis amongst some community services, and this can lead to hasty decisions about awarding custody of children to others. Clearly, the loss of children is devastating for the patient and even the fear that this may happen may precipitate secondary morbidity or relapse. While there will be situations where this may be temporarily or permanently justified, it is a major decision and should only be made after a series of other options are tried (Cowling, McGorry & Hay, 1995).

Patients requiring special consideration

There are some subgroups of patients requiring special consideration and some are briefly discussed below.

Treatment-resistant first-episode psychosis patients

Discussed more fully by Birchwood (see Chapter 9), our experience has been that response to treatment is commonly related to duration of illness rather than the severity of illness. Christison, Kirsch & Wyatt (1991), in an extensive review of alternative treatments for non-responsive psychotic patients, concluded that clozapine, adjunctive lithium and adjunctive benzodiazepines exert the best overall outcome. Psychological and social treatments are essential adjuncts and have an augmenting effect on the resolution of psychotic symptoms (Drury et al., 1996a,b).

Patients with complicating substance abuse disorders

Apart from the difficulties in differential diagnosis and assessment in patients with psychosis complicated by substance abuse, treatment is further complicated by the effects of these substances on medication use and difficulties in combining complementary management strategies to address both disorders adequately. Psychostimulants, hallucinogens, alcohol, and a number of other substances of abuse, e.g. marijuana, may precipitate or aggravate psychotic symptoms via their effects on neurotransmitter systems. Finally, medication compliance, social instability, relapse and rehospitalization are reportedly significantly worse in young mentally ill substance abusers (Drake & Wallach, 1989; Linszen, Dingemans & Lenior, 1994) (see also Chapter 13).

Patients with mental retardation

Mental retardation carries a higher risk for schizophrenia with rates being reported at 3% (Turner, 1989). Patients with even mild mental retardation are difficult to accommodate in mainstream psychiatric services due to their limitations in communication skills and functioning. Unusual behavioural problems are very common among people with mental retardation, e.g. self-mutilation and autistic behaviours. Physical and neurological disabilities, e.g. cerebral palsy and epilepsy, commonly complicate patients with moderate and severe mental retardation (Turner, 1989). Even if psychosis develops, it is usually more appropriate to manage these patients within a specialized service for mental retardation, including residential units with secondary consultation or community-based treatment (Royal College of Psychiatrists, 1986).

Conclusion

The effective initial management of a person's first episode of psychosis should improve outcomes and limit the impact of psychosis for patients and relatives, particularly in the short to medium term when vulnerability to the disabling effects of psychosis is at its peak. Early detection, comprehensive assessment and collaborative engagement in treatment have proven benefits and low-dose antipsychotic medication should be the norm. Addressing psychological factors and protecting the patient's developmental trajectory is essential to maximizing the potential for recovery.

References

Amador, X. F., Strauss, D. H., Yale, S. A., Flaum, M., Endicott, J. & Gorman, J. M. (1993). Assessment of insight in psychosis. *American Journal of Psychiatry*, **150**, 873–9.

Andreasen, N. C. (1984). *The Broken Brain: The Biological Revolution in Psychiatry*. New York: Harper & Row.

Angermeyer, M. C. & Kuhn, L. (1988). Gender differences in age at onset of schizophrenia: an overview. *European Archives of Psychiatry and Clinical Neuroscience*, **237**, 351–64.

Atakan, Z. (1995). Violence on psychiatric inpatient unit. What can be done? *Psychiatry Bulletin*, **19**, 593–7.

Baldessarini, R. J., Cohen, B. M. & Teicher, M. (1988). Significance of neuroleptic dose and plasma level in the pharmacological treatment of psychosis. *Archives of General Psychiatry*, **45**, 79–91.

Bleuler, E. (1950). *Dementia Praecox or the Group of Schizophrenias*. Translated by J. Zinkin. New York: International University Press.

Bowden, C. L., Calabrese, J. R., Wallin, B. A., Swan, A., McElroy, S. L., Risch, S. C. & Hirschfeld, R. M. A. (1995). Illness characteristics of patients in clinical drug studies of mania. *Psychopharmacology Bulletin*, **31**, 103–9.

Breier, A. & Strauss, J. S. (1983). Self control in psychotic disorder. *Archives of General Psychiatry*, **40**, 1141–54.

Carpenter, W. T. & Buchanan, R. W. (1994). Schizophrenia: reply. *New England Journal of Medicine*, **331**, 276.

Chadwick, P. D. & Lowe, C. F. (1990). Measurement and modification of delusional beliefs. *Journal of Consulting and Clinical Psychology*, **58**, 225–32.

Christison, G. W., Kirsch, D. G. & Wyatt, R. J. (1991). When symptoms persist: choosing among alternative somatic treatments in schizophrenia. *Schizophrenia Bulletin*, **17**, 217–45.

Cowling, V., McGorry, P. D. & Hay, D. A. (1995). Children of parents with psychotic disorders. *The Medical Journal of Australia*, **163**, 119–20.

Drake, R. E. & Wallach, M. A. (1989). Substance abuse among the chronic mentally ill. *Hospital and Community Psychiatry*, **40**, 1041–6.

Drury, V., Birchwood, M., Cochrane, R. & Macmillan, F. (1996a). Cognitive therapy and recovery from acute psychosis: a controlled trial. I. Impact on psychotic symptoms. *British Journal of Psychiatry*, **169**, 593–601.

Drury, V., Birchwood, M., Cochrane, R. & Macmillan, F. (1996b). Cognitive therapy and recovery from acute psychosis: a controlled trial. II. Impact on recovery time. *British Journal of Psychiatry*, **169**, 602–7.

Emsley, R. A., McCreadie, R. & Livingston, M. (1995). Risperidone in the treatment of first episode patients with schizophreniform disorder. Abstract presented at the 8th ENCP Congress, Venice, Italy, October, 1995.

Garety, P., Kuipers, L., Fowler, D., Chamberlain, F. & Dunn G. (1994). Cognitive behavioural therapy for drug resistant psychosis. *British Journal of Medical Psychology*, **67**, 259–71.

Häfner, H., Riecher-Rössler, A., Maurer, K., Löffler, W., Munk-Jorgensen, P. & Strömgren, E. (1989). How does gender influence age at first hospitalization for schizophrenia? A transnational case register study. *Psychological Medicine*, **19**, 903–18.

Heinrichs, D. W., Cohen, B. P. & Carpenter, W. T. (1985). Early insight and the management of schizophrenic decompensation. *Journal of Nervous and Mental Disease*, **173**, 133–8.

Hoyberg, O. J., Fensbo, C., Remvig, J., Lingjaerde, O., Sloth-Nielsen, M. & Salvesen, I. (1993). Risperidone versus perphenazine in the treatment of chronic schizophrenic patients with acute exacerbations. *Acta Psychiatrica Scandinavica*, **88**, 395–401.

Jackson, H. J., McGorry, P. D., Edwards, J. & Hulbert, C. (1996). Cognitively oriented psychotherapy for early psychosis (COPE). In *Early Intervention and Prevention in Mental Health*, ed. P. J. Cotton & H. J. Jackson, pp. 131–54. Melbourne: Australian Psychological Society.

Jackson, H. J., McGorry, P., Edwards, J., Hulbert, C., Henry, L., Francey, S.,

Maude, D., Cocks, J., Power, P., Harrigan, S. & Dudgeon, P. (1998). Cognitively oriented psychotherapy for early psychosis (COPE): preliminary results. *British Journal of Psychiatry* (Supplement) In press.

Kane, J. (1993). The use of higher dose antipsychotic medication. *British Journal of Psychiatry*, **164**, 431–2.

Keks, N., Kulkarni, J. & Copolov, D. (1989). Treatment of schizophrenia. *Medical Journal of Australia*, **151**, 462–57.

Kellner, C. (1995). Is ECT the treatment of choice for first break psychosis? (Editorial). *Convulsive Therapy*, **11**, 155–7.

Klein, D. F. & Davis, J. M. (1969). *Diagnosis and Drug Treatment of Psychiatric Disorders*. Baltimore: Williams and Wilkins.

Lieberman, J. A. (1993). Prediction of outcome in first-episode schizophrenia. *Journal of Clinical Psychiatry*, **54**, 13–17.

Lieberman, J., Jody, D., Geisler, S., Alvir, J. M., Loebel, A., Szymanski, S., Woerner, M. & Borenstein, M. (1993). Time course and biologic correlates of treatment response in first episode schizophrenia. *Archives of General Psychiatry*, **50**, 369–76.

Linszen, D., Dingemans, P. & Lenior, M. (1994). Cannabis abuse and the course of schizophrenic disorders. *Archives of General Psychiatry*, **51**, 273–9.

Loebel, A. D., Leiberman, J. A., Alvir, J. M. J., Mayerhoff, D. I., Geisler, S. H. & Szymanski, S. R. (1992). Duration of psychosis outcome in first episode schizophrenia. *American Journal of Psychiatry*, **149**, 1183–8.

Malla, A. K. & Norman, R. M. G. (1994). Prodromal symptoms in schizophrenia. *British Journal of Psychiatry*, **164**, 487–93.

Mason, P., Harrison, G., Glazebrook, C., Medley, I., Dalkin, T. & Croudace, T. (1995). Characteristics of outcome in schizophrenia at 13 years. *British Journal of Psychiatry*, **167**, 596–603.

McCandless-Glimcher, L., McKnight, S., Hamera, E., Smith, B. L., Peterson, K. A. & Plumlee, A. A. (1986). Use of symptoms by schizophrenics to monitor and regulate their illness. *Hospital and Community Psychiatry*, **37**, 929–33.

McElroy, S., Keck, P., Pope, H. & Hudson, J. (1992). Valproate in the treatment of bipolar disorder. Literature review and clinical guidelines. *Journal of Clinical Pharmacology*, **12**, 42S–52S.

McEvoy, J. P., Hogarty, G. E. & Steingard, S. (1991). Optimal dose of neuroleptic in acute schizophrenia: a controlled study of neuroleptic threshold and higher haloperidol dose. *Archives of General Psychiatry*, **48**, 739–45.

McEvoy, J. P., Apperson, L. J., Applebaum, P. S., Ortlip, P., Brecosky, J., Hammill, K., Geller, J. L. & Roth, L. (1989). Insight in schizophrenia. Its relationship to acute psychopathology. *Journal of Nervous and Mental Disease*, **177**, 43–7.

McGorry, P. D. (1992). The concept of recovery and secondary prevention in psychotic disorders. *Australian and New Zealand Journal of Psychiatry*, **237**, 3–17.

McGorry, P. D. & Kulkarni, J. (1994). Prevention and preventively oriented clinical care in psychotic disorders. *Australian Journal of Psychopharmacology*, **7**, 62–9.

Meltzer, H. & Okayli, G. (1995). The reduction of suicidality during clozapine treatment in neuroleptic resistant schizophrenics. *American Journal of Psychiatry*, **152**, 183–90.

Nordstrom, A. L., Farde, L., Wiesel, F. A., Forslund, K., Pauli, S., Halldin, C. & Uppfeldt, G. (1993). Central D2 dopamine receptor occupancy in relation to antipsychotic drug effects: a double-blind PET study of schizophrenic patients. *Biological Psychiatry*, **33**, 227–35.

Power, P. Elkins, K., Adlard, S., Curry, C., McGorry, P. D. & Harrigan, S. (in press). An analysis of initial treatment of first episode psychosis. *British Journal of Psychiatry*. (Supplement) in press.

Remington, G., Kapur, S. & Zipursky, R. B. (In press). Pharmacotherapy of first episode psychosis. *British Journal of Psychiatry* (Supplement).

Riecher-Rössler, A., Fätkenheuer, B., Löffler, W., Maurer, K. & Häfner, H. (1992). Is age of onset in schizophrenia influenced by marital status? *Social Psychiatry and Epidemiology*, **27**, 122–8.

Rothschild, A. J. Samson, J. A., Bessett, M. P. & Carter-Campbell, J. T. (1993). Efficacy of the combination of fluoxetine and perphenazine in the treatment of psychotic depression. *Journal of Clinical Psychiatry*, **54**, 338–42.

Royal College of Psychiatrists (1986). Psychiatric services for mentally handicapped adults and young people. *The Bulletin of the Royal College of Psychiatrists*, **10**, 321–2.

Spiker, D. G., Weiss, J. C., Dealy, R. S., Griffin, S. J., Hanin, I., Neil, J. F., Perel, J. M., Rossi, A. J. & Soloff, P. H. (1985). The pharmacological treatment of delusional depression. *American Journal of Psychiatry*, **142**, 430–5.

Stone, C. K., Garver, D. L., Griffiths, J., Hirschowitz, J. & Bennet, J. (1995). Further evidence of a dose response threshold for haloperidol in psychosis. *American Journal of Psychiatry*, **152**, 1210–12.

Szymanski, S. R., Masiar, S., Mayerhoff, D., Loebel, A., Geisler, S., Pollock, S., Kane, J. & Lieberman, J. (1994). Clozapine response in treatment-refractory first-episode schizophrenia. *Biological Psychiatry*, **35**, 278–80.

Szymanski, S. R., Tyrone, D. C., Gallagher, F., Erwin, R. & Gur, R. (1996). Course of treatment response in first-episode and chronic schizophrenia. *American Journal of Psychiatry*, **153**, 519–25.

Thomas, C., Bartlett, A. & Mezey, G. C. (1995). The extent and effects of violence among psychiatric in-patients. *Psychiatric Bulletin*, **19**, 600–4.

Turner, T. H. (1989). Schizophrenia and mental handicap: an historical review, with implications for further research. *Psychological Medicine*, **19**, 301–14.

Wadeson, H. & Carpenter, W. (1976). Impact of the seclusion room experience. *Journal of Nervous and Mental Disease*, **163**, 318–28.

Wehr, T., Goodwin, F., Wirz-Justice, A., Breitmaier, J. & Craig, C. (1982). 48-hour sleep-wake cycles in manic-depressive illness: naturalistic observations and sleep deprivation experiments. *Archives of General Psychiatry*, **39**, 559–65.

Weiden, P., Manewitz, A. & Dixon, L. (1989) Neuroleptic medication in schizophrenia. Presented at the International Congress of Schizophrenia Research, Santiago, May, 1989.

Wyatt, R. J. (1991). Neuroleptics and the natural course of schizophrenia. *Schizophrenia Bulletin*, **7**, 325–51.

Zemlan, F. P., Hirschowitz, J., Sautter, F. J. & Garver, D. L. (1984). Impact of lithium therapy on core psychotic symptoms of schizophrenia. *British Journal of Psychiatry*, **144**, 64–9.

8

Home-based treatment of first-episode psychosis

JAYASHRI KULKARNI

Introduction

The world-wide implementation of deinstitutionalization has led to the rapid growth of community-based psychiatric treatment. Many studies (Anthony, Buell & Sara, 1972; Bond, Miller & Krumweid, 1988; Braff & Lefkowitz, 1989; Dharwadkar, 1994) have focussed on models of community psychiatric care which are predominantly 'after-care' models designed to allow earlier discharge of patients from hospital and prevent readmission. Hoult's work (Hoult, 1984a,b, 1986; Hoult, Reynolds & Charbonneau-Powis, 1983) emphasized the clinical feasibility of managing acutely psychotic people in community settings. Stein & Test (1980) developed a model of assertive community living programmes for severely disabled, chronically unwell individuals with schizophrenia, while Wright, Hener & Shape (1989) outlined the large costs involved in the intensive management of patients recently discharged after prolonged periods in hospital.

In a recent review of home-based versus hospital-based care, Marks et al. (1994) conducted a controlled trial in which 92 patients were managed at home (daily living programme; DLP) and were compared with 97 patients initially managed in standard inpatient and, later, outpatient settings. The DLP model constituted a programme of problem-orientated activities aimed at improving patients' quality of life. Patients remained in the study for 18 months. One hundred and eighty nine patients were randomly allocated to DLP or standard inpatient care, with the patients being cared for mainly by psychiatric nurses using case management principles.

Sixty five per cent of all patients were potential new admissions, but the DLP programme was not orientated to deal with the specific problems facing individuals suffering from their first-episode of psychosis. At the nine-month mark of the study, 55% of DLP patients had been admitted at least once to hospital. The total number of admissions for DLP was 160, with 159 admissions being recorded for the control patients. This high number of admissions and comparability across both groups, suggests that the DLP model was not able adequately to maintain young psychotic people out of hospital. The DLP did decrease the duration of the admissions by 80% when the community team was responsible for discharge; and, overall, Marks et al., (1994) did find that the DLP group outcome was superior to that of the control group, in terms of psychotic symptom improvement, social adjustment, patient satisfaction and economic costs.

However, Marks et al. (1994) did not find any sustained long-term improvement, although the follow-up period was only 20 months. Three DLP patients suffering from depression committed suicide, and one man with paranoid schizophrenia killed a neighbour's baby. This led to considerable adverse publicity for the DLP intervention, and added to the resistance from authorities already encountered by the authors. Thornicroft & Breakey (1991) have also described community care as being unable to 'cure' serious mental illness, emphasizing the need for continuing long-term support. Again, Thornicroft & Breakey's work does not include a home-based programme specifically designed for the treatment of first-episode psychosis. While community psychiatric care aspects have been studied in both uncontrolled and controlled trials (Burns, Beardsmore & Bhat, 1993; Dick, Cameron & Cohen, 1985; Fenton, Tessier & Struening, 1979), the acute home-based treatment of young people suffering their first-episode of psychosis has not received much specific attention in the literature.

In view of the high prevalence of secondary morbidity, including depression and post-traumatic stress disorder (McGorry et al., 1991), in hospitalized recent-onset psychosis patients, it seems appropriate to adopt a preventive approach to secondary morbidity by managing the patient in a community setting if, and where, possible. Falloon (1992) discussed the home-based management of people identified as suffering from the prodromal symptoms of schizophrenia, emphasizing a stress management approach; however, Falloon did not routinely extend home-based clinical treatment to individuals experiencing an acute initial episode of psychosis.

By extending some of Falloon's work, and utilizing the principles of community psychiatric care, an integrated home-based management programme was developed for people suffering from their first episode of psychosis. The bulk of this chapter describes this home-based approach, with the aims of this approach including the effective treatment of the psychotic episode, the prevention of secondary morbidity, the rapid return of the patient to their usual lifestyle, the reduction in relapse rates, and the improvement in patients' quality of life and their satisfaction with the delivery of the clinical service.

Key factors in successful home-based management of first-episode psychosis

The success of a home-based approach in meeting the aforementioned aims depends on a number of factors pertaining to the individuals, their families and the treating team; these are now each discussed in some detail.

The individual

Severe psychotic illness in itself does not appear to present a barrier to successful home-based treatment. In fact, clinical experience suggests that it is the *dangerousness* of the symptoms expressed by the patient, rather than the *intensity* of these same symptoms, that appears to determine whether or not an individual will require hospitalization. Also, suicidal or homicidal thoughts and actions require thorough investigation and may mitigate against home-based treatment. Similarly, hostility directed towards family members and prompted by delusional material, requires equally careful assessment and might also rule out home treatment. Whether or not the identified patient has ready access to firearms or other weapons at home, needs to be thoroughly investigated and dealt with in the initial assessment of the individual. Indeed, clinicians need to perform regular ongoing risk assessments for suicidality and dangerous behaviour.

Illicit substance abuse is a serious problem, because of the role played by marijuana and amphetamine use in precipitating or perpetuating psychosis (see Chapter 13) (Linszen, Dingemans & Lenior, 1994; Martinez-Arevalo et al., 1994; Negrete, 1989; Thomas, 1993). The client's family need to be able to prevent the individual from having access to illicit drugs during the acute illness phase. Drug rehabilitation issues should be addressed by the treating team when the individual has recovered from acute psychosis.

The person's role in the family and issues of compliance with treatment need to be assessed to optimize home-based treatment. A shared illness model between patients, their families and the treating clinicians may be useful, but it is not always necessary for successful home-based treatment. It seems more useful for all parties concerned to agree on the management strategies and their implementation, rather than focussing intensely on understanding the possible reasons for the onset of psychosis.

The family

An early understanding of the person's family is of paramount importance in managing the acutely psychotic individual at home. Without the co-operation of a caring family, the home-based treatment approach is clearly a difficult, if not viable, alternative to inpatient care. Since the family are the constant primary carers in this model, assessment of their needs and capabilities are of great importance. To this end, a family rating scale (see Appendix 1), is currently being developed to assist in the rapid assessment of the family's ability to embark on home-based treatment. This scale focusses on several key areas with priority being given to assessment of the family's physical and emotional state and with special attention being given to sleep deprivation and signs of physical neglect in family members.

The families of hospitalized patients are generally given secondary importance in mental health delivery systems. In our model of treatment, the welfare and health of families are just as important to the treating clinicians as the needs of the identified client. So, for example, clinicians need to assess carefully those family members who have 'rostered' themselves on for 'night duty' at home and for how long they have been undertaking such 'tasks'. The family's work schedules, availability, and resources in terms of extended family/friends networks, are important ingredients in determining a successful outcome for home-based treatment. Poor current family interaction patterns and pre-existing family problems are difficulties that may be exacerbated during this phase. Paradoxically, in this model the presence of high family expressed emotion (Pai & Roberts, 1983) may be somewhat advantageous during the acute phase of illness. Provided the hostility and critical components are not pronounced, people with over-involved families tend to remain engaged in treatment and recover more quickly compared with people who have more distant, disengaged families.

Containment of the sick individual by the family is another major determinant of successful home-based treatment, and families may need to be given permission by the treatment team and empowered, for example, to confiscate the patient's car keys or take other similar actions, before treatment can commence. Disengaged families often experience difficulties in containing the individual because of splitting amongst the family members over the best course of action. Family burden issues may appear in the later phases of prolonged illness, but are related, at least in part, to the individual's rate and type of recovery, this again reinforcing the need for rapid, effective treatment of psychotic symptoms (Stirling et al., 1991).

The crisis intervention model is applicable in working with the families of first-episode psychosis patients in the initial stages of treatment. The implementation and explanation of clear management plans is very important, especially in view of the almost prototypic early family reactions of confusion, guilt, denial and emotional numbing. It is equally important for the family to receive an unambiguously clear message of favourable recovery and outcome from the treating team. Families and people suffering from psychosis are usually not familiar either with the management of psychiatric illness, nor with home-based treatment; therefore, the tasks for the treating team are to demystify both approaches for the family and sick individual (see also Chapter 14).

The treating team

Clinicians involved in home-based treatment need to understand and work within an entirely different framework from that found in hospital- or clinic-based practices. The treating team are 'guests' in the patient's home and, as such, need to respect that the power relationships are different. Loss of control over the working environment, lack of access to medical equipment, diminished access to other colleagues, and safety issues, are but some of the new challenges which confront the treating team and with which they need to cope. This type of work requires a great deal of flexibility from clinicians. Since clinicians must make many vital decisions about the person and the family's safety, as well as monitor diverse aspects of treatment, it is imperative that they are sufficiently experienced and confident in making independent decisions. All members of the multidisciplinary team, including medical staff, need to be able to function well in both their specialty roles and as generic community team clinicians. To illustrate this point:

> The team was asked to treat a 27-year-old woman with first-episode psychosis, and at the initial assessment clinicians had to assist with the management of her father who had recently suffered an acute myocardial infarction, deal with her extremely agitated mother, and negotiate with the electricity company to reinstate power that had been cut because of a 'failure to pay the bill'.

Staffing numbers need to be sufficient to allow the clinicians to visit the patient's home up to three times per day, when and if necessary, during the hyperacute phase. Our experience suggests that small specialist teams providing home-based treatment suffer from higher rates of 'burn-out' related to overwork. Instead, the incorporation of the ideals and goals of home-based treatment for first-episode psychosis into a larger, general community treatment team, allows greater flexibility of rostering and a better ability to provide intensive input. Careful rostering is required to overcome the potential problem of the patient and family being seen by too many different team members. Once a good therapeutic alliance has developed between the acutely psychotic individual, family members and clinicians, it is important to maintain continuity of care for at least six months to a year. Again, a larger team with the dual mandates for crisis intervention and continuing care, allows follow-up to take place with the same clinicians.

Confidentiality issues pose many problems for clinicians working within the home-based treatment model. Since the family are functioning as important primary carers, it is often difficult to maintain strict confidentiality with information received from the client. Also, therapeutic interactions usually take place in the family living areas and it is often difficult to create a private setting. However, if privacy is deemed to be the important ingredient in establishing rapport with the individual, then the clinician may conduct interviews in other parts of the home, or in outdoor settings. Again, flexibility is essential; the clinician needs to be able to balance the client's needs with the family's needs. These points are illustrated in the ensuing case study.

> A patient experienced hallucinations and delusions specifically related to his neighbours and was unable to discuss these symptoms in the context of the family home. Many subsequent sessions were conducted in a local fast-food restaurant, allowing some privacy for the individual. With his permission, the clinicians were able to describe his problems to his family and devise management strategies.

Good communication skills are an essential tool for the clinician because the client and family often have no other available sources of information, nor are they able to share experiences with others in a similar situation; therefore, they are virtually totally dependent on the team for information. Also, because families and clients are unfamiliar with mental health systems in general, and the home-based treatment model in particular, they require clear instruction from the clinicians so as to ensure the implementation of management strategies. Not only do management plans need to be clearly explained, but details of the clinicians' visiting times need to be stipulated; both are necessary factors in empowering the client and family – thereby optimizing the success of home-based treatment. In early intervention approaches, clinicians need to be pragmatic, not only in helping the client return to school or work, but also with regard to many other treatment issues. Since the person is living in his or her home environment, this often expedites an earlier return to normal activities, because the client, and others, are less likely to view the client as being 'sick'. Also, because most people equate hospitalization with severe illness, then having the client managed at home minimizes the emergence and entrenchment of the 'sick role'.

The treating team may need to monitor progress quickly at school or work. This means that during the recovery period, team visits should be organized around the client's time commitments. Acting on the client's behalf, the treating team takes up issues with employers or schools, typically much earlier than would occur with hospitalized patients. Early attention to these issues frequently reduces the prospect of the client losing his or her job or of study being compromised; however, it is important that this contact is ongoing and that employers and educators are apprised of, and updated as to, the client's progress. Again, in order to provide the best advocacy for the client, confidentiality issues should be balanced with the need to educate employers about illness and management issues. These points are illustrated in the following case study.

> David is a 20-year-old man who worked in a ceramics factory and developed psychosis over three months. He believed that his workmates had been plotting against him and he heard them talking about him. David became increasingly isolative and one day he threatened his supervisor with physical violence because he believed that his supervisor was spreading rumours about his being homosexual. David was successfully treated at home over a period of three weeks. During this time, David gave permission for the clinicians to meet with his employer and explain his symptoms. Since David was keen to return to work quickly, a meeting was held between his employer, his supervisor and David, with David's key clinician advocating on his behalf and providing general information about psychosis. Good recovery was emphasized and the incident between

David and his supervisor was discussed. David chose to discuss his illness with some workmates and, on his return to work, he received good support from them.

Another important task for the treating team is to ensure that all aspects of management are covered. In hospital or clinic settings, there are usually well-established protocols for assessment and treatment which are frequently followed in a reflex manner by clinicians. In the home-based treatment model where flexibility is an important key, management plans need to be clearly formulated and highlighted for clinicians, carers and clients alike. While the task in hospitals has often been to break down the rigid structures and allow individuals more freedom and flexibility, in the home-based treatment model the clinicians' task is to introduce some structure for carers and individuals in order to optimize a successful outcome.

Specific management strategies for home-based treatment of first-episode psychosis

The 'package' approach

As previously stated, in embarking on home-based treatment for the first-episode of psychosis, all parties require some structure to the management plan. One way of providing carers and clients with a better idea of what to expect has been the development of a treatment package. This is an operating, written timetable, which outlines step-by-step treatment plans and approximate timelines. In hospital settings, clinicians may have the right to answer a carer's questions about a client's probable length of stay with a 'wait and see' response. But in the client's home, the alteration of the power structure compels clinicians to deliver more definite answers. The provision of a working timetable helps to impart a clearer sense of control over the illness for both client and family. There is comfort in having a sense of 'closure' to the illness by timetabling recovery and post-acute follow-up periods. A written package also assists the treating team in ensuring that steps are not forgotten. All packages are formulated with the client and carers, and are individualized. The language used is non-jargonistic, and a tangible treatment schedule often offers hope when carers and clients are grappling with the intangible concept of psychosis. Pragmatism and optimism are essential ingredients in successful home-based treatment. An example of a package is given in Tables 8.1 to 8.4 with the tasks and

Table 8.1. *The tasks and foci of the immediate or crisis phase**

Steps	Tasks and foci of this phase
1	Formulation and delivery of the individual package
2	The provision of a clear visiting schedule by the treatment team
3	Medication (usually sedative) for the client initially, then choose an appropriate antipsychotic
4	Blood tests, x-rays – to check physical health
5	Assessment of troubling symptoms
6	Discussions with the family for the twin purposes of helping the family to cope, and of gathering information about the client prior to their illness
7	Get to know client and family
8	Corresponding need for the client and family to get to know and trust the clinicians
9	Liaise with client's general practitioner

* The average duration of this phase is 2–7 days.

Table 2. *The tasks and foci of the acute phase**

Steps	Tasks and foci of this phase
1	Medication – monitor type and dose of antipsychotic drug Treating team to initially administer medication, then hand over to family. Family members are given both verbal and written instructions on medication administration
2	Monitoring of the patient's pulse, blood pressure and response to medication conducted by the team
3	Discussions with family and client about the nature of psychosis and how medications work. Clinicians respond to family's needs on type and quantity of information
4	Deal with issues of leave from work and organize certificates
5	Discuss family tasks

* The average duration of this phase is 7–10 days.

foci for each of the four phases of treatment being stipulated in each table. These phases are labelled the immediate or crisis phase, the acute phase, the recovery phase, and the follow-up phase. Each of these four phases corresponds to Tables 8.1, 8.2, 8.3, and 8.4, respectively.

While an obvious criticism of a package as shown in Tables 8.1 to 8.4 is that it is simplistic and perhaps overly optimistic, it still provides a framework upon which special individual and personal needs can be

8 HOME-BASED TREATMENT OF FIRST-EPISODE PSYCHOSIS

Table 8.3. *The tasks and foci of the recovery phase**

Steps	Tasks and foci of this phase
1	Discussion with the family and client about how to prevent relapses and early recognition
2	Client to take responsibility for medication. Medication times to be worked out again
3	Number of drugs to be simplified and discussion of when medication can be tapered off – usually about six months from now
4	Discussion about when to return to work and a visiting schedule to be organized

* The average duration of this phase is 14–20 days.

Table 8.4. *The tasks and foci of the follow-up phase**

Steps	Tasks and foci of this phase
1	Discuss progress in terms of work and relationships
2	Watch for relapses – and deal with any
3	Special training – related to socializing at work
4	Discussions with family about how they are coping
5	Tapering off medication and monitoring outcome

* The average duration of this phase is 6–12 months.

built. Along with the package, the clinicians undertake many supportive psychotherapeutic strategies to educate the client and family, all the time aiming for a rapid recovery.

Medication management

In the hyperacute or crisis phase, there is usually an urgent need to reduce anxiety quickly by sedating the patient. This is an especially important step in allowing the anxious and vigilant family to rest and 're-group'. Sedating benzodiazepines, such as temazepam, are very useful in this phase and can be used during the day if necessary, as well as at night. Once physical investigations have been performed and the decision to use an antipsychotic medication is made, then the correct choice of antipsychotic drug is very important. In the home-based treatment model, there is a pressing need to prevent any dangerous side-effects since constant clinical monitoring is not available. Routinely, the treating team needs to carry emergency kits of anticholinergic medications with intravenous and intramuscular injection equipment, as well as other emergency medications and resuscitation equipment. Antipsychotics which possess a gentle onset of action and yield fewer side-effects are superior to drugs which carry a high risk of extrapyramidal side-effects. The newer antipsychotic medications, such as risperidone, are useful because they carry a lower risk of side-effects. A regular dose of diazepam offers useful adjunctive treatment in the early days of treatment. As with all first-episode psychotic patients, the medication regimen should begin at very low doses and be titrated gradually. However, it is important to provide the client with rapid relief from troubling psychotic symptoms. An older antipsychotic drug such as chlorpromazine, can be useful because of its sedating property, but in the home treatment setting it should be prescribed at night, in order to overcome postural hypotension.

In the home-based treatment model it is imperative that the clinicians provide the family and clients with education about the medications, since it is the latter who will be faced with dealing with any resultant problems. Clear guidelines about the response times, side-effects and doses of medications, need to be given. These guidelines should preferably be set out in writing as well as verbally communicated to the client and family. If a high-potency neuroleptic is being used, then prophylactic anticholinergics may be advisable for the first few weeks. Emergency instructions and contact numbers should be given at the first visit. The least possible number of drugs should be used to avoid confusion. Moreover, it is advisable that in the early phase of treatment, the clinicians on the treating team should actually administer the medication and then hand this task over to the family who, eventually, will hand over the responsibility, in turn, to the client. The timing of medication administration can be flexible and should fit in with the client's lifestyle. A sense that there will be some endpoint to drug treatment should be discussed with the client and carers from the beginning of the intervention. This often prevents the sense of the client being given a 'life sentence' on medication being communicated to the family and client. If this positive expectation is not communicated to the family and client, then medication non-compliance may result.

Physical investigations

In the home-based treatment model, it may be more difficult to obtain access to pathology services in order to perform blood tests for haematological, renal, hepatic, illicit substance and electrolyte measures. However, it is important not to overlook the need for both physical examinations and investigations to be conducted, in order to exclude underlying organic disease and to establish baselines for the future as discussed in Chapters 6 and 7. Many private pathology services offer home-based blood and urine testing and should be used if possible. General practitioners (GPs) are routinely contacted by the treatment team very early in the home treatment of a young psychotic person. GPs can provide information about the client's physical health, as well as linking the team and the patient with local pathology services. It should also be possible, ideally in co-operation with the GP, to organize specialized tests, such as a CT brain scan or an MRI scan for the client, on an outpatient basis. The timing and explanations involved in detailing such procedures should be handled carefully, and must involve the family as well. Initially, vital signs monitoring should be conducted by the treatment team clinicians at every visit, and then less frequently according to the client's needs; that is, if changes are made to medication regimens or there are alterations in the client's physical state.

Psychoeducation

Optimism and pragmatism seem to be the keys to successful psychoeducation in the home-based treatment setting. It is imperative that clear instructions about medication and illness are provided to all family members and clients. Multimedia presentations are preferable, as again it must be stressed that the family and client have no other 'peers' from whom to learn about the illness or its management. Myths about psychosis which are damaging, or which may lead to noncompliance with treatment, need to be identified and refuted. Generally, it is more effective overall, to work gently along with the family and client, rather than attempting to enforce the clinicians' models or perspectives dogmatically. Finally, the illness phase needs to be considered when discussing important issues, and clinicians have to be prepared to repeat information at different times to the client and family.

Psychosocial issues

When the client is treated at home, there is often a more rapid reintegration into the community with little resultant secondary morbidity, such as post-traumatic stress disorder or depression; these are more often related to hospitalization issues. The rapid re-integration may mean that the client is eager to return to normal activities, and not keen to participate in formal recovery programmes. Under such circumstances, it may be counterproductive to provide introspective programmes to review the course of the client's illness or putative precipitating factors, particularly if the client is keen to deny the psychotic illness and proceed with his or her life. The home-based treatment model lends itself to encouraging the individual to use denial as a recovery style, at least in the shorter term (McGorry, 1992), although the effect of this on longer-term outcome measures of relapse and symptom exacerbation are yet to be determined.

If clients require specific skills training, or have other socialization needs, then general community resources may be more suitable than specific psychiatric day programmes. This is in keeping with the general ethos of home-based treatment of downplaying the seriousness and potential chronicity of psychosis, but rather adopting the view that psychosis is a treatable and temporary illness. As a 'safety net' preventive strategy, clients should be provided with contact phone numbers for access to clinicians, even after they have been discharged from the programme.

Hospital support for the treatment of first-episode psychosis clients at home

While attempting to manage first-episode clients at home, it is important to monitor continually the progress made by the client, as well as the stress experienced by both the carers and client. If the clinicians believe that carers are not able to undertake, or continue, home-based treatment, then hospitalization should not be viewed as constituting 'failure.' The community treatment team then has the opportunity to work with the client and family to facilitate a non-traumatic hospitalization. Voluntary, short-term hospitalization may afford a useful alternative. The community team can provide support and education for the family while the client is in hospital, and this may assist in arriving at a better outcome for all concerned.

A well integrated hospital and community service allows easier access to inpatient beds and earlier discharge for intensive community follow-up. If staff are familiar with both settings, then continuity of care and the follow-through of management plans can be implemented and better ensured.

Results of a pilot study of home-based treatment of clients with first-episode psychosis

A pilot study of 18 first-episode psychosis patients (11 males, 7 females) managed at home by the Adult Community Treatment Team (ACTT) of Dandenong Hospital in Victoria, Australia, was conducted between

June 1994 and December 1994 (Fitzgerald & Kulkarni, 1998). All patients were referred to ACTT during the six-month study period. Four of the 18 patients were hospitalized. The average age of the 11 male patients was 20.0 ($SD = 2.2$) years. All 11 were single and were living with their family of origin. By contrast, the average age of the seven female patients was 29.1 ($SD = 4.2$) years. Four of the female patients were living with their family of origin, while three were married – each was living with her spouse and children.

In terms of the DSM-IV (APA, 1994) diagnoses accorded to the 11 male patients, seven received diagnoses of schizophrenia or schizophreniform disorder, three schizoaffective disorder, and one bipolar disorder–manic phase. For the females, two received diagnoses of schizophrenia or schizophreniform disorder, two schizoaffective disorder, and three bipolar disorder–manic phase.

With regard to drug and alcohol use, of the 11 males, seven used cannabis, three used amphetamines, two opiates, one used cocaine, and two had used more than 30 grams of alcohol per day for the past three months. (Because some of the males were polydrug abusers, the number of drugs endorsed exceeds $n = 11$). On the other hand, only one of the seven females used drugs or alcohol at all, this person admitting to regular cannabis use.

Psychopathology ratings completed at the first visit showed that the mean 18-item Brief Psychiatric Rating Scale (BPRS) score (Overall & Gorham, 1962) was 38 ($SD = 6.2$) points; the mean Scale for the Assessment of Positive Symptoms (SAPS) score (Andreasen & Olsen, 1982) was 41 ($SD = 8.3$) points; and the mean Scale for the Assessment of Negative Symptoms (SANS) score (Andreasen & Olsen, 1982) was 31 ($SD = 12.3$) points. The maximum daily antipsychotic drug dose in chlorpromazine equivalents ranged from 50 mg to 400 mg. The mean daily dose was 182 ($SD = 89$ mg) chlorpromazine equivalents (which in turn is equal to approximately 4 mg haloperidol). A wide range of neuroleptics was used including chlorpromazine ($n = 8$), thioridazine ($n = 1$), haloperidol ($n = 2$), trifluoperazine ($n = 1$), and risperidone ($n = 6$). Nine patients (seven males, two females) did not accept the treating team's model of illness, although all carers accepted the illness model presented by the team.

In terms of outcome, eight patients (four males, four females) had recovered within 26 days of involvement by the ACTT. Recovery was measured by a significant decrease (greater than, or equal to, a 20-point fall) in SAPS scores, subjective reports by the client and carer, plus a return to their previous occupation. Six patients made good recoveries using these criteria between 26 and 42 days of ACTT involvement. Quality of Life ratings (Heinrichs, Hanlon & Carpenter, 1984) completed pre- and post-treatment for these 14 patients showed a significant rise of 43.3 points. Follow-up over a ten-month period to date, has revealed that one patient suffered a relapse, and this person was treated at home.

The four patients (three males, one female) who required hospitalization were compared with the successfully home-treated group on several measures. There were no significant differences in terms of the BPRS, SAPS, or SANS scores at first or subsequent visits. No differences were found in terms of: medication doses or types, illicit substance use, economic situation, or acceptance of illness models. A clear difference was found in the subjective rating made by the clinicians at first visit of the family's capacity to cope and provide care. While a formal family assessment tool was not used, clinicians rated families on a scale from 1 to 10 on the family's state of anxiety, availability, supportiveness and pre-existing problems. Scores closer to 10 suggested that familes accorded such scores were very capable, when compared with scores closer to 1, which suggest that those lowly-rated families were experiencing great difficulties in coping. When these scores were compared between the groups, there was a significant difference ($p = 0.013$), with the hospitalized group having significantly lower family rating scores. While the sample size is very small and unevenly distributed, this finding concurs with the clinicians' view that a key factor in whether or not home-based treatment is successful depends on the abilities of the family carers. Severity of illness, acceptance of illness models, economic circumstances, and medication regimes, did not seem to influence location of treatment although, again, one needs to be mindful of the very small sample size.

This pilot study was conducted at a time when the model of home-based treatment for first-episode psychosis was at a very early developmental stage. We are continuing to assess and improve our programme. The study measures are crude and the treatment strategies are still in evolution. Fundamentally, the ACTT is a general community psychiatric team comprising 16 staff members who have accumulated five years of experience as a team, working in home-based and boarding-house settings with psychotic clients who are usually chronically disabled. Staff members include three medical staff, two psychologists, one social worker and ten psychiatric nurses. The ACTT provides a 24-hour service, seven days per week. The focus on first-episode patients enables the team to make full use of their already well-developed community psychiatry skills and experience, as well as allowing the team to further develop these skills with a specialist focus.

Dissemination of the goals and strategies for managing first-episode patients was by informal and formal education sessions, and all members of the ACTT were given the opportunity to manage first-episode clients. In this way, the special issues related to the first-episode group were highlighted to the whole team, rather than setting up a small, specialist team. A larger study is continuing, with particular attention being paid to a longer-term follow-up.

Conclusion

Home-based treatment of the patient with first-episode psychosis presents the clinician with several challenges which if met, can provide the patient with excellent outcomes. The careful assessment of carers and individuals, the ongoing monitoring of their progress, and the adoption of flexible treatment approaches, are keys to success in this model. Clinician anxiety is often higher because of the lack of control over the location of the treatment setting, but the resulting decrease in stigma and secondary morbidity for the individual represents a rewarding counter-balance. The home-based treatment model epitomises a number of goals which all clinicians strive to achieve in the optimal treatment of first-episode psychosis. Home-based treatment provides care in a free and familiar environment, empowers the client and carers, emphasizes the need for clinicians to work in close collaboration with the individual and family, necessitates careful and minimal medication regimens, and offers a rapid return to normal lifestyles.

References

American Psychiatric Association (1994). *Diagnostic and Statistical Manual*, 4th edn., DSM-IV. Washington, DC: American Psychiatric Association.

Andreasen, N. C. & Olsen, S. (1982). Negative vs positive schizophrenia: definition and validation. *Archives of General Psychiatry*, **39**, 789–94.

Anthony, W., Buell, G. J. & Sara, S. (1972). The efficacy of psychiatric rehabilitation. *Psychological Bulletin*, **78**, 447–56.

Bond, G. R., Miller, L. D. & Krumweid, R. D. (1988). Assertive case management in three CMHCs: a controlled study. *Hospital and Community Psychiatry*, **39**, 411–8.

Braff, J. & Lefkowitz, M. (1989). Community mental health treatment: what works for whom? *Psychiatry Quarterly*, **51**, 119–34.

Burns, T., Beardsmore, A. & Bhat, A. V. (1993). A controlled trial of home based acute psychiatric services. *British Journal of Psychiatry*, **163**, 49–61.

Dick, P., Cameron, L. & Cohen, D. (1985). Day and full time psychiatric treatment – a controlled comparison. *British Journal of Psychiatry*, **147**, 246–9.

Dharwadkar, N. (1994). Effectiveness of an assertive outreach community treatment program. *Australian and New Zealand Journal of Psychiatry*, **28**, 244–9.

Falloon, I. R. H. (1992). Early intervention for first episodes of schizophrenia: a preliminary exploration. *Psychiatry*, **55**, 4–15.

Fenton, F. R., Tessier, K. & Struening, E. L. (1979). A comparative trial of home and hospital psychiatric care. One year follow-up. *Archives of General Psychiatry*, **36**, 1073–9.

Fitzgerald, P. & Kulkarni, J. (in press). Home-based management of patients with first-episode psychosis. *British Journal of Psychiatry*. (Supplement).

Heinrichs, D. W., Hanlon, T. E. & Carpenter, W. T. (1984). The Quality of Life Scale: an instrument for rating the schizophrenic deficit syndrome. *Schizophrenia Bulletin*, **10**, 388–98.

Hoult, J. (1984a). Schizophrenia: a comparative trial of community orientated and hospital orientated psychiatric care. *Acta Psychiatrica Scandinavica*, **69**, 359–72.

Hoult, J. (1984b). Community orientated compared to psychiatric hospital orientated treatment. *Social Science and Medicine*, **18**, 1005–10.

Hoult, J. (1986). Community care of the acutely mentally ill. *British Journal of Psychiatry*, **149**, 137–44.

Hoult, J., Reynolds, I. & Charbonneau-Powis, M. (1983). Psychiatric hospital versus community treatment: the results of a randomised trial. *Australian and New Zealand Journal of Psychiatry*, **17**, 160–7.

Linszen, D. H., Dingemans, P. M. & Lenior, M. E. (1994). Cannabis abuse and the course of recent onset schizophrenic disorders. *Archives of General Psychiatry*, **51**, 273–9.

McGorry, P. D. (1992). The concept of recovery and secondary prevention in psychotic disorders. *Australian and New Zealand Journal of Psychiatry*, **237**, 3–17.

McGorry, P. D., Chanen, A., McCarthy, E., Van Riel, R., McKenzie. D. & Singh B. S. (1991). Post-traumatic stress disorder following recent-onset psychosis: an unrecognised post-psychotic syndrome. *Journal of Nervous and Mental Disease*, **179**, 253–8.

Marks, I. M., Corolly, J., Muijer, M., Audini, B., McNamee, G. & Lawrence, R. E. (1994). Home-based versus hospital based care for people with serious mental illness. *British Journal of Psychiatry*, **165**, 179–94.

Martinez-Arevalo, M. J., Calcedo-Ordonez, A. & Varo-Prieto, J. R. (1994). Cannabis consumption as a prognostic factor in schizophrenia. *British Journal of Psychiatry*, **164**, 679–81.

Negrete, J. (1989). Cannabis and schizophrenia. *British Journal of Addiction*, **84**, 349–51.

Overall, J. E. & Gorham, D. R. (1962). Brief Psychiatric Rating Scale. *Psychological Reports*, **10**, 799–812.

Pai, S. & Roberts, E. J. (1983). Follow-up of study of schizophrenic patients initially treated with home care. *British Journal of Psychiatry*, **143**, 447–50.

Stein, L. I. & Test, M. A. (1980). Alternative to mental hospital treatment:

1. Conceptual model, treatment program and clinical evaluation. *Archives of General Psychiatry*, **37**, 392–7.

Stirling, J., Tantum, D., Thomas, P., Newby, D., Montague, L., Ring, N. & Rowe, S. (1991). Expressed emotion and early onset schizophrenia: a one year follow-up. *Psychological Medicine*, **21**, 675–85.

Thomas, H. (1993). Psychiatric symptoms in cannabis use. *British Journal of Psychiatry*, **163**, 141–9.

Thornicroft, G. & Breakey, W. (1991). The Costar Program: improving patients' networks. *British Journal of Psychiatry*, **159**, 245–9.

Wright, R. G., Hener, J. R. & Shape, J. (1989). Defining and measuring stabilisation of patients during 4 years of intensive community support. *American Journal of Psychiatry*, **146**, 1293–8.

Appendix 1. Dandenong Hospital Department of Psychiatry

Pilot community treatment family resources scale
Carer version

	High			Low	
Given your relative's current state, what do you believe is the level of risk for self harm or harm to others?	5	4	3	2	1
What level of confidence do you have that your relative will accept taking medication?	5	4	3	2	1
What level of confidence do you have that your relative can be successfully treated at home?	5	4	3	2	1
What level of confidence do you think professionals have in your relative being successfully treated at home?	5	4	3	2	1

8 APPENDIX 1

Staff version

	Low			High	
What is the carer's level of availability to care for the client at home? (e.g. capacity to take time off work, to draw on extended family)	1	2	3	4	5
What reserves of coping ability does this family possess at this time?	1	2	3	4	5

	a great deal			not at all	
To what extent do you feel that carers are able to organize and take charge of this situation?	5	4	3	2	1
To what extent are carers committed to having the client treated at home?	5	4	3	2	1
To what degree have the family's normal routines been disrupted by the client's behaviour?	5	4	3	2	1
To what extent are the family in agreement with health professionals about what is wrong with the client?	5	4	3	2	1

	not well				well
How well does the client usually get on with the family?	1	2	3	4	5

Mandatory community treatment indicators
Staff version

	High			Low	
What is the risk of self harm or harm to others?	5	4	3	2	1
What degree of confidence is there that the client will accept medication?	5	4	3	2	1
What level of confidence do carers have in the client being successfully treated at home?	5	4	3	2	1
What level of confidence do you as a professional have in the client being successfully treated at home?	5	4	3	2	1

9

Early intervention in psychosis: the critical period

MAX BIRCHWOOD

Introduction

Interventions in psychosis, whether biological or psychosocial, have generally been blind to issues pertaining to age of onset and phase of illness. Such neglect reflects the dominance of the two main paradigms of care. In the first paradigm, treatment is provided within the context of *acute crisis care* and further attempts *to achieve prophylaxis*. Rehabilitation is the second paradigm which sometimes arises from a failure of the first. *Rehabilitation* involves focusing on the amelioration of disabilities, occasionally within a framework of relative asylum (Birchwood & Macmillan, 1993). Community outreach models frequently involve a blend of these two approaches. Both of these paradigms are rooted in the Kraepelinian nosological framework and, while long-term follow-up studies demonstrate the heterogeneity of outcomes in psychosis, they do appear, at first sight, to support the two paradigms. For instance, between one-third and one-half of patients have either single or multiple episodes with little or no residual symptoms, whereas the remainder have multiple episodes with varying, and often increasing impairment (Hegarty et al., 1994). Thus, the early phase of psychosis may be viewed as a period during which it is possible to determine which path an individual is likely to follow. A radically different view is gaining currency which argues that the personal and social context of psychosis is a major influence, and that the early phase of psychosis is a 'critical period' in the long-term trajectory of psychosis with major implications for secondary prevention. In this chapter, I will outline the core elements of the concept, review evidence for this proposition, and describe a prototype of intervention appropriate to the 'critical period'.

Critical periods

Prospective follow-up studies of first-episode psychotic patients

The bulk of follow-up studies of psychosis have reported on samples of convenience which are inevitably drawn from those maintaining contact with services: thus, a distorted picture, biased towards chronicity, may be evident. First-episode studies are not without their own problems: for example, determining their epidemiological representativeness is one issue which has been demonstrated only in the 'Determinants of Outcome in Severe Mental Disorder' study (DOSMD) (Jablensky et al., 1992), and there are the perennial problems related to comparability of measures, sampling, and density of follow-up, all of which constrain generalization (Hegarty et al., 1994). On the other hand, it is also true that if findings from follow-up studies are so sensitive to methodology and context, then this itself brings into question whether general conclusions can be drawn. However, the follow-back studies and the prospective studies do permit key hypotheses to be tested and certain conclusions to be drawn. Since we are concerned with a supposed critical period of early psychosis, in this section I will focus only on first-episode prospective studies. Similar reviews have been undertaken by Ram et al. (1992), Warner (1994) and Hegarty et al. (1994), all of which will be referred to as appropriate. The studies are summarized in Table 9.1 and will be discussed under the following headings.

The pre-neuroleptic era

The studies of Stephens (1978), Bleuler (1978) and, to a degree, Wing (1966) bear on this important and intriguing area: was the outcome for schizophrenia one of remorseless chronicity before the neuroleptic era? The answer to this is undoubtedly in the negative. First-episode studies in the era of institutional care do not suffer from epidemiological bias: nearly all first-episode patients were admitted to hospital and were unlikely to be 'camouflaged' within the community for appreciable periods (Ram et al., 1992). Twenty-three per cent of Bleuler's (1978) sample had recovered after 20 years and a further 20% showed long-term symptoms of mild severity: for the majority this was not a barrier to re-employment. Thirty-five per cent showed stable chronic symptoms and a further 30% continued to undulate between illness and well being. After treatment, Stephens' (1978) patients were followed up from between 1948 and 1951 for ten years or more. Twenty-four

Table 9.1. Prospective follow-up studies of first-episode psychosis

Study	Subjects	Inclusion criteria	Follow-up	Measures/criteria	Patterns of course/outcome
Biehl et al. (1986)	n = 70 (see Schubart et al., 1986)			Assessment schedule	Poor: 35%
Eaton et al. (1995)	n = 90 First episode: 1978–80	PSE; ICD-9 Repeated annually	10 years	—	
Helgason (1990)	n = 107 Iceland: 1966–67	ICD-9	21 years		Died: 23/107 No or minor symptoms (no treatment) – 8%; Minor symptoms – 22%; moderate symptoms – 50%; severe symptoms – 21%
DOSMD: Jablensky et al. (1992)	n = 1379 12 centres 10 countries	PSE/CATEGO	2 years	DAS	Mild (1 episode, no symptoms) = 39% Intermittent – relapsing = 21% Severe – unremitting = 39%
Johnstone et al. (1986, 1990)	n = 236 First admissions in defined catchment area	CATEGO 'S' by PSE	2 years	Relapse/re-admission	Relapse: 60%, No relapse: 40%

Study	Sample	Diagnosis	Follow-up	Outcome measures	Outcome
Mason et al. (1995)	n = 67 First episode 1978–80	ICD-9	13 years	DAS GAF	No or mild symptoms: 49% No relapse in recent 2 years: 80% Good or fair social outcome: 55% Employed in last two years: 37% Independent community living: 97% Living alone: 28% Receiving treatment: 76%
Schubart et al. (1986)	n = 70	PSE/ICD-9	2 years	DAS	Good adjustment: 26% Intermediate: 39%
Scottish Schizophrenia Research Group (1988, 1992)	n = 49 4 hospitals, first admissions	RDC	5 years	Re-admission 'Overall outcome' Kraweicka scale	37% 'well' 47% re-admitted 38% psychotic symptoms at follow-up 23% employed
Shepherd et al. (1989)	n = 49 First admission over 18 months in semi-rural area	PSE/CATEGO	5 years	PSE, DAS	1 episode, no impairment: 22%

per cent had 'recovered', whereas 30% were 'improved'; overall, 50% were rated as having *improved* relative to their first discharge. John Wing's (1966) five-year follow-up of patients admitted to three British mental hospitals in 1956 showed that nearly 50% had an excellent prognosis requiring little attention from psychiatric aftercare or rehabilitation services. A further 38% were asymptomatic in the last six months of their follow-up. While we would not have known the employment status of those individuals without the interruption of psychosis, the Wing study paints a much more optimistic picture about the capabilities of those affected than is often the case. In fact, Bleuler's (1978) impression was that few of his patients completely recovered without some vestige of their illness remaining but, despite this, many were able to resume employment.

Without doubt, these studies used different diagnostic procedures, measures and follow-up periods; yet despite this, their results paint a similar picture and add strength to the conclusion that untreated schizophrenia is not a deteriorating and inevitably socially disabling disorder; in excess of one-third can recover symptomatically, and a further one-third can function quite independently without intensive community outreach.

Neuroleptics were not widely used until the late 1950s, in fact towards the end of the follow-up period in the Wing (1966) and Stephens (1978) studies. The Bleuler (1978) sample was treated almost entirely within the pre-neuroleptic era and the sample was subject to minimal attrition. It is salutary to be reminded about the type of treatment provided by Bleuler's clinic in Switzerland, particularly as fully 60% of his patients recovered 20 years after their first-episode – sufficient for them to be able to return to work and to support themselves. This figure is far in excess, for example, of that reported by Kraepelin (1896) from his hospital in Munich – he labelled only 12% of his patients as 'social recoveries'. As Warner (1994) has explained, Bleuler's account of his treatment methods from the first decade of the twentieth century, reads like a model of those introduced half a century later as part of the social psychiatry revolution of post-war Europe. Bleuler de-emphasized institutional methods, advocating a high threshold for admission and rapid discharge. He championed active community rehabilitation, returning the patient to his own family or, where this was not possible, to a substitute family: 'Idleness facilitates the predomination of the complexes over the personality, whereas regulated work maintains the activity of normal thinking' (p. 11); thus, return to an appropriate occupation was vital according to Bleuler to promote well-being, although faultless performance could not be expected. Minimizing work stress, family troubles, or a sense of failure, were all part of Bleuler's philosophy of care. Warner (1994) argues that '...the modern pessimistic view of the untreated course of schizophrenia may have developed because the introduction of anti-psychotic drugs in the 1950s and their subsequent universal employment in the treatment of psychosis has masked what was previously known about the natural history of the illness' (p. 11). Warner also considers that *excessive* treatment with neuroleptics may have exacerbated disability consistent with recent findings (Schooler, 1994).

Nevertheless, the meta-analysis of follow-up studies by Hegarty et al. (1994) does point to an improvement in outcomes during the 1960s when neuroleptics were widely used: however, it should not be assumed that all the favourable outcomes we see today are solely attributable to neuroleptics – continuous care, support and community-based rehabilitation are potent influences on outcome. The WHO cross-cultural studies, for example, demonstrated favourable outcomes in cultures with extended family networks (Jablensky et al., 1992), despite the lesser use of neuroleptic drugs. In the classic review of the North American follow-up studies conducted in the neuroleptic era, McGlashan (1988) observed that ... 'schizophrenia may be quite malleable to prolonged environmental/psychosocial perturbations...; these have negative potential when applied too intensively or ambitiously, but positive potential if applied steadily in a supportive rehabilitative mode in the context of stable and supportive community care' (p. 538). Studies from the pre-neuroleptic era caution against excessive pessimism about schizophrenia and excessive optimism about the efficacy of neuroleptic drugs.

These studies from the pre-neuroleptic era must be set against recent work, reviewed later in this chapter and elsewhere in this book, suggesting that early neuroleptic treatment can prevent or minimize later symptoms, for example, arising from relapse. For example, Waddington, Youssef & Kinsella (1995) followed-up 88 long-term residents in an Irish psychiatric hospital, many of whom had experienced decades of initially untreated psychosis (mean = 17 years) prior to the introduction of neuroleptics in Ireland. They found that the longer the duration of psychosis prior to the introduction of neuroleptics, the greater the poverty of speech at the 'end state' (when the average age was 66 years), and the more continuous neuroleptic treatment had to be. The point to be made here is that untreated psychosis is not inevitably 'Kraepelinian', particularly where it is positively managed in a community context. Earlier and ongoing neuroleptic treatment may enhance the outcome, but to assume that the illness course would otherwise be chronic and remorseless would seem to be erroneous.

Clinical and social outcomes

In their seminal paper, Strauss & Carpenter (1977) demonstrated that clinical recovery was not a prerequisite for social recovery; in fact, they reported substantial desynchrony between, for example, residual symptoms and social functioning, the correlations being no greater than 0.50. Normal processes as well as abnormal ones contribute to social functioning and social readjustment (Birchwood, Hallett & Preston, 1988) and the first-episode studies follow the same general rule. The correlation between symptoms and functioning is of the same order (Shepherd et al., 1989), with social outcome in the early phase being better than might be expected in the light of clinical outcome alone. Thus, Shepherd et al. (1989) demonstrated that 30% of their patients showed moderate to severe social impairment, whereas 70% experienced multiple episodes and/or residual symptoms over the first five years. Mason et al. (1995) echo this point: 'the status of symptoms may have little relevance to every day social functioning' (p. 602). Schubart et al. (1986) and the linked study of Biehl et al. (1986) examined the course of social disability over the first five years using the WHO Disability Assessment Schedule (WHODAS) (WHO, 1988). Neither baseline clinical symptoms, nor age or gender, predicted social outcome at five years; only WHODAS scores at six months predicted outcome at one, two, three, and five years. Like Strauss & Carpenter, they found that the best predictor of social outcome was an *earlier* measure of social functioning. Similarly, the 'Suffolk County' follow-up study of Bromet et al. (1996) followed up 96 people with a first-episode of DSM-III-R (APA, 1987) schizophrenia and found that the best predictor of functioning at six months was premorbid functioning, although functioning at six months was highly correlated with level of symptomatic remission by this time. Clearly, the onset of psychosis and the level of early remission can act like a 'main effect' depressing social functioning, and it may be expected that improving early clinical outcome will enhance early social functioning; however, there are multiple influences on social functioning (e.g. social opportunities and individual psychological reaction to the onset of psychosis). Thus, both 'naturalistic' and 'formal' psychosocial interventions will be essential to restore social functioning and improve quality of life.

The relationship between the 'acute' and 'residual' symptoms

What is the nature of the relationship between acute and residual positive symptoms? Only two of the prospective studies took sufficiently frequent and dense follow-up measures to address this question. The pattern of course from the five-year follow-up of Shepherd et al. (1989) in England is presented in Figure 9.1.

Thirty-five per cent of the patients in Shepherd et al.'s sample revealed a pattern of repeated relapse and an increasing incidence of persisting, drug-resistant psychotic symptoms between episodes; a further 35% also had several episodes but no residual symptoms. This finding is consistent with the view that repeated relapse *can* drive chronicity among a significant proportion of patients but, of course, a general increase in illness severity may underlie both. The Madras study (Eaton et al., 1995; and Thara et al., 1994) only reported whether patients experienced complete or incomplete remissions although, as with the British study (Shepherd et al., 1989), the researchers found a clear differentiation between those with, and without, residual symptoms following a relapse. After ten years, only 9% of the Madras sample were recorded as having positive symptoms, and this compares, for example, with 40% of the 600 patients followed up after two years in the developed countries in the DOSMD study (Jablensky et al., 1992). This astonishingly low rate of residual symptoms is paralleled by the low rate of relapse; on average, patients experienced only two episodes over the ten-year follow-up period.

What can be said with certainty is that 'residual' symptoms arise as a result of the resistance of early phase acute symptoms to treatment which may increase with relapse. Therefore, in considering the management of residual symptoms (whether through pharmacological or cognitive means), we have argued for a focus on improving recovery from the acute episode in the early phase (Drury et al., 1996).

The 'plateau effect'

Bleuler's classic follow-up study (Bleuler, 1978) observed that patients reach a plateau of psychopathology and disability early in the course of illness, which of course, is contrary to the Kraepelinian (Kraepelin, 1896) notion of progressive psychopathology. This was neatly illustrated in the report from the Washington cohort of the International Pilot Study of Schizophrenia (Carpenter & Strauss, 1991) which followed up patients two years, then 11 years, after the episode of inclusion. Table 9.2 summarizes the results for all patients as well as for the subsample who were functioning initially at a lower level on the Level of Functioning Scale (Carpenter & Strauss, 1991). It is apparent that the early deterioration among many of the patients stabilized by two years and fully 75% of the patients showed no change in relapse, social contacts, occupational functioning and residual symptoms between two and 11 years. Indeed, amongst those patients struggling after two

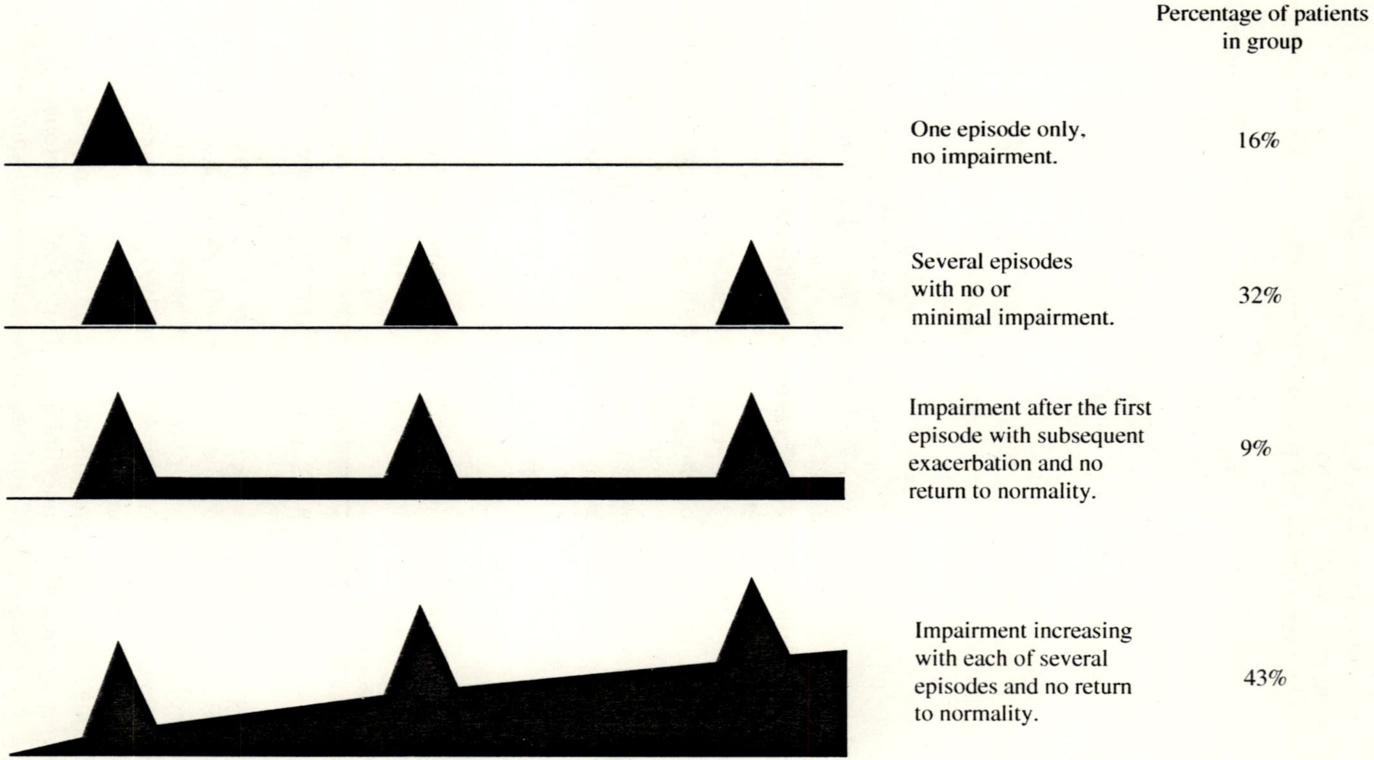

	Percentage of patients in group
One episode only, no impairment.	16%
Several episodes with no or minimal impairment.	32%
Impairment after the first episode with subsequent exacerbation and no return to normality.	9%
Impairment increasing with each of several episodes and no return to normality.	43%

Figure 9.1. Five-year outcome following a first presentation of schizophrenia (adapted from Shepherd et al., 1989).

Table 9.2. *Two- versus eleven-year outcome in schizophrenia*

Variable	Better %	Same %	Worse %
1. All patients			
Hospitalization	11	89	0
Social contacts	12	71	18
Employment	12	71	18
Symptoms	9	85	6
2. Patients functioning 'poorly' at inclusion			
Hospitalization	80	20	0
Social contacts	36	46	18
Employment	36	55	9
Symptoms	21	79	0

years, one-third showed *improvement* by 11 years, suggesting a relenting of the biosocial process – a notion taken up by Courtney Harding and her colleagues (Harding, Brooks & Ashikaga, 1987) in their Vermont study of chronic 'back ward' patients released into the community and followed up many years later.

Generally, the prospective first-episode studies have not addressed this 'plateau' hypothesis: this requires a truly prospective design with multiple follow-up points. The one exception was the unique investigation conducted by Thara et al. (1994) and Eaton et al. (1995) in the city of Madras, which followed along a cohort of 90 first-episode schizophrenic patients monthly for ten years; there was very little attrition. They discovered a steep decline in the prevalence of both the positive and negative syndromes during the first year of follow-up and the prevalence of subjects with either positive or negative symptoms stabilized to about 20–25% after two years; and, as Thara et al. and Eaton et al. indicate, two years has been accepted as the standard threshold for chronicity prior to the era of community mental health care. Thara, Eaton and colleagues found no evidence for an increase in negative symptoms later in the course of the illness and, in fact, once two years had elapsed, the prevalence of negative symptoms was relatively low. There was, however, a small tendency for an increase in the proportion of the cohort with both positive *and* negative symptoms from some time in the third year, through to the tenth year. There was no evidence for the substitution of positive by negative symptoms, and these two groups of symptoms were moderately independent, both cross-sectionally and prospectively, underlining the notion that we should be thinking in terms of groups of symptoms rather than 'parcels' of schizophrenic disorder. Harrison et al. (1996) present an analysis of the Nottingham, UK, Centre sample of the first-episode schizophrenic cohort which is part of the DOSMD study (Jablensky et al., 1992; Mason et al., 1995) and bears upon the plateau hypothesis. They examined the relationship between short-term (two years) and long-term (13 years) trajectories of outcome when established predictors were controlled for. The established predictors were summarized in their baseline (onset) model which was developed to maximize prediction at year 2; this included (under ICD-10) (WHO, 1992) male gender, less acute onsets, never married, and duration of untreated psychosis (DUP) greater than six months. The addition of information about the two-year course type to the baseline model substantially increased prediction of outcome at 13 years in terms of social activity and psychopathology, but not hospitalization or employment. The course type was a binary classification: complete or near complete remission at two years; versus 'continually psychotic', more than one relapse and/or residual personality change, with the latter predicting an unfavourable outcome.

The Madras and Nottingham studies provide the strongest evidence yet for the concept of the plateauing of psychopathology and disability in the early course of psychosis. This conclusion is supported by less robust data from other centres: for example, from the Agra Centre of the IPSS (Dube, Kumar & Dube, 1984) and from other follow-up studies (Achte et al., 1986; Huber et al., 1980). Collectively, these data support McGlashan's view (McGlashan, 1988) that deterioration, though variable, does occur in the pre-psychotic period and early in the course of psychosis (whether treated or untreated), but this will stabilize between two and five years and may even relent among those who initially deteriorate most.

Early relapse in schizophrenia

The definitions of remission and relapse range across the studies. The Scottish Schizophrenia Research Group (1988) defined good outcome as the patient experiencing no readmissions and no positive symptoms or negative symptoms at follow-up. Sixty-one per cent of patients experienced a 'good' outcome at one year, with this falling to 37% by two years accompanied by a 47% rate of readmission. The Northwick Park study (Johnstone et al., 1986) defined relapse as the development of psychotic features (as described by clinicians or relatives) leading to admission. At the end of two years, only 35% of patients were considered to be relapse free; however, this sample included many patients who had participated in a trial of maintenance neuroleptic medication. Shepherd et al. (1989) found that 22% of their first-admission sample had not relapsed after five years (i.e. 78% relapse rate). A study conducted in inner-city Birmingham, UK (Birchwood, Macmillan & Smith, 1992) found a one-year readmission rate of 35%, rising to 50% after the second year. The DOSMD study (Jablensky et al., 1992) reported that in developed countries, an average of 39% of patients experienced only one episode and only mild or no impairment after two years. A one year follow-up of patients with DSM-III-R (APA, 1987) schizophrenia and other psychoses was conducted in Amsterdam, Holland, by Linszen, Dingemans & Lenior (1994). Using standard ratings and careful operational criteria for relapse, Linszen and colleagues found that in the region of 23% of patients suffered a relapse within one year, despite the high degree of medication compliance amongst the patients.

There are so many predictors of early relapse that were not controlled for in these studies that it makes it difficult to draw a meaningful figure for the 'true' one- and two-year relapse rates. At one extreme, we find the Madras study (Thara et al., 1994; Eaton et al., 1995) reporting an average of only two relapses over ten years, whereas 60% of patients in the Northwick Park study (Johnstone et al., 1986) had relapsed within two years.

In view of the interplay of so many prognostic variables and the heterogeneity of the populations studied, it is best to summarize these data in terms of confidence intervals. Although limited, these studies do suggest a one-year relapse rate of between 15% and 35%, with a benchmark figure of 25%, and rising to between 30% and 60% over two years, with a benchmark figure of 40%, rising to up to 80% within five years. These results, derived from the first-episode studies, are broadly consistent with the findings of the meta-analysis of long-term follow-up studies of schizophrenia by Hegarty et al. (1994), which concluded that 40.2% of patients with schizophrenia had a favourable outcome. It is worth re-emphasizing the point that clinical–symptomatic recovery is not an absolute prerequisite for social recovery; while it would be incorrect to assume orthogonality between these two dimensions, it may be helpful from a clinical point of view to distinguish between them, since different kinds of interventions will be required to promote social recovery.

Long-term outcome

In the Nottingham study Mason et al. (1995), found that after 13 years, 49% of patients had no or mild symptoms, whilst 55% had good or fair social outcome as measured by the WHODAS (WHO, 1988). Nearly 40% of patients were employed in the two years prior to the 13-year follow-up; however, only 17% of the patients showed complete recovery (this being defined as patients exhibiting no symptoms, no disability and receiving no treatment). These data are consistent with follow-up studies conducted in the UK over shorter periods of time. The Scottish Schizophrenia Research Group (1988) reported that 46% of their patients had no active symptoms after five years; and Shepherd et al. (1989) reported that 57% of their first-admission patients had no or minimal impairment after five years – this result being consistent once again with the *plateau* effect discussed earlier. Mason et al. (1995) also compared their results with Bleuler's (1978) very long-term outcome data conducted in the preneuroleptic era; using Bleuler's original criteria, they found remarkable similarities, with perhaps a marginally better outcome occurring over the shorter follow-up period of the Nottingham study.

Although there are no truly very long-term prospective studies of first-episode psychosis, the available data do seem to support the conclusions of reviews of the outcome literature by Hegarty et al. (1994), McGlashan (1988) and Warner (1994); that is, while complete recovery is relatively rare, up to one-half achieve a favourable clinical and social outcome, with higher figures being reported in some cultures (Eaton et al., 1995). The meta-analysis of Hegarty et al. (1994) emphasizes that these figures will differ according to the diagnostic criteria adopted. Thus, the DSM-III-R (APA, 1987) and DSM-IV (APA, 1994) definitions require a minimum of six months of illness (including prodromal or residual symptoms), i.e. they include a built-in chronicity requirement, and find that less than 30% will be substantially improved, whereas using broader criteria such as ICD-10 (WHO, 1992) which requires one month's duration of illness for a diagnosis of schizophrenia, the proportion showing substantial recovery rises to, on average, 46.5%. The circularity inherent in building in a chronicity criterion to a definition has been noted by many other authors (e.g. Warner, 1994) and reflects the influence of Kraepelinian doctrine. The problem from the perspective of this chapter is that with so many factors affecting prognosis, the pathways to chronicity will be many and varied; to define a subgroup within the psychotic spectrum as having a poor outcome and give them a diagnosis, rather assumes some kind of homogeneity of outcome, when in fact the reverse is likely to be the case. This is particularly unhelpful from the point of view of early intervention where the manipulation of prognostic variables early in the course of attention is our focus.

Suicide

Suicide is a tragic but common early outcome of people with schizophrenia but tends to be a neglected feature of outcome studies, often subsumed within attrition statistics (Caldwell & Gottesman, 1990). While exact figures are difficult to establish, the percentage of those with schizophrenia who commit suicide ranges between 8% and 15% (Caldwell & Gottesman, 1990), and risk factors, such as youth, male gender, higher IQ or educational attainment, have been identified (Drake et al., 1985; see also Chapter 12).

Risk factors for suicide were investigated by Westermeyer, Harrow & Marengo (1991) in their study of 586 first-episode and early phase RDC-defined schizophrenic, 'other' psychotic and non-psychotic disordered patients. Rates of suicide were 8.8% for schizophrenia, 7.2% for 'other' psychosis, and 4% for depression. The predictors of suicide suggested two themes: failed expectations (with predictors including high IQ, good premorbid functioning, and high premorbid attainment), and fear of mental disintegration (with predictors including the presence of early relapse or disability). In view of the findings from the Madras and Nottingham studies, that longer-term difficulties will be apparent by two years, it might be expected that by then patients will also have developed an awareness of the constraints and limitations upon their functioning. Thus, Westermeyer et al. (1991) found that, of those who committed suicide, two-thirds had done so by six years following the first-episode, leading the authors to label it as a 'critical period' of suicide risk. The suicide literature is covered in more depth elsewhere in this book (see Chapter 12). I shall argue later in this chapter, however, that patients' appraisals of the meaning of psychosis and the implications for the self, are active early in the course of psychosis and provide new meaning to the problems of comorbidity, including depression and suicidal thinking.

Predictors of outcome

Social and family contacts

Low levels of non-family social contacts are associated with early relapse (Johnstone et al., 1990), general poor early outcome (Beiser et al., 1988, 1989), and poor occupational functioning (Johnstone et al., 1992); however, social contact, social competence and features of the illness such as negative symptoms, are difficult to disentangle conceptually. The link between premorbid functioning and outcome suffers a similar problem. Nevertheless, higher educational attainment was linked to delayed relapse in the Northwick Park study (Geddes et al., 1994). Birchwood et al. (1992) found isolation from family a major risk factor for early (12-month) relapse in an inner city sample in Birmingham,

UK, and the patients from Indian backgrounds who stayed with their families revealed a lower rate of relapse/readmission.

High expressed emotion (EE) in close relatives is a robust predictor of relapse (Bebbington & Kuipers, 1994) but its predictive efficacy with first-episode patients is weaker (Linszen et al., 1996) or non-existent (Johnstone et al., 1986; Stirling et al., 1991). Recent studies of EE in first-episode patients (Stirling et al., 1993) support previous assertions (Birchwood, 1992) that EE is not a family 'trait', but a much more fluid characteristic. Stirling and colleagues reported a metamorphosis of the components of EE (emotional over-involvement to criticism) during the first 12 months after first treatment, and suggest that there are processes at play in the family interior linked to relatives' emotional adaptation to the appearance of psychosis in their offspring. The EE work is discussed in more detail in Chapter 14.

Gender and age at onset

Like many follow-up studies, the first-episode studies consistently find that males have a generally poorer outcome (Beiser et al., 1988; Eaton et al., 1995; Geddes et al., 1994; Scottish Schizophrenia Research Group, 1992), and that early age of onset is associated with more severe illness in many studies (e.g. Soni, Tench & Routledge, 1994), although there were some exceptions (Ram et al., 1992).

Depression

The presence of affective symptoms has long been held to be associated with favourable outcome (McGlashan, 1988); however, this finding has recently been challenged. Depression in the context of a non-affective psychosis is common (DeLisi, 1990) with point prevalence figures varying from 17.5% (Mason et al., 1995) to 30% (Harrow et al., 1995). Depression and suicidal thinking is often the cause of crisis and readmission (Shepherd et al., 1989), and has been shown to be predictive of later relapse (Johnson, 1981) and suicide (Roy, 1986). The Northwick Park study (Johnstone et al., 1986) found that subjective feelings of depression and hopelessness at first admission predicted earlier first readmission; on the other hand, the presence of depressive delusions (i.e. suggestive of an affective psychosis) was associated with better early outcome. The presence of hopelessness has been shown to be a critical factor in suicide prediction (Drake et al., 1985) and it is precisely this variable which has been linked to early relapse in the Northwick Park study (Johnstone et al., 1986).

Symptoms

The presence of early negative symptoms is predictive of poor early- (Beiser et al., 1988; Beiser, Iacono & Erickson, 1989; Scottish Schizophrenia Research Group, 1988), and long-term (Eaton et al., 1995) outcome. For some patients, negative symptoms may represent a proxy variable for a different neurodevelopmental process linked to low genetic risk, soft neurological signs, and male gender (Johnstone et al., 1992; Pilowsky, Kerwin & Murray, 1993).

Depressive delusions were associated with a low rate of early relapse in the Northwick Park study (Johnstone et al., 1986), whereas depression and hopelessness were linked to a higher rate of early relapse (see above). It might be argued that depressive delusions are indicative of affective psychosis which carries a more benign outcome; hopelessness, on the other hand, is indicative of vulnerability to recurrent depression which has been linked to early relapse (Johnson, 1981).

Drug abuse

Potentially half of patients entering psychiatric treatment have significant drug and alcohol histories (Mueser et al., 1990) and the reason for this comorbidity has been the subject of recent concern. The relationships are numerous and complex (Ram et al., 1992); for example, to what extent are substances used to cope with psychotic symptoms?; to what extent does use or abuse precipitate onset in vulnerable individuals and bring forward in time the onset of psychosis?; under what circumstances does a history of abuse, or the quantity, frequency or variability of use, operate as a prognostic sign, whether positive or negative? Both in relation to the issue of onset and of relapse, disentangling cause and effect will be difficult to establish. In relation to the question of onset, the recent study by Hambrecht & Häfner (1996) reveals a complex picture which will require further clarification. Conversely, a recent study by Linszen et al. (1994) described in detail in Chapter 13, has gone some way to help clarify the relationship between relapse and cannabis use during the early course of recent-onset schizophrenia.

This study strongly suggests that use and abuse can significantly affect the timing, if not the probability, of relapse. Only intervention studies would be able to address this issue definitively, although the implications for treatment and care are clear (see also Chapter 13).

Neuroleptic medication

Controlled trials of maintenance neuroleptic medication are rare in first-episode psychosis: only three have been reported hitherto. Kane

(1983) found that seven of eight patients in a placebo-treated group relapsed at a mean of 18 weeks, compared with one of eight patients on active maintenance fluphenazine who relapsed at the 25th week. The Scottish Schizophrenia Research Group (1988) found an advantage for active treatment, and good initial response to neuroleptics was a predictor of lower relapse rate. The best controlled study is again the Northwick Park study (Johnstone et al., 1986), in which 54 first-episode schizophrenic patients were assigned to drug treatment and 66 to placebo under double-blind conditions. The impact of this manipulation was significant, but marginal, compared to trials involving consecutive admissions: 60% of patients on placebo relapsed over two years versus 40% on active medication. The impact of medication was much less than, for example, another variable monitored in this study, the duration of untreated psychotic illness (DUP; see below). A subsequent analysis found that those with a short pre-treatment duration of untreated illness (< 1 year) and who received active medication, had a poorer occupational outcome than those who received placebo, suggesting that early neuroleptic use (two years post-first-episode) can exact a price in occupational terms. Given that 40% of patients functioned well on placebo over the two years, this finding emphasizes the importance of predicting who is likely to relapse (and therefore likely to need medication). It also highlights the need for further research into the use of low-dose medication and complementary methods of relapse prevention. The discontinuation of medication in those with a short duration of illness should be considered, together with the use of an 'intermittent' or 'targeted' medication paradigm in which treatment is provided at the earliest sign of relapse (Birchwood, 1995).

Untreated illness

Despite the profound and distressing changes which accompany a first episode of psychosis, it is surprising that the time to first presentation and treatment is highly variable (this issue has been considered already in Chapter 3). Considered collectively, a range of studies from North America, Europe and Australia show an average DUP, or a treatment lag, of approximately one year in the case of schizophrenia and related psychoses. However, in all of these studies the standard deviation was generally greater than the mean and, where reported, the median was much less than the mean (e.g. mean of 74 weeks compared with a median of 20 weeks in the study by McGorry & Singh, 1995). This suggests a significant effect of outliers with very long durations, and one should note that approximately a quarter of the Northwick Park sample had treatment lags in excess of one year. In this study, Johnstone et al. (1986) found that the longer time to presentation was associated with increasing complications of frank psychotic illness, including severe behavioural disturbance and family difficulties (often involving multiple failed attempts to access appropriate care), and life-threatening behaviour (Humphries et al., 1992). These findings underline the fact that individuals were in need of urgent treatment.

Two studies have demonstrated a close link between the DUP and the early course of schizophrenia. Johnstone et al. (1986) found that those patients taking longer than one year to access and exit services revealed a greatly increased (by a factor of 3) relapse rate over the following two years, when compared with those with a briefer DUP. The variable 'DUP' emerged as the strongest predictor of relapse, greater than the impact of maintenance medication, which was also manipulated in this study (active versus placebo). Loebel et al. (1992) examined a first-episode sample using a standardized treatment and assessment protocol, and found that both the time to remission and the degree of remission were closely related to DUP when other prognostic variables were controlled (gender, age at onset, mode of onset, premorbid adjustment). Wyatt (1991) has suggested that delayed initiation of neuroleptics is associated with treatment resistance; thus, less complete recovery from the first episode due to delayed presentation could be the result of biological change related to a putative toxic effect of the psychosis, which might account for the raised risk of relapse in the Northwick Park study (Johnstone et al., 1986) and the delayed and less complete remissions in the Loebel et al. study. Vulnerability models have been invoked to help explain the problem of heterogeneity of outcome in schizophrenia (Zubin & Spring, 1977): I would propose that some of the variance in vulnerability may have its origins in events surrounding the first episode, in particular untreated psychosis. Also, during this period, significant psychosocial decline or stagnation can occur (Jones et al., 1993) and, at this crucial time of educational and vocational development, limits on long-term recovery may be set that some have argued can have long-term prognostic implications (McGlashan, 1988; Warner, 1994).

However, the relationship between DUP and early outcome remains circumstantial. Understanding the reasons for this variable but long duration of untreated illness is crucial in determining the direction of causality and the potential for reducing delay. The Loebel et al. (1992) study found no relationship between DUP and age at onset, mode of onset, premorbid adjustment, or severity of illness. Male gender, however, was associated with longer DUP and also earlier age at onset of illness. Loebel and colleagues comment that families may exhibit a greater tolerance for disturbed behaviour in male adolescents. Perhaps an even more likely explanation is that families have greater difficulty in recognizing psychopathology in males and, accordingly, delay seeking help for them. Among males in particular, longer DUP is linked to a longer prodrome (Loebel et al., 1992). Thus, the transition from poor premorbid state to 'at-risk mental state', and on to frank psychosis, may be difficult to discern, and may lead to delay in recognition and acceptance of psychopathology. McGorry et al. (1996) found a significant correlation between duration of prodrome and untreated psychosis, thus supporting this possibility. A second factor concerns the pathways to care (see Chapter 3). A study in Birmingham (Birchwood et al., 1992) reported that longer DUP was documented among those living alone in the inner city (usually African-Caribbeans and whites), compared with those living in a family setting. Patients of South Asian origin were nearly always resident with their family and showed a correspondingly shorter period of untreated illness (14 weeks) than the sample as a whole (30 weeks). This study hypothesized that as the African-Caribbean group were living alone at onset and took a longer time to access services, this increased the likelihood of judicial agencies becoming engaged, compared with the South Asian group who were more likely to access care via GPs. Johnstone et al. (1986), in noting the relationship between long duration of untreated illness and multiple failed attempts to access care though GPs, suggest that one reason for delay may be due to the difficulty of, or lack of training among, GPs in recognizing psychosis. Other reasons might include a reluctance on the part of GPs to refer on in ambiguous cases, or point to 'collusion' between the GP and family, driven in turn by the difficulty close relatives may experience in facing up to the possibility that their child is suffering from psychosis. In this respect, the fear and stigma associated with severe mental illness among patients and their supporters should not be underestimated (Perkins & Moodley, 1993).

The critical period concept: summary and evaluation

The challenging of the assumption underlying the Kraepelinian doctrine has provided fertile ground for the growth of early intervention concepts and strategies. The acceptance of the heterogeneity of psychosis, the concept of stress vulnerability, and the introduction of effective interventions, have together provided the setting conditions for a more optimistic view of the treatment of psychosis, and schizophrenia in particular. There are parallels here with changes which have occurred in oncology where early detection and intervention are seen as central to effective treatment. For similar changes to occur in psychosis, we require clarity about *what* we are preventing and *how*. We introduced the concept of the 'critical period' (Birchwood & Macmillan, 1993; Birchwood, McGorry & Jackson, 1997) with this aim in mind. The concept of early intervention does not assume heterogeneity; in fact, early intervention is as compatible with the concept of dementia praecox as it is with breast cancer. Here, we are proposing something different about this early phase of psychosis which we believe contains important therapeutic implications.

In previous presentations of the concept we have included only the post-first-treatment period as our putative critical period; although the onset of treatment marks a major event in the early development of psychosis, however, it is perhaps artificial to separate the period of untreated psychosis from the post-first-treatment phase as they may well have some continuity in the processes involved. For example, if it is proposed that exposure to psychosis is toxic in some way, then this will apply equally to the post-treatment phase as to the pre-treatment phase.

There are three propositions essential to the concept of the 'critical period'.

(1) Mental and social deterioration, if it occurs, is non-linear

The prospective studies have shown that, for many, there is a rapid period of progression of psychosis prior to, and following, the first presentation. There is a well-documented prodromal period plus untreated psychosis of varying duration linked to underachievement in psychosocial domains (Jones et al., 1993). The evidence for the risk of early progression is strong – the risk of relapse, for example, is high within two years, and nearly three-quarters of patients can expect to relapse within five years. Bleuler's early studies, and taken together with the recent high quality studies from Madras and Nottingham, provide compelling evidence that the course type is predictable by year 3 (including on average, the 12 months of DUP), with a stabilization of the absolute level of morbidity. This fact is probably not lost on patients themselves; suicide risk is particularly high during this early phase, especially following a relapse.

The therapeutic implication of this lies in its clarification of a time scale for early intervention. The first three years of (treated and untreated) illness offer a window of opportunity to prevent, or limit, this potential decline. Intervention efforts after the plateau of morbidity has been reached will face a greater challenge than that implemented at the first episode; however, the extent to which the damage is *irreversible* following the achievement of the plateau, is of crucial significance and is an interesting research question.

If the therapeutic implications of this are to be realized, then it must first be demonstrated that intervention *can* change the early course of psychosis, leading to a lower plateau of morbidity than would otherwise have been the case. An interesting research question then arises: if the 'grip' is then relaxed, will the individual deteriorate to another plateau or, conversely, will the improvements require *relatively* little maintenance? This in part will turn on whether the interventions inhibit the development of 'toxic' influences which, in their absence, will follow their natural course (e.g. neurobiological changes which are the consequence of relapse), or conversely introduce 'healthy' influences which introduce a virtuous circle. There is likely to be a combination of these two processes and, again, this poses an interesting research question.

(2) The critical period witnesses the ontogeny of significant variables
Here we argue that the biological, psychosocial and cognitive changes which are influential in the course of psychosis are not 'given' but actively develop during this period. The possibility of a biological toxicity was first raised by Wyatt (1991). Pretreatment exposure to psychosis has been suggested by Wyatt as a key factor, but also the incidences of relapse, treatment resistance and episodes of untreated psychosis *following* the first treatment should also contribute to this theoretical toxicity. The prevention and the minimization of relapse and the focus on early treatment resistance will be key therapeutic objectives here.

There is evidence that the family influences on relapse are also active during this period. The metamorphosis of components of expressed emotion as we have seen, occurs in one direction (emotional over-involvement to criticism) and suggests the operation of a process consistent with recent concepts that EE should be viewed as a state, not a trait, characteristic. The results of the Amsterdam study (Linszen et al., 1996) failed to find any additional benefits of behavioural family intervention in the context of an individual case management approach. Therapeutically, the content of family intervention may need to change to reflect this flux of family relationships, with a key therapeutic objective being the prevention of negative attitudes in the relationships. In this context it is perhaps not surprising that the Amsterdam First-episode Family Intervention study failed to find any additional benefits to standard family intervention when delivered in the context of needs-led case management. In fact, this study demonstrated negative reactions in some families, particularly families characterized as low EE, suggesting the operation of a different process; for example, those involving early adjustment patterns centred around loss and mourning (Birchwood, 1992; Linszen et al., 1996).

Although a poorly researched area, there is a developing literature on the psychological adaptation to the onset of psychosis (Jackson & Birchwood, 1996; Jackson et al., 1996) (see Chapter 10). We believe that there are early developmental processes here which have implications for the prevention of long-term secondary difficulty, particularly depression and suicide.

There are two broad models of the individual response to psychosis: the *trauma* and the *evaluative* models. The *trauma* model focusses on the role of psychosis and the circumstances of its management as an event, posing a threat to the physical and psychological well-being of the individual and its sequelae, e.g., post-traumatic stress (McGorry et al., 1991). Traumatic beliefs (e.g. 'the world is not a safe place', 'people cannot be trusted') have been studied in other contexts but their relevance to psychosis has only recently begun to be addressed (Jackson & Birchwood, 1996; Jackson et al., 1996; see Chapter 10), and the potential links with social avoidance and withdrawal are apparent.

The *evaluative* model focusses directly on the beliefs or appraisals of the meaning of psychosis for the individual. One aspect focusses on the meaning of the diagnosis for the individual's identity and concept of self and social position. The second concerns the individual's model of the illness itself; for example, within a health belief framework (Budd, Hughes & Smith, 1996).

We have investigated early developmental changes within the evaluative framework which concern the perceived impact on the patient's social position and identity, and their relationship with depression and suicidal thinking (Birchwood & Iqbal, 1998).

Whereas cognitive theory argues that the lowering of self-regard has early origins, recent ideas based on social ranking and power from ethology (e.g. Price et al., 1994) argue that certain situations are likely to be depressogenic where they are perceived to embody *loss* (e.g. acceptance of a forced and subordinate role); *humiliation* (events which undermine the person's rank, attractiveness or status); and *entrapment* in which the situation prevents the individual from moving forward and achieving desired goals or roles, and thus affirming an identity. In our previous work (Birchwood et al., 1993) we established that depression was linked to evaluation of loss (e.g. 'I am capable of little of value as a result of my illness'), humiliation (e.g. 'I cannot talk to people about my illness'), and entrapment (e.g. 'I am powerless to influence or control my illness'). In a recent prospective study involving patients in early psychosis (Birchwood & Iqbal, 1998) it was found that changes, particularly in the appraisal of entrapment, anticipated changes in depressed mood and suicidal thinking in a sample of patients in the early phase of psychosis. The appraisal of entrapment itself changed over time, but was preceded in many instances by a compulsory admission which was seen by the individual to provide 'hard evidence' for the perception that they were entrapped by a malignant illness and an omnipotent agency (e.g. psychiatric services). These appraisals were less plastic as time progressed, suggesting that they were laid down in this early phase. The 'sealing over' strategy (see also Chapter 10) measured in the course of this prospective study, was linked to both traumatic and evaluative beliefs, particularly the sense of entrapment in a relapsing psychotic illness and the internalization of the negative social stereotypes of mental illness. Thus, although patients attempt to 'seal over', they do so because the appraisal of psychosis embodies a denigration of the self which is painful and which patients attempt to suppress through the 'sealing' process.

The therapeutic implication is that cognitive therapy should focus on these developing appraisals in the early phase of psychosis (Birchwood & Iqbal, 1998) which address directly the problems of depression and suicidal thinking. This might include the use of group techniques to rebut the challenge to social status (Drury et al., 1996).

(3) The desynchrony between clinical and social functioning begins in early psychosis

While symptoms and social functioning are clearly not orthogonal, the prospective studies, including those in early psychosis, emphasize their desynchrony on cross-sectional evaluation. The studies of Biehl et al. (1986) and Schubart et al. (1986) emphasize continuity within each domain, such that the best predictor of social functioning after five years is an earlier measure of the *same* characteristic. From a therapeutic point of view it should not be assumed that improvements in social and community functioning can be 'bought' by a focus on symptoms alone. Early intervention may best be conceived as a process involving three domains: symptoms, and psychosocial and psychological functioning, each requiring attention independent of the other. The domains clearly interact; for example, improvements in vocational functioning may enhance self-esteem and promote social engagement which may reduce vulnerability to relapse.

The results of the DOSMD study (Jablensky et al., 1992) have confirmed earlier findings that socio-cultural influences can affect early outcome for schizophrenia, and the follow-up study of first-episode schizophrenia in Madras (Eaton et al., 1995) suggests the apparent early advantage for developing countries is maintained after ten years. This is consistent with the view that sustained early intervention can affect the long-term trajectory of psychosis. Changing the early course of psychosis will be no easy task as the variables at play are numerous; the critical period hypothesis suggests that multimodal intervention strategies will be essential and need to be sustained over at least two years. These strategies are considered below.

Overview of interventions in the critical period

Reducing delay

It has been argued that in excess of one-third of first-episode psychotic patients experience a lengthy period of untreated illness which may have long-term consequences, much of which is, in principle at least, preventable (Birchwood & Macmillan, 1993; Helgason, 1990). Reducing these delays will require a clear understanding of the factors affecting delay; these are considered at length elsewhere in the book (see Chapter 3).

Relapse prevention

Relapse is one factor which appears to underpin developing treatment resistance and early disability (Shepherd et al., 1989). As we have seen, some 40% of first-episode schizophrenics relapse within two years, rising to 80% within five years (Shepherd et al., 1989). Maintenance medication is of proven prophylactic efficacy (Kane, 1989) but placebo-controlled follow-up studies of first episodes of schizophrenia are very rare; the Northwick Park study (Johnstone et al., 1986) found that 60% of patients on placebo and 40% on active medication relapsed within two years; thus 40% did not relapse even though they were not on active medication. Therefore, it is important to predict who will do well without, and who will fare badly in spite of, maintenance medication. The apparently lower dose of neuroleptic required in the acute treatment study by McEvoy, Hogarty & Steingard (1991), for the sub-sample of first-episode cases compared to the multiple-episode cases of schizophrenia, suggests that 'lower' dose maintenance medication may be adequately prophylactic for this group.

This is important in view of the finding in the Northwick Park study that among those with short pretreatment psychotic illnesses, better outcome in occupational terms was associated with placebo prescription (Johnstone et al., 1990). Intermittent strategies offer no clear-cut advantage over conventional paradigms (Herz et al., 1991); however, there is evidence that low dose and targeted strategies combined can adequately control relapse, compared with low and standard doses alone (Marder et al., 1987; Marder, 1994). This may prove to be a helpful approach with a substantial proportion of first-episode (drug naïve) patients and deserves careful study. Cannabis abuse has also been linked to early relapse in recent-onset schizophrenia (Linszen et al., 1994) with clear therapeutic implications.

The early detection of impending relapse presents a further opportunity for relapse prevention, since it is now understood that psychotic relapse describes a process with a modal period of 2–4 weeks in which changes in cognition, emotion and perception metamorphose into frank psychotic symptoms (Birchwood, 1995). These early symptoms have been characterized as 'prodromal' (importing the biomedical concept) and have led to numerous studies attempting to establish the sensitivity and specificity of 'early signs', with some, albeit modest, success (Birchwood & Drury, 1995). The logical consequence of this model is that intervention informed by the presence of early signs is viewed as a means of 'primary' prevention of relapse. Recent thinking has moved towards the view that prodromes are not discrete but are continuous with relapse and best thought of as 'early or minor relapse', and there may be several prodromes prior to a full relapse; thus, early identification and intervention may be thought of as a form of secondary prevention (Birchwood, 1995).

We should be thinking, therefore, of reducing the duration and severity of relapse as well as its incidence. After all, as we have seen earlier in the book, the duration of psychotic symptoms is as harmful as its incidence. A second consequence of this model questions the assumption that prodromes are templates against which to compare each patient's mental state. Like relapse itself, the 'prodromes' should show between-subject variability, but also within-subject temporal stability. It is for this reason that we introduced the concept of the 'relapse signature' – a personalized set of early symptoms which may include core or common symptoms, together with symptoms unique to each patient. If a patient's early relapse signature can be identified, then it may be expected that the predictive power of 'prodromal' symptoms may be increased, although it must be recognized that individuals may move into and out of early relapse, and also that the process might be 'spontaneously' aborted for psychological, psychosocial or biological reasons (Birchwood, 1995).

With this in mind, the prevention of relapse using 'early signs' methodology should be considered as a form of secondary prevention, reducing the severity and frequency of symptoms. Gaining an image of the relapse signature will be important through careful interviewing of the client and family; Figure 9.2 gives one such example for a patient labelled KF. This may not be a straightforward task after the first episode, as the process of development and presentation at the first episode is potentially protracted and confusing.

At least an hypothesis about the relapse signature should be developed and a strategy worked out in advance. This should include the following elements. First, the client, family and keyworker should be armed with this information and a clear route of access to the service rehearsed. Second, an intermediate 'alert' state should be identified in which changes in mental life and behaviour suggestive of relapse, lead to *increased contact* and support of the client and family; this should involve closer surveillance of mental state. This may be sufficient in many instances but will enable the keyworker to determine at close quarters whether the changes appear 'relentless and remorseless' and require further action. Third, a package of early intervention strategies should be implemented. These will include an individualized targeted dose of neuroleptic medication, stress management and cognitive therapeutic strategies aimed at emerging psychotic symptoms (Birchwood, 1995; Chadwick, Birchwood & Trower, 1996). Figure 9.3 shows the impact in one case. We have recently concluded a trial of this approach (Birchwood, 1995), and provisional results show a marked reduction in the rate of relapse, and duration of psychosis in the experimental group (Birchwood & Drury, 1995). A recent study by Marder (1994) reports the outcome of a similar strategy in which patients maintained on low doses (5–10 mg every two weeks) of fluphenazine decanoate received active or placebo supplementation depending on the onset of prodromes. A reduction of relapse in the second year was reported, although the specificity of a prodrome for relapse was not high; however, the occurrence of a prodrome was a good marker of a patient at high risk of ultimate exacerbation, this being consistent with the concept of the prodrome as an 'at-risk mental state' (Yung et al., 1996).

Family intervention is a further option for relapse prevention (Kavanagh, 1992), although the predictive efficacy of high expressed emotion among first-episode patients is somewhat weaker (Birchwood, 1992), possibly because harmful, stressful relationships may take some

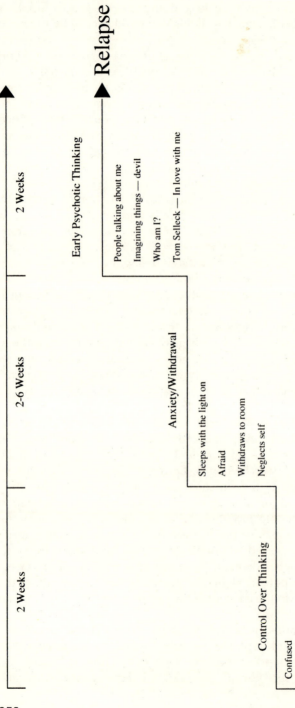

Figure 9.2. Early signs and symptoms of a relapse: KF.

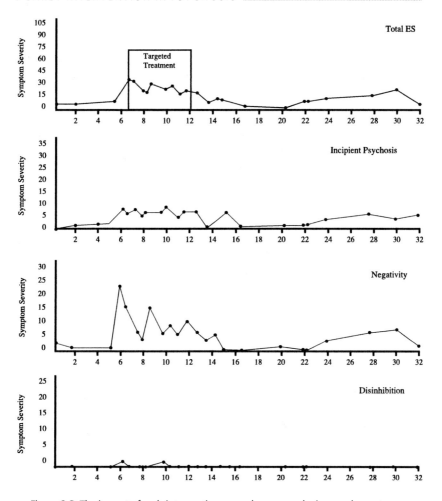

Figure 9.3. The impact of early intervention procedures on early signs and symptoms.

time to evolve (Stirling et al., 1991) and may account for a failure of family intervention to control early relapse (Linszen et al., 1996). The development of a strategy to prevent the development of harmful criticism and hostility is indicated – one which will require a clear understanding of the genesis and early development of expressed emotion (Birchwood, 1992).

Cognitive therapy in the early psychological adjustment to psychotic illness

As we have seen, the psychological well-being of patients following the first diagnosis of schizophrenia is not a well-researched topic, yet there is considerable evidence that the problems of early adjustment can have serious consequences. Suicide is one such consequence, and is by no means usually a direct consequence of psychotic thinking (Caldwell & Gottesman, 1990). Risk factors such as awareness of the deteriorative effects of illness in the context of good premorbid adjustment (Cotton, Drake & Gates, 1985), and fear of mental deterioration (Drake et al., 1985), are well established. Chronic depression arising out of the acute episode (Johnson, 1981) has similar correlates, including hopelessness, perceived loss of control over illness, and the absorption of the negative stereotypes of mental illness (Birchwood et al., 1993). Short-term traumatic reactions to acute, particularly first, psychotic episodes have been documented during the recovery phase, including depression (McGlashan & Carpenter, 1976) and post-traumatic stress disorder (McGorry et al., 1991); both have links with the experience of illness and the circumstances of its management (see Chapter 10). Poor premorbid psychological and social adjustment are well documented in schizophrenia, and the developing concept of self and identity are likely early casualties. Adjusting to the onset of psychosis will require cognisance of developmental stage in addition to *specific* issues of adjustment to psychosis (e.g. trauma, loss, fear of relapse, etc.).

Denial of illness is a frequently used defensive manoeuvre which has its own costs (e.g. drug non-adherence); acceptance of illness, on the other hand, can lead to pessimism and loss of self-efficacy (Birchwood et al., 1993; Warner et al., 1989). What kind of adjustment should be the aim? We have argued that a central feature should be the blame-free acceptance of illness, together with the encouragement of a sense of mastery over illness through education and inculcating strategies of control (see Birchwood & Tarrier, 1994). Facing up to the reality of the disorder, yet at the same time avoiding 'engulfment' in the chronic patient role, will require more than the provision of information and skills; an ongoing supportive therapeutic relationship will be needed to assist the client's passage into psychological well-being (Frank & Gunderson, 1990).

There are some very specific implications for cognitive therapy arising from the evaluative model discussed earlier in the prevention and management of depression, hopelessness and suicidal thinking. In summary, empirical and theoretical work has confirmed the relationship between the symptoms of depression/hopelessness/suicidal ideation, and the cognitive appraisals of *self and psychosis* (loss, humiliation and entrapment), *self and symptoms* (e.g. the power and malevolence of voices), and the implications for *self-evaluation* (failure, worthlessness). Cognitive therapy is ideally suited to focus on these appraisals (Chadwick et al., 1996). For example, interventions have been developed which enhance control over psychotic relapse (Birchwood, 1995); change the appraisals of the power and authority of voices (Chadwick & Birchwood, 1995); and change patients' beliefs about the self and psychosis in the course of recovery from acute psychosis (Drury et al., 1996) – all of which have impacted on depression. Our experience of implementing cognitive therapy in acute psychosis has suggested that appraisals of self and psychosis are more accessible during the acute crisis (Birchwood & Drury, 1995) and should start during this period.

The theme of the cognitive therapy is therefore focussed on key appraisals of self and psychosis, aiming to challenge and put them to the empirical test. These appraisals include: *entrapment in psychotic illness* (beliefs about psychosis as a malignant and uncontrollable illness, and beliefs about the power and malevolence of auditory hallucinations); *loss and humiliation* (belief that the individual has lost all valued goals and roles, and is capable of little of value and is devalued by others); *causal attribution* (a belief that psychosis arises as a result of a defect of the self or personality); and *self-evaluative beliefs*, particularly regarding worthlessness and failure. The *entrapment* belief may be addressed in two ways. First, patients can be trained in methods of detecting and controlling early signs of relapse (Birchwood, 1995) in the context of psychoeducation about psychosis as an external stressor which can be brought under a patient's control. Individuals are debriefed about the events leading up to the onset of psychosis, and helped to identify possible triggers. Second, key beliefs about the power of voices should be challenged and tested (Chadwick & Birchwood, 1994), including related persecutory beliefs. *Negative self-evaluation* can be addressed in two ways. First, individual sessions can be conducted using cognitive therapy to challenge negative self-evaluations together with goal setting in valued interpersonal and achievement domains. Secondly, a group intervention can be conducted such as the one we employed in our trial of cognitive therapy for acute psychotic symptoms. This included those elements unique to the individual to necessarily rebut any challenge to the individual's social status (Drury et al., 1996).

Early social recovery

Prior to the first treatment, prodromal changes can impact heavily on interpersonal and vocational relationships (Jones et al., 1993) and cause damage to, and shrinkage of, the social network for many young people (Hirschenberg, 1985). Social isolation is a known prognostic factor in psychosis (Jablensky et al., 1992) and 'tracks' long-term outcome (McGlashan, 1988). While there are few guidelines for developing interventions in this area (Jackson & Edwards, 1992), community-oriented care involving assertive outreach, can improve the quality and quantity of the social network (Thornicroft & Breakey, 1991). Returning to, or establishing, a work pattern can become increasingly difficult with the passage of time without work; and the diagnosis of schizophrenia makes such a prospect doubly difficult (Warner, 1994). Normal pathways to employment can be frightening and overwhelming for people with psychosis and may require specific co-operation between health, social services and employment agencies, in order to facilitate the pathway and to guard against relapse.

Managing early treatment resistance

After five years, up to 50% of patients will experience residual, treatment-resistant symptoms (Shepherd et al., 1989). These have long-term prognostic implications; for example, a recent long-term follow-up study by Harrow et al. (1995) found that where 'delusions are found in a schizophrenic patient after the acute phase they are likely to recur or persist over the next 2 to 8 years' (p. 102).

According to Harrow and colleagues, long-term treatment resistance has its origins in the critical period; thus, efforts to focus directly on this might be repaid over the long term. Clozapine is used increasingly with treatment-resistant symptoms of a more protracted nature and may find useful application earlier than is usually considered.

Cognitive therapy, which has been widely employed in the treatment of neurotic disorders, has found recent application and early success with psychotic symptoms (Chadwick et al., 1996; Garety, Kuipers & Fowler, 1994; Kingdon & Turkington, 1994). The approach involves the direct engagement of the delusional beliefs (including delusions about voices), and examining the inferences and evaluations patients make about situations (e.g. voice activity) which are linked to delusional thinking by using intellectual challenges and empirical tests.

For reasons outlined above, our approach to treatment resistance has focused on the acute psychotic episode as the origin of residual symptoms or treatment resistance. We believe that this is the most appropriate setting to implement CT as we hypothesize that delusional thinking is encapsulated by a need to reject otherwise stigmatizing labels and ethnosemantic constructs of madness which, because of fragile self-esteem, individuals are unable to resist (Birchwood & Drury, 1995).

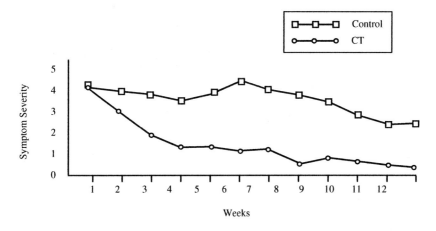

Figure 9.4. The impact of CT intervention on recovery from acute psychosis.

During the acute phase we believe that the individual is psychologically more accessible and defenses more permeable.

The cognitive therapy (CT) (see Drury et al., 1996) programme we use incorporates the following elements:

(1) Individual CT involving the eliciting of evidence for delusional beliefs, including beliefs about hallucinations, and subsequent challenging of that evidence. This is conducted in an atmosphere of 'collaborative empiricism' following the development of a sound therapeutic relationship.
(2) Group CT in groups of three to five clients. The aim of this group was to promote universality and to identify and find value and acceptance among a group of young people with similar problems. The solidarity of the group enabled them to highlight and challenge the cultural stereotypes of mental illness and to acquire a degree of control over psychotic illness.
(3) Family engagement. This had two aims: first, to counsel families against expecting quick cures or solutions, and to understand and collaborate with the CT approach.

The results (Drury et al., 1996) revealed a speedier and more complete recovery from acute psychosis (see Figure 9.4) which was maintained at nine months follow-up in a sample of young, psychotic patients (average age was 29 years).

We believe that CT should not be viewed as a 'treatment' but as part of the process of recovery. Recovery can be most effectively negotiated when the individual is aware of his or her active role in managing the future course of illness, and when his or her strengths are harnessed to bring about a process of change and personal growth. This can protect the person from the damaging effect of stigma, and increase the likelihood of a satisfactory readjustment of the individual's roles and goals, and reaffirmation of identity.

Concluding remarks

In the UK the nomination of a keyworker or case manager to support individuals with a serious mental illness is predicated upon the client having multiple or complex needs, usually defined in terms of a risk of harm to self or others. If the early intervention paradigm becomes part of the landscape of community care, this definition will need to be broadened to include risk of future deterioration *because* the individual has experienced a first psychotic episode. If indeed this is a critical period, it will be required to demonstrate that the early outcome can be improved significantly and, ideally, if the grip is relaxed, such improvements would require *relatively* little maintenance. Only properly conducted randomized controlled trials with a long follow-up period can satisfactorily address this question. Truly the era of secondary prevention in psychosis has begun.

References

Achte, K., Lonnqvist, J., Juusi, K. Piirtola, O. & Niskanen, P. (1986). Outcome studies on schizophrenic psychoses in Helsinki. *Psychopathology*, **19**, 60–7.

American Psychiatric Association (1987). *Diagnostic and Statistical Manual*, 3rd edn, revised. Washington, DC: American Psychiatric Association.

American Psychiatric Association (1994). *Diagnostic and Statistical Manual*, 4th edn. Washington, DC: American Psychiatric Association.

Bebbington, P. & Kuipers, L. (1994). The predictive utility of expressed emotion in schizophrenia: an aggregate analysis. *Psychological Medicine*, **24**, 707–18.

Beiser, M., Erickson, D., Fleming, J. A. E. & Iacono, W. G. (1993). Establishing the onset of psychotic illness. *American Journal of Psychiatry*, **150**, 1349–54.

Beiser, M., Fleming, J. A. E., Iacono, W. G. & Lin, T. (1988). Refining the diagnosis of schizophreniform disorder. *American Journal of Psychiatry*, **145**, 695–700.

Beiser, M., Iacono, W. G. & Erickson, D. (1989). Temporal stability in major mental disorders. In *The Validity of Psychiatric Diagnosis*, ed. L. N. Robins & J. E. Barrett, pp. 77–98. New York: Raven Press.

Biehl, H., Maurer, K., Schubart, C., Krumm, B. & Jung, E. (1986). Prediction of outcome and utilisation of medical services in a prospective study of first onset schizophrenics: results of a prospective five-year follow-up study. *European Archives of Psychiatry and Neurological Sciences*, **236**, 139–47.

Birchwood, M. (1992). Family factors in psychiatry. *Current Opinion in Psychiatry*, **5**, 295–9.

Birchwood, M. (1995). Early intervention in psychotic relapse: cognitive approaches to detection and management. *Behaviour Change*, **12**, 2–19.

Birchwood, M. & Drury, V. (1995). Using the crisis. In *Emergency Mental Health Services in the Community*, ed. M. Phelan, G. Strathdee & G. Thornicroft, pp. 116–48. Cambridge, UK: Cambridge University Press.

Birchwood, M. & Iqbal, Z. (in press). Depression and suicidal thinking in psychosis. In *Outcome and Innovation in Psychological Treatment of Schizophrenia*, ed. T. Wykes, N. Tarrier, & S. Lewis. Chichester, UK: Wiley.

Birchwood, M. & Macmillan, F. (1993). Early intervention in schizophrenia. *Australian and New Zealand Journal of Psychiatry*, **27**, 374–8.

Birchwood, M. & Tarrier, N. (1994). *The Psychological Management of Schizophrenia*. Chichester, UK: Wiley.

Birchwood, M., Hallett, S. & Preston, M. (1988). *Schizophrenia: An Integrated Approach to Research and Treatment*. Harrow, Essex, UK: Longman.

Birchwood, M., Macmillan, F. & Smith, J. (1992). Early intervention. In *Innovations in the Psychological Management of Schizophrenia*, ed. M. Birchwood & N. Tarrier, pp. 115–46. Chichester, UK: Wiley.

Birchwood, M., Cochrane, R., Macmillan, F., Kucharska, J. & Cariss, M. (1992). The influence of ethnicity and family structure on relapse in first episode schizophrenia: a comparison of Asian, Caribbean and White patients. *British Journal of Psychiatry*, **161**, 783–90.

Birchwood, M., Mason, R., Macmillan, F. & Healy, J. (1993). Depression, demoralisation and control over psychotic illness. *Psychological Medicine*, **23**, 387–95.

Birchwood, M., McGorry, P. & Jackson, H. (1997). Early intervention in schizophrenia. (Editorial). *British Journal of Psychiatry*, **170**, 2–5.

Bleuler, M. (1978). *The Schizophrenic Disorders: Long Term Patient and Family Studies*, translated by S. Clements. New Haven: Yale University Press.

Bromet, E. J., Jandorf, L., Fennig, S., Lavelle, J., Kovasznay, B., Ram, R., Tanenberg-Karant, M. & Craig, T. (1996). The Suffolk County Mental Health Project: demographic, premorbid and clinical correlates of 6–month outcome. *Psychological Medicine*, **26**, 953–62.

Budd, R. J., Hughes, I. C. T. & Smith, J. A. (1996). Health beliefs and compliance with antipsychotic medication. *British Journal of Clinical Psychology*, **35**, 393–7.

Caldwell, J. & Gottesman, I. (1990). Schizophrenics kill themselves too. *Schizophrenia Bulletin*, **16**, 571–90.

Carpenter, W. & Strauss, J. (1991). The prediction of outcome in schizophrenia. V: Eleven year follow-up of the IPSS cohort. *Journal of Nervous and Mental Disease*, **179**, 517–25.

Chadwick, P. & Birchwood, M. (1994). Challenging the omnipotence of voices: a cognitive approach to auditory hallucinations. *British Journal of Psychiatry*, **164**, 190–201.

Chadwick, P. & Birchwood, M. (1995). A cognitive approach to auditory hallucinations. In *Cognitive–Behavioural Interventions in Psychosis*, ed. G. Haddock & P. Slade, pp. 71–85. London: Routledge.

Chadwick, P., Birchwood, M. & Trower, P. (1996). *Cognitive Therapy for Hallucinations, Delusions and Paranoia.* Chichester, UK: Wiley.

Cotton, P., Drake, R. & Gates, C. (1985). Critical treatment issues in schizophrenics. *Hospital and Community Psychiatry*, **36**, 534–6.

DeLisi, L. (1990). *Depression in Schizophrenia.* Washington, DC: American Psychiatric Press.

Drake, R., Gates, C., Cotton, P. & Whittaker, A. (1985). Suicide among schizophrenics: who is at risk? *Journal of Nervous and Mental Disease*, **172**, 613–17.

Drury, V. (1994). Recovery from acute psychosis. In *Psychological Management of Schizophrenia*, ed. M. Birchwood & N. Tarrier, pp. 23–51. Chichester, UK: Wiley.

Drury, V., Birchwood, M., Cochrane, R. & Macmillan, F. (1996). Cognitive therapy and recovery from acute psychosis: A controlled trial. *British Journal of Psychiatry*, **169**, 593–601.

Dube, K., Kumar, N. & Dube, S. (1984). Long-term course and outcome of the Agra cases in the International Pilot Study of Schizophrenia. *Acta Psychiatrica Scandinavica*, **170**, 170–9.

Eaton, W., Thara, R., Federman, B., Melton, B. & Liang, K-Y. (1995). Structure and course of positive and negative symptoms in schizophrenia. *Archives of General Psychiatry*, **52**, 127–34.

Frank, A. & Gunderson, J. (1990). The role of the therapeutic alliance in the treatment of schizophrenia: relationship to course and outcome. *Archives of General Psychiatry*, **47**, 228–36.

Garety, P., Kuipers, L. & Fowler, D. (1994). Cognitive behavioural therapy for drug-resistant psychosis. *British Journal of Medical Psychology*, **67**, 259–71.

Geddes, J. R., Black, R. J., Whalley, L. J. & Eagles, J. M. (1994). Persistence of the decline in the diagnosis among first admissions to Scottish hospitals from 1969 to 1988. *British Journal of Psychiatry*, **163**, 620–6.

Hambrecht, M. & Häfner, H. (1996). Substance abuse and the onset of schizophrenia. *Biological Psychiatry*, **40**, 1155–63.

Harding, C. M., Brooks, G. W. & Ashikaga, T. (1987). The Vermont longitudinal study of persons with severe mental illness. II: Long-term outcome of subjects who retrospectively met DSM-III criteria for schizophrenia. *American Journal of Psychiatry*, **144**, 727–35.

Harrison, G., Croudace, T., Mason, P., Glazebrook, C. & Medley, I. (1996). Predicting the long-term outcome of schizophrenia. *Psychological Medicine*, **26**, 697–705.

Harrow, M., MacDonald, A. W., Sands, J. R. & Silverstein, M. L. (1995). Vulnerability to delusions over time in schizophrenia and affective disorders. *Schizophrenia Bulletin*, **21**, 95–109.

Hegarty, J. D., Baldessarini, R. J., Tohen, M., Waternaux, C. & Oepen, G. (1994). One hundred years of schizophrenia: a meta-analysis of the outcome literature. *American Journal of Psychiatry*, **15**, 1409–16.

Helgason, L. (1990). Twenty years follow-up of first psychiatric prevention for schizophrenia: what could have been prevented? *Acta Psychiatrica Scandinavica*, **81**, 231–5.

Herz, M., Glazer, W., Mostert, M., Sheard, M., Szymanski, H., Hafez, H., Mirza, M. & Vana, J. (1991). Intermittent vs maintenance medication in schizophrenia. *Archives of General Psychiatry*, **48**, 333–7.

Hirschenberg, W. (1985). Social isolation among schizophrenic out-patients. *Social Psychiatry*, **20**, 171–8.

Huber, G., Cross, G., Schuttler, R. & Linz (1980). Longitudinal studies of schizophrenic patients. *Schizophrenia Bulletin*, **6**, 592–5.

Humphries, M., Johnstone, E., Macmillan, J. & Taylor, P. (1992). Dangerous behaviour preceding first admissions for schizophrenia. *British Journal of Psychiatry*, **161**, 501–5.

Jablensky, A., Sartorious, N., Emberg, G., Anker, M., Korten, A., Cooper, J. & Bertelson, A. (1992). Schizophrenia: manifestations, incidence and course in different cultures. A World Health Organization Ten Country Study. *Psychological Medicine*, Monograph Supplement 20.

Jackson, C. & Birchwood, M. (1996). Early intervention in psychosis: opportunities for secondary prevention. *British Journal of Clinical Psychology*, **35**, 487–502.

Jackson, H. J. & Edwards, J. (1992). Social networks and social support in schizophrenia. In *Schizophrenia: An Overview and Practical Handbook*, ed. D. Kavanagh, pp. 275–92. London: Chapman & Hall.

Jackson, H. J., McGorry, P. D., Edwards, J. & Hulbert, C. (1996). Cognitively oriented psychotherapy for early psychosis (COPE). In *Early Intervention and Prevention in Mental Health*, eds. P. Cotton & H. Jackson, pp. 131–54. Melbourne: Australian Psychological Society.

Johnson, D. (1981). Studies of depressive symptoms in schizophrenia. *British Journal of Psychiatry*, **139**, 89–101.

Johnstone, E. C., Crow, T. J., Johnson, A. L. & Macmillan, J. F. (1986). The Northwick Park Study of first episode schizophrenia: I. Presentation of the illness and problems relating to admission. *British Journal of Psychiatry*, **148**, 115–20.

Johnstone, E. C., Macmillan, J. F., Frith, C. D., Benn, D. K. & Crow, T. J. (1990). Further investigation of the predictors of outcome following first schizophrenic episodes. *British Journal of Psychiatry*, **157**, 182–9.

Johnstone, E., Frith, C., Crow, T., Owen, D., Done, D., Baldwin, E. & Charlette, A. (1992). The Northwick Park Functional Psychosis Study: diagnosis and outcome. *Psychological Medicine*, **22**, 331–46.

Jones, P. B., Bebbington, P., Foerster, A., Lewis, S. W., Murray, R. M., Russell, A., Sham, P. C., Tone, B. K. & Wilkins, S. (1993). Premorbid social underachievement in schizophrenia: results from the Camberwell Collaborative Psychosis Study. *British Journal of Psychiatry*, **162**, 65–71.

Kane, J. M. (1983). Low dosage medication strategies in the maintenance treatment of schizophrenia. *Schizophrenia Bulletin*, **9**, 528–31.

Kane, J. M. (1989). The current status of neuroleptics. *Journal of Clinical Psychiatry*, **50**, 322–8.

Kavanagh, D. (1992). Recent developments in expressed emotion and schizophrenia. *British Journal of Psychiatry*, **160**, 601–20.

Kingdon, D. G. & Turkington, D. (1994). *Cognitive–Behavioural Therapy of Schizophrenia*. Brighton, UK: Erlbaum.

Kraepelin, E. (1896/1987). Dementia Praecox. In *The Clinical Roots of the Schizophrenia Concept*, ed. J. Cutting & M. Shepherd, pp. 13–24. Cambridge, UK: Cambridge University Press.

Linszen, D., Dingemans, P., Van der Does, J., Nugter, A., Scholte, P., Lenior, R. & Goldstein, M. J. (1996). Treatment, expressed emotion and relapse in recent onset schizophrenia. *Psychological Medicine*, **26**, 333–42.

Linszen, D., Dingemans, P. & Lenior, M. (1994). Cannabis abuse and the course of schizophrenic disorders. *Archives of General Psychiatry*, **51**, 73–9.

Loebel, A. D., Lieberman, J. A., Alvir, J. M. J., Mayerhoff, D. I., Geisler, S. H. & Szymanski, S. R. (1992). Duration of psychosis and outcome in first episode schizophrenia. *American Journal of Psychiatry*, **149**, 1183–8.

Marder, S., Van Putten, T., Mintz, J., McKenzie, J., Labell, M., Faltico, G. & May, R. (1987). Low and conventional dose maintenance therapy with fluphenazine decanoate. *Archives of General Psychiatry*, **44**, 518–21.

Marder, S. R. (1994). Fluphenazine vs placebo supplementation for prodromal signs of relapse in schizophrenia. *Archives of General Psychiatry*, **51**, 280–7.

Mason, P., Harrison, G., Glazebrook, C., Medley, I., Dalkin, T. & Croudace, T. (1995). Characteristics of outcome in schizophrenia at 13 years. *British Journal of Psychiatry*, **167**, 596–603.

McEvoy, J. P., Hogarty, G. E. & Steingard, S. (1991). Optimal dose of neuroleptic in acute schizophrenia. *Archives of General Psychiatry*, **48**, 739–45.

McGlashan, T. (1988). A selective review of North American long-term followup studies of schizophrenia. *Schizophrenia Bulletin*, **14**, 515–42.

McGlashan, T. & Carpenter, W. (1976). Post-psychotic depression in schizophrenia. *Archives of General Psychiatry*, **33**, 231–9.

McGorry, P. D. (1992). The concept of recovery and seondary prevention in psychotic disorders. *Australia and New Zealand Journal of Psychiatry*, **26**, 3–18.

McGorry, P. D., Chanen, A., McCarthy, E., Van Riel, R., McKenzie, D. & Singh, B. (1991). Post-traumatic stress disorder following recent onset psychosis. An unrecognised postpsychotic syndrome. *Journal of Nervous and Mental Disease*, **179**, 253–8.

McGorry, P. Edwards, J., Mihalopoulos, C., Harrigan, S. M. & Jackson, H. J. (1996). EPPIC: an evolving system of early detection and optimal management. *Schizophrenia Bulletin*, **22**, 305–26.

McGorry, P. & Singh, B. (1995). Schizophrenia: risk and possiblility. In *Handbook of Studies on Preventative Psychiatry*, ed. B. Raphael & G. D. Burrows, pp. 491–514. Amsterdam, The Netherlands: Elsevier Science.

Mueser, K. T., Bellack, A. S., Morrison, R. L. & Wade, J. H. (1990). Gender, social competence, and symptomatology in schizophrenia: a longitudinal analysis. *Journal of Abnormal Psychology*, **9**, 138–47.

Perkins, R. E. & Moodley, P. (1993). The arrogance of insight. *Bulletin of the Royal College of Psychiatrists*, **17**, 233–4.

Pilowsky, L. S., Kerwin, R. W. & Murray, R. M. (1993). Schizophrenia: a neurodevelopmental perspective. *Neuropsychopharmacology*, **9**, 83–91.

Price, J., Sloman, L., Gardner, R., Gilbert, P. & Rohde, P. (1994). The social competition hypothesis of depression. *British Journal of Psychiatry*, **164**, 309–15.

Ram, R., Bromet, E. J., Eaton, W. W., Pato, C. & Schwartz, J. E. (1992). The natural course of schizophrenia: a review of first-admission studies. *Schizophrenia Bulletin*, **18**, 185–207.

Roy, A. (1986). Suicide in schizophrenia. In *Suicide*, ed. A. Roy, pp. 128–47. Baltimore: Williams and Wilkins.

Schooler, N. R. (1994). Deficit symptoms in schizophrenia: negative symptoms versus neuroleptic-induced deficits. *Acta Psychiatrica Scandinavica*, **380**, (Supplement), 21–6.

Schubart, C., Krumm, B., Biehl, H. & Schwartz, R. (1986). Measure of social disability in a schizophrenic patient group: definition, assessment and outcome over 2 years in schizophrenic patients of recent onset. *Social Psychiatry*, **21**, 1–9.

Scottish Schizophrenia Research Group (1988). The Scottish First Episode Schizophrenia Study. V: One year follow-up. *British Journal of Psychiatry*, **152**, 470–6.

Scottish Schizophrenia Research Group. (1992). The Scottish First Episode Schizophrenia Study: VIII: Five year follow-up: clinical and psychosocial findings. *British Journal of Psychiatry*, **161**, 496–500.

Shepherd, M., Watt, D., Falloon, I. & Smeeton, N. (1989). The natural history of schizophrenia: a five-year follow-up in a representative sample of schizophrenics. *Psychological Medicine*, Monograph Supplement 15.

Soni, S. D., Tench, D. & Routledge, R. C. (1994). Serum abnormalities in neuroleptic-induced akathisia. *British Journal of Psychiatry*, **165**, 669–72.

Stephens, J. H. (1978). Long-term prognosis and follow-up in schizophrenia. *Schizophrenia Bulletin*, **4**, 25–47.

Stirling, J., Tantum, D., Thonks, P., Newby, D. & Montague, L. (1991). Expressed emotion and early onset schizophrenia. *Psychological Medicine*, **21**, 675–85.

Stirling, J., Tantam, D., Newby, D., Montague, L., Ring, N. & Rowe, S. (1993). Expressed emotion and schizophrenia: the ontogeny of EE during an 18 month follow-up. *Psychological Medicine*, **23**, 771–8.

Strauss, J. & Carpenter, W. T. (1977). Prediction of outcome in schizophrenia. III: Five year outcome and its predictors. *Archives of General Psychiatry*, **34**, 159–63.

Thara, R., Henrietta, M., Joseph, A., Rajkumar, S. & Eaton, W. (1994). Ten- year course of schizophrenia – the Madras longitudinal study. *Acta Psychiatrica Scandinavica*, **90**, 329–36.

Thornicroft, G. & Breakey, W. (1991). The COSTAR Programme. 1: Improving social networks of the long-term mentally ill. *British Journal of Psychiatry*, **159**, 245–59.

Tien, A. Y. & Eaton, W. W. (1992). Psychopathological precursors and sociodemographic risk factors for the schizophrenic syndrome. *Archives of General Psychiatry*, **49**, 37–46.

Waddington, J. L., Youssef, H. A. & Kinsella, A. (1995). Sequential cross-sectional and 10-year prospective study of severe negative symptoms in relation to duration of intitially untreated psychosis in chronic schizophrenia. *Psychological Medicine*, **25**, 849–57.

Warner, R., Taylor, D., Powers, M. & Hyman, J. (1989). Acceptance of the mental illness label by psychotic patients: effects on functioning. *American Journal of Orthopsychiatry*, **59**, 398–409.

Warner, R. (1994). *Recovery from Schizophrenia: Psychiatric and Political Economy*, 2nd edn. London: Routledge.

Westermeyer, J. F., Harrow, M. & Marengo, J. T. (1991). Risk for suicide in schizophrenia and other psychotic and non-psychotic disorders. *Journal of Nervous and Mental Disease*, **179**, 259–66.

Wing, J. K. (1966). Five year outcome in early schizophrenia. *Proceedings of the Royal Society of Medicine*, **59**, 17–18.

World Health Organization (1988). Psychiatric Disability Assessment Schedule. Geneva: World Health Organization.

World Health Organization (1992). *Manual of the International Classification of Diseases, Injuries and Causes of Death*, 10th rev. edn. Geneva: World Health Organization.

Wyatt, R. J. (1991). Neuroleptics and the natural course of schizophrenia. *Schizophrenia Bulletin*, **17**, 325–51.

Yung, A., McGorry, P., McFarlane, C. A., Jackson, H. J., Patton, G. C. & Rakkar, A. (1996). The prodromal phase of first episode psychosis: past and current conceptualisations. *Schizophrenia Bulletin*, **22**, 283–303.

Zubin, J. & Spring, B. (1977). Vulnerability: a new view of schizophrenia. *Journal of Abnormal Psychology*, **86**, 103–26.

10
Recovery from psychosis: psychological interventions

HENRY J. JACKSON, JANE EDWARDS, CAROL HULBERT AND
PATRICK D. MCGORRY

Background

Until the late 1950s, psychodynamically oriented psychotherapy was considered to be the therapy of choice for the psychoses. This approach lost general currency because of two major factors: the successful introduction of neuroleptic medication in the 1950s and the empirical demonstration that psychodynamically oriented psychotherapy was comparatively ineffective in treating people suffering from schizophrenia (Gunderson et al., 1984; May, 1968). Essentially, where implemented, only drug treatment exerted a differential and superior effect; psychodynamically oriented treatments effected only marginal improvements (e.g. May, 1968). Neuroleptic medication became the mainstay of treatment in the psychoses, but with increasing recognition that not all individuals experienced complete remission from their symptoms, and that many suffered from problems in various life domains, even when their positive psychotic symptoms were brought under complete or partial control. The flaw with the thinking underpinning both psychoanalytically and biologically based research was 'reductionism'. One model stressed the 'psychological'; the second, the 'biological'.

The 1960s to the 1980s heralded the emergence of the behavioural paradigm and its application to the problems of psychiatric patients. Aggressive, bizarre, and acting out behaviours were targeted and evaluated using single-subject experimental designs whilst group-based methods were used to train social and independent living skills (Bellack & Hersen, 1979; Scott & Dixon, 1995) and deliver psychoeducational family therapy and patient psychoeducation (Falloon, 1985;

Kavanagh, 1992a, b) (see Note 1, page 297). Although there were some notable successes, particularly regarding family psychoeducation (Dixon & Lehman, 1995; Falloon, 1985; Kavanagh, 1992a, b; Scott & Dixon, 1995) and, to a lesser extent, social skills training (see Halford & Hayes, 1991; Smith, Bellack & Liberman, 1996), issues have arisen with regard to poor generalization to real life community settings and instability of maintenance effects (Halford & Hayes, 1991; Smith et al., 1996), as well as the capacity of 'real world' services to implement the expertise in everyday practice (Kavanagh, 1992b).

In more recent times, we have seen what can be described as a third phase of therapeutic endeavour, one that we believe constitutes a sea-change in terms of how we conceptualize the accessibility of the psychotic individual to psychotherapeutic intervention; the emergence of cognitively oriented approaches in treating affective and anxiety disorders (Beck et al., 1979; Beck & Emery, 1985) and, more recently, their application to the problems experienced by those suffering from schizophrenia (see Note 2, page 297). Three types of interventions are subsumed under the cognitive rubric: first, those which aim to address information-processing deficits (Green, 1993) in order to improve problem-solving skills or skills acquisition (see Liberman, Kopelowicz & Young, 1994); and, second, those which aim to reduce delusions and hallucinations and/or alleviate suffering in those experiencing the same (e.g., Bentall, Haddock & Slade, 1994; Chadwick, Birchwood & Trower, 1996; Fowler, Garety & Kuipers, 1995; Tarrier, 1992). The third group of cognitive approaches are those which focus on the person and his or her construal of the disorder, the disorder's impact on the self, and the adaptation of the self in the wake of a psychotic disorder. Jackson et al. (1996, 1998), Perris (1989), Strauss and Davidson (Davidson & Strauss, 1992, 1995; Strauss, 1994) and, arguably, Hogarty et al. (1995), are proponents of this therapeutic perspective.

Since Green's (1993) work in cognitive remediation is primarily aimed at assisting skills-type training and its application involves an elaboration of the behavioural approach (paradigm) it is not considered further here (see Note 3, page 297). In this particular book chapter, we have chosen to focus exclusively on the latter two of these three major emergent areas: the adaptation of the self in the wake of psychosis and the psychological treatment of positive symptoms.

The self and psychosis

There have been very few researchers who have focused on the issue of self in psychosis from a non-psychodynamic or non-psychoanalytic stance. Some work has been undertaken in this regard by Perris, Strauss and Davidson, and Hogarty. Their work, despite primarily focussing on multiple-episode patients, seems highly relevant to working with individuals with first-episode psychosis.

Carlo Perris

Attachment theory, short-term psychodynamic and cognitive therapeutic principles, contained within the meta-theory of constructivism, comprise the theoretical underpinnings of the approach developed by Perris (Perris, 1989; Perris & Skagerlind, 1994). Some of the core ingredients in his therapy are: an emphasis on the importance of the uniqueness of every individual; a recognition that every person '...has the potential to influence his/her own condition; at least to a certain degree' (Perris, 1992, p. 138); an emphasis on working with the healthy side of the individual; and an emphasis on respecting, maintaining and improving the person's autonomy and competence.

The therapeutic techniques are those of basic cognitive psychotherapy, but therapy is flexible with regard to treatment length, dose, choice and timing of interventions. Therapy is '...carried out at various levels and with different goals in mind' (Perris & Skagerlind, 1994, p. 65). Thus, therapy can range from molecular to molar approaches, i.e. from the detection of basic cognitive deficits and their 'remediation' through self-instructional training, to the modification of delusional and hallucinatory experiences, through to cognitive rehabilitation and the promotion of interpersonal competence. The therapy is not aimed at the reduction or elimination of symptoms *per se*. Rather: 'The ultimate aim of the therapy, however, is to help the patient in the discovery of dysfunctional schemata, or working models which have contributed in determining his/her feelings and in ruling his/her behaviour, and eventually correct them' (Perris, 1992, p. 140).

John Strauss and Larry Davidson

John Strauss and his colleague Larry Davidson are long-standing advocates of a life-context model which views the *person* in psychosis as being able to affect their own developmental trajectory and outcomes (Davidson, 1992; Davidson & Strauss, 1992, 1995; Strauss, 1994). Dissatisfied with both biological and psychoanalytic models, they and their colleagues have examined the ways in which individuals may be able to engage in constructive activity to improve their own functioning, noting that illness may not always be a hindrance to growth: illness can change the person's world view and not always detrimentally

(Davidson & Strauss, 1995). Breier and Strauss (1983, 1984) studied the ways in which people with schizophrenia attempted to control their symptoms, how they utilized social relationships in the process of recovery, and attempted to recover a sense of self-efficacy which had been lost during psychosis (see also Bandura, 1977, 1986). Our work in developing cognitively-oriented psychotherapy for early psychosis (COPE: EPPIC, 1998) has been informed by their reports, particularly their emphasis on the person as an active agent in his or her own destiny.

Gerard Hogarty

Hogarty et al. (1995) have described personal therapy (PT) as a phase-oriented psychotherapy for schizophrenia which assumes that a disease or similar biological dysfunction underpins the clinical presentation, and that complete cerebral integrity should not be assumed – instead it is assumed that patients are at least transiently compromised with regard to cognitive functioning, e.g. abstraction and problem-solving. Hogarty and colleagues provide a broad package of skills in their treatment regimen and, in this regard, they are trying to treat the whole person. Traditional behavioural techniques of modelling, rehearsal, practice, feedback and homework are utilized in imparting or building skills. Cognitive strategies such as coping are taught and the influence of the patient on others (e.g. the family) is examined. The formation of a treatment alliance and the provision of psychoeducation conducted within individual and group sessions are given initial priority, along with active advocacy of the patient by the therapist, as are the establishment and maintenance of low but effective medication for maximal benefit but with no or minimal side-effects.

In their 1995 publication Hogarty et al. briefly comment on two studies involving n's of 91 and 54 being conducted but subsequently, at three years' assessment, have found an advantage for PT for those patients residing with families (but not for those without families) in preventing relapse (Hogarty et al., 1997a) and in promoting personal and social adjustment (Hogarty et al., 1997b). In fact, effect sizes for social adjustment favoured PT quite markedly at years 2 and 3.

Searching for a new paradigm

The shortcomings of the neo-Kraepelinian paradigm (Andreasen, 1984; Robins & Guze, 1970) have been extensively documented, as has the lack of consideration of schizophrenia (or psychosis more broadly defined) as a psychological disorder (Bentall, 1990; Healy, 1990, 1993; McGorry, 1992, 1994,1995; Sass, 1992, 1994). The limitations include the variable course of the disorder, i.e. the course is not inevitably deteriorating; the fact that a proportion of clients suffer a single episode only; that not all clients reveal structural brain changes; that not all have poor outcomes; that psychosis is broader and more inclusive of other disorders than schizophrenia; and that the specific diagnoses of schizophrenia, and bipolar or schizoaffective disorder are neither clear nor stable in the first episode (Fennig et al., 1994; Jackson et al., 1996). Since one may be able to positively affect both course and outcome, there is a need to deliver treatment at the earliest available opportunity (McGorry, 1992; McGlashan & Johannessen, 1996). We need to develop a model which allows for a psychological dimension but equally acknowledges a biological basis for the disturbance (Coursey, 1989; Coursey, Keller & Farrell, 1995).

Over more than a decade, our research group has been developing guidelines for a preventively oriented therapy aimed at assisting first-episode psychotic clients to adapt in the wake of the first psychotic episode, preventing or alleviating secondary morbidity and subsequent episodes/relapses. The therapy is based explicitly on two additional principles which run contrary to the neo-Kraepelinian model, namely: that the needs of first-episode clients are not the same as those with more established or chronic forms of illness; and that maximal and carefully tailored therapeutic input in the first 2–5 years may have powerful downstream effects (Birchwood & Macmillan, 1993; Birchwood, McGorry & Jackson, 1997; McGorry, 1992, 1995).

Our theoretical underpinnings for this therapy have derived from a variety of approaches including trauma theory, attributional theory, social psychology, social learning theory (in particular self-efficacy theory), cognitive therapeutic principles, and life-span development. This apparent congeries of approaches can be subsumed under the metatheory of constructivism. The nub of the constructivistic approach is that humans actively create and construe their personal representational model of the world (Bruner, 1986; Guidano, 1987; Kelly, 1955; Mahoney, 1991; Neimeyer & Mahoney, 1995). Yet, our approach is best dubbed 'critical constructivism', for it accepts the real constraints placed upon the person by the world, culture, and biology (see Note 4, page 297). This approach stands in marked contrast to more radical constructivistic approaches such as solipsism (Sass, 1992, 1994) or the post-modern approach (Gergen, 1994) which would deny such 'assumed' constraints. Two aspects of critical constructivism are worthy of underscoring. The first is the emphasis on the self, and the second is the emphasis on the developmental context which, naturally, is instrumental in shaping the former (Mahoney, 1991). Both aspects are highly relevant to the person with first-break psychosis.

The self

The self is regarded as relatively coherent, but one that is dynamic and pluralistic (Mahoney, 1991; Markus & Nurius, 1986; Singer & Salovey, 1993). Michael Mahoney (1991) has described four core concepts of self: these pertaining to the formation of identity, the expression, range and modulation of emotion, the expression and modulation of power, and a reality orientation – the latter referring to the person becoming increasingly aware of the demands of the world and others. One can draw upon the concept of possible selves (Markus & Nurius, 1986) to see that illness and its aftermath may affect the individual's concept of him- or herself as they are, as they wished to be (the positive self), and the self they fear they might become (feared or undesired self) (Ogilvie, 1987). The key issue here is that the recovering clients may panic, recognizing that with the onset of illness or 'breakdown' they might not achieve their 'hoped for selves' and fearing that they might become a 'mental patient'.

Development

Gould (1978), Erikson (1950), and Levinson (1986) have described the various broad conceptual developmental phases and challenges facing the individual as they move along the lifespan course, with Levinson (1986) nominating the years 17–22 as the period of early adult transition (see Note 5, page 297). During this momentous period, major developmental tasks are to individuate from the family, to develop and expand on one's interests, hobbies and skills, to discover and experiment with one's sexuality, to form and maintain relationships, including those of an intimate kind, and to move towards taking up employment or further study opportunities. During this period the person is moving from preceding developmental periods to a new phase when he or she is expected, and expects, to assume more self-control over their lives and be less dependent upon external regulation. Adolescence and early adulthood are periods when the person can flex his or her muscles, so to speak, and demonstrate some control in certain domains, by testing limits within the environment, with this sense of self-efficacy and power being of critical importance to self-regulation. The peer group becomes more important with mutual peer interactions helping form the person's social self – the person learning to mesh with others and at times to subjugate oneself; but also learning both to lead others, as well as to individuate from them.

During such a critical life phase, sustained obstacles to forming such a broad raft of skills across various life domains may interfere with future adult development (Schulz & Heckhausen, 1996; Sugarman, 1986). Any significant upheaval (e.g. launching a career) poses a major threat to the self, and may detrimentally affect the person and the realization of developmental tasks. Psychosis could be understood to constitute significant upheavals as even 'minor psychiatric' disorder can compromise these developmental tasks (Kessler et al., 1995).

Impact of the psychosis on self and development

The effects of the psychosis on the self and development may be potentially cataclysmic, causing derailment, truncation, deflection or paralysis of the person's developmental trajectory. Psychosis has the potential to change or alter the person's usual way of construing themself, their environment and their future, and the devastation is further potentiated where the person is relatively young and developmentally 'immature'. This means in practice that the individual may reduce his or her movement towards independence from the family, and reduce their striving towards self-acceptance and integration of the various parts of self. Positive risk-taking or growth, which at the most superficial level might include trying out new clothes, music, hairstyles, etc., is likely to be inhibited. Substance abuse could become entrenched. Study habits and motoric skills acquisition could be affected, as could self-esteem. In short, all of this is likely to interfere with identity formation, attenuate the ability to exert power (establish self-efficacy), and interfere with emotional expression and modulation. Naturally, where instability or poor functioning has clearly long preceded any evidence of psychosis or its prodromata in the adolescent, then the psychosis and its consequences may be even more traumatic, leading to more chaotic sequelae and trajectories in which it is harder for helpers to intercede (Gleick, 1994). Of course, many of these features can be seen in those people who are chronically unemployed, where there is derailment for other reasons (e.g. social, economic), leading to the same secondary effects. It may be the case that much deficit functioning may represent *indirect*, not *direct*, sequelae of the 'disorder'.

Discussion of developmental factors necessarily entails consideration of personality factors (Millon, 1996). Although the consensus is that personality does not stabilize until somewhere around the age of 30 years (McCrae & Costa, 1990), there is agreement amongst clinicians and researchers that long-standing differences in 'temperament' are manifest between people (e.g. Cloninger et al., 1993) and the same holds true when people develop 'character traits' during the adolescent period (Cloninger et al., 1993). Conceivably, personality styles or traits could be affected directly by the psychosis and the person's response to it, especially if the person experiences psychosis in adolescent years, further impeding the person's subsequent developmental trajectory, via a potentially pathoplastic process, whereby the psychosis and pre-existing personality style become inextricably and irrevocably entwined with one another (Hulbert, Jackson & McGorry, 1996).

Rationale for intervention and implications for the self

The perceptions of the clients of themselves, and their attitude towards the disorder *per se*, may be instrumental in determining how they will cope with the illness, and may well influence their mid- to longer-term outcomes. We have argued elsewhere that, by intervening early in the psychotic episode, we may be better able to help the client to preserve a sense of self (i.e. *identity*) and preserve or increase the person's sense of *power* or self-efficacy (Jackson et al., 1996). We further suggest that it may be possible to influence the course of the disorder and minimize relapse, disabilities, handicaps and secondary morbidity if we can intervene early and comprehensively in the first-episode (Jackson et al., 1996).

We view the promotion of adaptation to an initial psychotic episode as the major aim of therapy and consider psychoeducation alone (McGorry, 1992, 1995) too narrow a strategy alone to promote this aim. Secondary morbidity is viewed as an expression of the individual's failure to adapt, whether this occurs *de novo*, or is a heightened expression of premorbid personality traits. The aim is to help the individual to come to terms with the illness, to maintain self-esteem and prevent demoralization and self-stigmatization, to assist the person in asserting some control over his or her environment and future, and to promote recovery.

However, given the relative youth of the clients who first present with psychosis, then it is not an ideal 'achievement' if recovery means that clients return to the 'biopsychosocial space' or developmental phase they occupied two years prior to the emergence of the psychosis. Optimally speaking, persons need to recover to the point in their developmental trajectory where they would have been if they had not become psychotic. This is consistent with the 'growth' model advocated by Davidson and Strauss (1992, 1995). Nevertheless, at this point in time, research is unable to inform us as to the appropriate timing and rate of recovery and 'catch-up'. This remains a clinical decision with few available evidence-based guidelines. We do not want to push too hard and perhaps precipitate a psychotic relapse. In some cases, clinicians may have to accept new trajectories.

Cognitively-oriented psychotherapy for early psychosis (COPE)

There are four phases to the COPE approach. The initial assessment phase overlaps with the second – the therapeutic alliance or engagement phase. Adaptation of the self in the wake of the initial psychotic episode forms the focus of the third phase. In the fourth phase the target is the alleviation or prevention of secondary morbidity, e.g. depression, post-traumatic stress disorder, and social phobia. These phases are neither necessarily discrete nor ironclad; nor do they represent an inevitably unfolding sequence. In fact, there is overlap with shifting occurring from one phase to another, although for clarity's sake, and to facilitate communication, we present them as discrete phases.

Assessment

This encompasses a broad range of domains, from symptom measurement to impact on self and others. Domains to be covered during the assessment phase include: symptoms and onset of disorder; the person's explanatory model and level of insight; their functioning in various domains both before, during, and after the psychotic episode; their descriptions of their possible selves which embody the person's goals, values and aspirations (Markus & Nurius, 1986; Murray, 1938); and their methods of coping. Details of the assessment are to be found in the therapists' manual (EPPIC, 1998). We find that assessment usually takes up to three sessions to complete adequately.

In asking questions, it is important to keep in mind that the client may not consider that he or she has an 'illness'. Therefore, it is appropriate to use the person's language in describing the episode, with phrases such as 'losing it' or 'out of it' being substituted for clinical terminology (Jackson et al., 1996). Repeated mental state examinations are necessary throughout the course of therapy because of fluctuations in symptom levels and types.

In assessing psychotic clients, the therapist must develop a good sense of the client's attributions about themselves in relation to the world, the past and the future. This assessment must extend further than an analysis of the so-called conscious automatic thoughts described by clients to uncover the themes, attribution styles, schemas, scripts and feelings which underpin these so-called automatic thoughts. Besides using careful direct questioning, supplementary ways of accessing these themes over time might be via diaries, autobiographical methods, self-monitoring sheets, empty chair technique, writing essays, or the use of a cassette tape-recorder or video-camera.

Traditional cognitive therapy techniques may be useful in identifying cognitive distortions, in this case 'labelling', 'magnification' and 'dichotomous thinking', yet this does not constitute the whole therapy for the psychotic population (Beck et al., 1979).

Once the therapist is clear about the client's thoughts and feelings about his or her current situation and their view of *present self*, the therapist should then explore the client's view of their *past selves*, that is, as the client saw himself or herself prior to the emergence of the illness, their view of their functioning, their aspirations, etc. Finally, one then needs to explore the map the client has drawn, understanding how the client now views the *present* and *future selves* in various domains and how they believe those *selves* have changed and why. The method here is to see how the illness has distorted or changed views of the *future expected and ideal selves*. There is, of course, the problem of the retrospective illusion, the person seeing their past as being better than it actually was in reality, and also of their *ideal self* being totally illusory and unlikely to occur.

The therapeutic alliance

Within the general psychotherapy field, there has been renewed interest in the therapeutic relationship (Binder & Strupp, 1997; Luborsky et al., 1985, 1997). Weinberger's (1995) recent review records the therapeutic alliance as being one of five factors which have emerged as strong predictors of outcome independent of the specific therapy employed, with the other four being expectations, confronting problems, mastery, and attribution of outcome. Mohr's (1995) review re-emphasized the importance of therapist characteristics as being associated with negative outcomes, namely, lack of empathy, underestimation of the severity of the client's problems, negative countertransference, poor techniques, high concentrations of transference interpretations, and disagreement with the client about the therapy process.

Collaboration in therapy is imperative and we would certainly endorse the above-listed factors. However, there are factors additional to the aforementioned ones, which are more specific to our client group of interest. If we turn to desirable therapist characteristics, these include flexibility, emotional atunement, and a strong knowledge of developmental and life-cycle issues.

The clients themselves may be compromised neurocognitively, although such deficits may be temporary. Most clients will have had no experience of therapy, little or no idea of what is expected of them, and little idea of what they can expect from therapy. They may not be used to meeting one-to-one and talking about their feelings and concerns. A key factor to remember is that these individuals frequently have a reduced awareness of illness (Amador et al., 1991) and are not necessarily 'help-seekers'; in many cases, they have been forced into treatment by the severity of their disorder. One factor favouring the development of a therapeutic alliance is the ability of the client to take an objective stance in relation to self (Sandler et al., 1970) – a skill these young people may need time to acquire.

These individuals may also experience difficulty in establishing a therapeutic alliance because of their experience of an involuntary admission and/or imposed treatment via a community treatment order, and past experience with trust within the family. In fact, trust is a major issue, with mistrust posing a potential stumbling block to effective therapy. During the untreated period of their illness, these young psychotic individuals may have been looked at askance, been humiliated, ridiculed, or actively rejected by the people around them. For a therapist to sit with them and be prepared to listen empathically to them, may be a novel experience for the individual – one viewed suspiciously for a time. Persevering with the individual is imperative, signalling that someone is interested in listening to him or her and attempting to understand *them*, not only their symptoms, onset and course, but also their strivings, aspirations, ideals and fears. This may indicate to the client that the therapist is investing in them as *a person* – a person who is not merely the sum of their symptoms. What needs to be communicated to the client is that the therapist does have that person's best interests at heart, is someone who sees them as inherently worthwhile, and will be supportive and accommodating, rather than harangue, lecture, criticize or patronize them.

The person with psychosis is vulnerable and fragile. Gently exploring a panoply of issues during the assessment phase may be apposite, benefiting client and therapist alike. For the client who has sealed over, or the difficult or reluctant client, then the assumption of a more oblique tactical approach may prove more productive. In the latter instance, offering assistance with practical problems, e.g. dealing with a friend, or helping them contact a utilities company to re-establish a phone or gas connection. That is, for these clients, we need to do something *for* them, not *to* them. In this way, trust may be gained and the work begun, although it does take time to rebuild trust in such clients.

Some clients may be worried that the therapist can read their mind and is thinking negatively about them. This is not necessarily an example of a passivity phenomenon, but is commensurate with their stage of development, and their lack of experience of both therapy and psychiatry. They are at a developmental period when peer social influences and the maintenance of 'social face' are highly salient and important factors. From our clinical experience, most will be concerned about stigma and appearing foolish to the therapist. One needs to be patient and, as mentioned previously, to start with where the client is at by perhaps focussing the session material around the problems clients raise, in order to keep them engaged in the therapeutic process.

Engagement will be assisted by the calm acceptance of psychotic material and by careful attention to non-verbal and verbal communication, as well as to the client's current relational capacity. Therapy may at times be experienced by the currently or recently psychotic client as intense and highly intimate, and therefore as anxiety provoking. At these times it may be necessary to agree to change the focus or to shorten the session. In working with individuals with depressive or negative symptoms, the therapist will need to assiduously avoid mirroring the client's negative or apathetic attitude. The therapist should manifest an attitude of cautious optimism and consistently reinforce the view that the client can influence the course of the disorder. Appropriately used, humour can normalize and enliven the interaction between the therapist and client, encouraging in the client the notion that he or she is accepted and is engaged in a collaborative endeavour.

Adaptation: shoring up the self

Model of adaptation

A theoretical model for COPE intervention is displayed in Figure 10.1. In this model the psychosis may or may not be triggered by external events which may be appraised as traumatic, or the psychosis itself may be appraised as traumatic (Jeffries, 1977; Lundy, 1992; Williams-Keeler, Milliken & Jones, 1994). The appraisal process itself will be affected by a number of factors. These will include the individual's pre-existing level of productive and non-productive coping skills/resources, such as whether they enlist social support, and focus on solving a problem (Lazarus & Folkman, 1984; for measures see Folkman & Lazarus, 1988; Frydenberg & Lewis, 1997), their general attributional style, e.g. as embodied in Seligman's (1991) concept of learned optimism and Bandura's (1977, 1986) self-efficacy concept, the underlying complexity, coherence and stability of the self-concept, including the person's core schemas/beliefs (Beck, Freeman & Associates, 1990; Mahoney, 1991), and their possible selves (representing themes, goals, strivings and aspirations: Markus & Nurius, 1986; Murray, 1938; Singer & Salovey, 1993), temperament/personality features (Cloninger et al., 1993; McCrae & Costa, 1990, 1997), and the level of pre-existing supports (e.g. family and social) in their environment, all of which may increase the person's resilience and increase the likelihood of recovery. Although not shown in Figure 10.1, the model would propose that 'true' secondary morbidity results from failed adaptation but that associated comorbid conditions may be worsened by the aforementioned factors via the appraisal and coping processes.

Other vulnerability factors which could potentially affect the person's appraisal of the psychotic experience and their ability to effect change, would include the age at which the psychosis is first experienced, and their developmental stage (Erickson, 1968), with the latter represented in Figure 10.1 as a third dimension. This developmental dimension would include a wide variety of spheres: physical–motor, cognitive, emotional, academic–occupational, social, intimate–sexual and leisure–hobbies.

The model presented in Figure 10.1 indicates that COPE focusses not only on helping the individual to challenge their appraisal processes of the psychosis and themselves, including their evaluation of their own self-worth (Birchwood & Iqbal, 1998; see also Chapter 9), but also on bolstering the person's coping responses/resources (Lazarus & Folkman, 1984; McGorry, 1992). The model draws attention to some other factors. The first is that COPE may focus to some extent on premorbid issues, e.g. the goals or possible selves which a person has, or attempt to help them understand and 'soften' unhelpful aspects of their general attitudinal style, e.g. pessimism, or personality traits, e.g. extreme prefectionism (Blatt, 1995), or core schemas/beliefs using more schema-oriented therapy (e.g. Young, 1994). Finally, a positive environment is important in promoting recovery. This includes health, mental health, social, family and work settings.

Assessment of issues relevant to adaptation
Initially, the clinician should attempt to identify and understand the client's explanatory model and level of insight. We have found a semi-structured interview, developed by Greenfeld et al. (1989), to be useful in this regard but have found the repertory grid (Fransella & Bannister, 1977; Kelly, 1955) to be especially useful for gaining a visual representation of how clients see themselves in relation to how they were in the past, and where and how they see themselves in the future. Grids are also useful in determining whether a given person holds entrenched and stereotypical beliefs about people with mental illness and those with medical illness, such as AIDS, diabetes and cancer, e.g. 'All people with mental illness are physically dangerous', or is engaging in invidious comparisons between himself and members of his peer group, e.g., 'John has gone on with his studies and I haven't'. It is important to remember that clients are members of the community too and, as such, frequently share the typical prejudicial stereotypes of the general

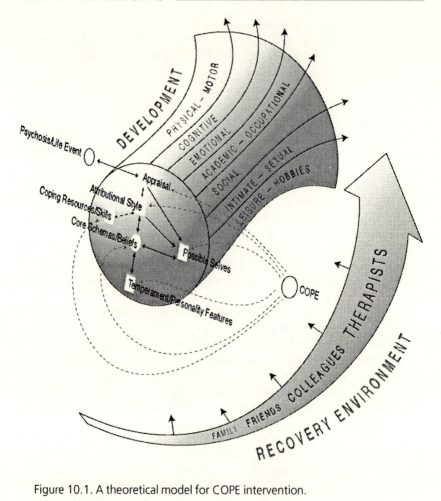

Figure 10.1. A theoretical model for COPE intervention.

community. Other approaches involving videos (Ioannides & Hexter, 1994), films, books, computerized material and questionnaires are useful, not only in initial interactive assessments, but in monitoring therapy progress and outcome.

A second important focus is on the possible selves, both positive and feared or undesired (Markus & Nurius, 1986; Ogil vie, 1987). We need to be able to gauge both the client's awareness of his or her illness (Amador et al., 1991) and the extent to which the person's positive possible selves (which encapsulates their goals and aspirations) have been distorted by the psychosis, and continually monitor both factors over time.

Goals of therapy for adaptation

The goals of therapy are to help the person: in searching for some meaning in the psychotic experience; to master the experience; and to protect their self-esteem which may have been damaged, or at the very least threatened by the psychotic experience. Protection of the viability of the positive possible selves is imperative; the complete suffusion or saturation of identity with feared possible negative selves, e.g. 'the chronic mental patient', is to be avoided (Jackson et al., 1996). Engulfment or entrapment by psychosis is particularly likely if the client has a family member with a chronic psychiatric illness, e.g. schizophrenia, or is admitted to a 'standard' inpatient unit with chronic psychotic patients. The longer-term goal is to enable the person to make a positive adaptation to the onset of the disorder, to play an active role in illness self-management if the disorder is persistent or prolonged (i.e. to promote self-efficacy), and to maintain the best possible quality of life in the context of the disorder.

Goals and therapy

Therapy for promoting adaptation The framework for our approach is modelled on that described by Davidson and Strauss (Davidson, 1992; Davidson & Strauss, 1992, 1995; Strauss, 1994). In the initial phase (phase 1: labelled 'discovering the self'; Davidson, 1992; Davidson & Strauss, 1995) we attempt to assist the individual in recognizing that he or she possesses the capacity to realize their potential, and we attempt to instil hope that 'things can be different'.

The second phase (phase 2: labelled 'taking stock of the self'; Davidson, 1992; Davidson & Strauss, 1995) involves a number of interventions/strategies. First, we regard psychoeducation as the key strategy within a broader psychotherapeutic endeavour. On the other hand, we do believe that this needs to be delivered to clients according to their mental state and so we provide psychoeducation on an individual interactive basis and tailored to 'where the person is at'. Clients, no matter how much they might attempt to deny their problems, are almost always bewildered to some extent by what is occurring to them and they are desirous of some explanation. Videos, information sheets, booklets, and visual tools, e.g. diagrams, are used as the basis for interactive discussion about psychosis. Typically, certain points are made. For example, information is provided about the nature of the disorders emphasizing the stress–diathesis model (Zubin & Spring, 1977); we inform clients that disability and poor quality of life are not inevitable, supplying them with information about the long-term outcome studies and generally emphasizing more positive outcomes.

Optimism and hope are introduced early in the piece; we tell clients that we believe they will recover at some point from this disorder, and this holds irrespective of the level or phase of their disorder or disability in early psychosis. In noting that specific subtype diagnoses, e.g. bipolar disorder, may be unstable in the first-episode, we tend to tell our clients that we believe they have a 'psychotic' disorder rather than give them a specific label such as 'bipolar disorder'. A strong emphasis is given as to how the self may be useful in aiding recovery, noting that individuals can influence the course and outcome of the disorder by learning coping and stress management approaches, recognizing early warning signs, enlisting social support, and pursuing their goals. Detailed descriptions of our psychoeducation approach are to be found in EPPIC (1997, 1998) and McGorry & Edwards (1997).

Second, we have found that detoxifying stereotypes is frequently necessary. To do this, we may use the repertory grid focussing one-by-one on the labels which clients may have identified as toxic. Questions can be asked of the individuals: 'what do you think about people with mental illness?', 'Why do you think this?', 'How did you arrive at this conclusion?'. Cognitive approaches can be used to examine the belief, look for the evidence, and look at alternatives. Role models, videos and consumer consultants are also very helpful in providing challenges to the clients' 'toxic' stereotypes.

Third, we focus on cognitive and coping work as it pertains to the person's present and future life. The therapist helps the individual to identify his or her strengths and limitations in assessing possibilities and planning for new projects or directions, or in planning for the return to projects and goals disrupted by the illness. In most cases, the COPE therapist will need to help the person to strengthen and broaden their coping repertoire, e.g. by highlighting the person's own coping strengths in other areas and by providing information about other coping methods derived from the literature, psychoeducational material and first-person accounts regarding coping mechanisms found to be helpful by others. Peers, self-help groups, mentors, other consumers, or psychoeducational groups may also be helpful in suggesting other coping methods.

Growth is important and the resumption of old 'positive' activities and the pursuit of new goals is an important focus of COPE work. Barriers to change or 'movement' need to be identified with, for example, loss of confidence and social withdrawal being very common. Cognitive approaches are fundamental to gently challenging the person's beliefs, e.g. 'I can't go back to my football'; 'Now I have schizophrenia I will not be able to work again'; 'I won't ever be able to go out with Jill again'.

Generally, in working cognitively with the person, there are three foci of interest: the distortions in thinking – the so-called cognitive errors; the thematic content which of course may be plainly wrong or unhelpful; and how these distortions combine with the thematic content to link-up with similar or different distorted thoughts to affect positive and feared possible selves and evaluations of self-worth (including sexual self-worth, a topic little discussed in the context of psychosis). Role-plays, diaries, and guided imagery with time projection, may all prove useful adjuncts to cognitive therapy by assisting the client to contemplate new courses of action or resuming established activities consonant with positive selves.

The third phase (phase 3: labelled 'putting the self into action'; Davidson, 1992; Davidson & Strauss, 1995) is where the therapist encourages and helps the person to both implement some change and assess the outcome. Positive outcomes are important but the individual must feel that the achievements are their own and that the outcomes reflect their actual capabilities. Some of the planned activities might be small scale in nature, e.g. making an arrangement to go out with old friends, and others might be bigger in scope, e.g. contacting an employer to ask for one's job back, or resuming studies for a degree, or studying for a car licence. Even if the person is in remission, with little or no neurocognitive impairment, recovery can be difficult, but not impossible. If the client has persistent impairment, recovery is even more difficult, but can be potentiated with a staged cognitive–behavioural therapy approach.

Cognitive approaches, coping skills, role-plays and guided imagery, together with therapeutic and mobilized social supports, are important in assisting the person to initiate and maintain behavioural change. The following vignette provides some indication of the issues and therapeutic work undertaken in adaptation phases 2 and 3:

> Toni was a 26-year-old sales assistant, admitted to EPPIC following a rapid onset of positive symptoms. She showed a good recovery and was apparently compliant with medication. Attending all her COPE sessions, she displayed an initial difficulty in identifying her issues and concerns. She was living at home, the only child of older migrant parents. It transpired that she had never dated and had only limited social contacts with her workmates. Despite recovering well, her parents remained very protective of her, the experience of the psychotic episode merely exacerbating the pre-existing parent–daughter relationship pattern. The parents appeared to discourage

> any socializing by Toni other than that initiated by themselves. Toni, herself, was ambivalent about both returning to work and resuming socializing. Major issues identified in therapy were Toni's concern at having to explain her absences to her work colleagues combined with her lack of assertiveness in dealing with her parents, her self-stigmatization, and her difficulty in comprehending what had happened to her. The treatment approach taken by the COPE therapist involved psychoeducation, the identification of dysfunctional beliefs, role-plays, and graded task assignments involving Toni separating somewhat from her family to pursue her own interests and goals, and feeling (and thinking!) both justified and able to do so.

Finally, the fourth phase (phase 4: 'appealing to the self'; Davidson, 1992; Davidson & Strauss, 1995) involves the therapist assisting the client to increase the sense of self, and distance him- or herself somewhat from negative aspects of their social environment (e.g. community stigma). Therapists can now focus on the individual's accomplishments during the recovery period and use cognitive techniques to help the person to challenge their social fears. The positive work established in phases 2 and 3 needs to continue. The focus is on realizing the functional self by increasing competence and power, and assisting identity formation.

It may be more appropriate to use more behavioural approaches for less introspective, 'unaware', high denial, or demoralized clients to change negative assumptions about community attitudes, for example. An *in vivo* exposure approach, labelled by us as 'action COPE', involves challenging the assumptions and fears in a graded manner by setting up real-life experiences, e.g. visiting the hairdresser, or meeting an old friend in a café. With the aid of the therapist, new and more positive cognitive schemas can be developed to replace negative assumptions but subsequent to some behavioural action. This is a reversal of phases 2 and 3 as described earlier in this section.

Secondary morbidity

Psychopathology of secondary morbidity
People recovering from psychosis may present with a range of 'associated' or 'comorbid' syndromes, e.g. depression, panic attacks, social phobia, post-traumatic stress disorder, alcohol and drug abuse, obsessive–compulsive disorder, insomnia, and so on (e.g. Bermanzohn, Porto & Siris, 1997; Bland, Newman & Orn, 1987; Henry et al., 1997a; Hulbert, McGorry & Jackson, 1997; Mooney & Pica, 1997; Strakowski et al., 1993).

The hierarchical approach to diagnosis allows comorbidity and secondary morbidity to be glossed over, and prevents the recognition and treatment of those conditions with treatments that have proven efficacious in other contexts, even though those treatments may need to be modified for the psychotic person.

Disentangling pre-existing conditions from current psychosis, even when the latter is successfully treated, may be very difficult. Such discriminations involve complex judgments, and various factors may further confuse such assessments. These traits or symptoms may exist prior to the episode but are exacerbated or precipitated by the psychosis to a stage where they are clinically meaningful. Then again, if the psychosis takes an insidious form, and perhaps if both the psychosis and drug abuse develop in parallel, then arguably the psychosis, drug abuse, and personality development may interact in a pathoplastic manner to produce a postpsychotic personality disorder (for a full discussion of this with regard to psychosis and personality disorder see Hulbert, Jackson & McGorry, 1996). Bermanzohn, Porto & Siris (1997) have proffered the term 'associated psychiatric disorders' to obviate the need to ponder these difficult-to-render distinctions. We have taken the somewhat more utilitarian view that, if the condition appears to be secondary to the psychosis according to the chronological sequence reported by client and informant (if available) alike, and appears to be secondary to failed adaptation or coping with the psychosis, then it should be a focus for therapeutic attention (see also Jackson et al., 1996). Also, these secondary conditions may not necessarily achieve full-blown disorder status, but we would argue that all subthreshold forms are worthy of treatment, as they will interfere, to some extent at least, with the recovery process.

The types and prevalences of these 'associated' or 'secondary' conditions are little studied in first-episode psychotic samples and, although there are in existence various reports (e.g. Strakowski et al., 1993), they do not represent formally constituted large-scale epidemiological studies which could satisfactorily and convincingly ascertain the incidence and prevalence figures for these conditions irrespective of a given setting. Nevertheless, in the EPPIC service which covers a *specified* catchment area, we have found a number of these conditions to be not uncommon. For example, our experience in EPPIC has been that both depression and social phobia are highly prevalent in this population (Henry et al., 1997a; Mooney & Pica, 1997). In the acute phase of psychotic illness, depression may resolve with the psychosis. If it persists or surfaces later, then it is deserving of treatment. Frequently this does not happen, and 'postpsychotic depression' is neglected.

For those who report social phobia *subsequent* to the psychosis, it can be understood in terms of social threat, and humiliation, due to a self-stigmatization process, remembering, of course, that the client is part of the general community at large. Frequently they share with that latter group stereotypes of the mentally ill, for instance that 'once mentally ill always mentally ill', and that the same people 'are dangerous physically, socially incompetent and lazy'. Therefore, it is not surprising, that in the wake of a psychotic episode, clients may be avoidant of social situations, particularly intimate ones, where they may be the focus of attention. Naturally, in a number of cases, the person's social anxiety may be an exacerbation of pre-existing schizotypal personality traits, or avoidant personality traits.

Post-traumatic stress disorder (PTSD) may occur, either in response to the hospitalization process, such as being forcibly restrained, or involuntarily admitted to hospital and exposed to other psychotic patients, being thrown in the back of a police van or ambulance, losing one's rights, and so forth (McGorry et al., 1991), or the psychosis itself may be experienced as traumatic (Jeffries, 1977; Williams-Keeler, Milliken & Jones, 1994). Also, OCD can present; in our experience it is not one of the more common conditions. In contrast, in a study with *chronic schizophrenic* patients, Bermanzohn et al. (1997) reported that nearly 30% of their small sample ($n = 37$)met the full criteria for OCD, a very high rate for this disorder.

As with the now familiar stereotype of the Vietnam veteran, alcohol and drugs may be used to excess in an effort for the person to: control their intrusive thoughts or alleviate anxiety produced by residual psychotic symptoms; deal directly with residual positive or negative symptoms, attempting to obtain an immediate effect from blotting them out from awareness; deal with their social anxiety, depressive thoughts and resulting emotional experiences; or it can present antecedent to the psychosis and be a precipitant for the same (e.g. Mueser et al., 1998).

Assessment of secondary morbidity
Assessment of secondary conditions necessitates the identification of all the relevant parameters such as onset (not always possible), severity, intensity, preoccupation, and the disability associated with the condition. If we take one example, that of secondary social phobia construed by us in this context as akin to self-stigmatization, then the therapist would be interested in determining which particular situations cause difficulty for the client, whether there are specific people the individual avoids, or whether the formality of an occasion or prominence of the client in a social context, is integral to exacerbating their social anxiety. Of course, the fact that the person is returning to their community following their first psychotic episode, perhaps after exhibiting embar-

rassing behaviour during their illness, may in itself be driving their social anxiety.

In a sense it is the underlying preoccupations and thematic content that we are concerned with in identifying psychopathology. These combine with the personality features and demoralization, threat, loss of power, loss of self-efficacy, and humiliation to lead to the development and maintenance of secondary morbidity.

Helping clients in the identification of automatic thoughts, cognitive distortions (e.g. magnification, fortune-telling, selective abstraction, etc.; for more details, see Beck et al., 1979; Beck & Emery, 1985; Beck, Freeman & Associates, 1990), dysfunctional beliefs and their linkage to affective expression, is of paramount importance. Again, if we take the case of secondary social phobia, typical dysfunctional cognitive schemata are: 'John will never want to see me again, now that I have come out of hospital'; 'My friends will never want to party with me again'; and 'people all know that I am abnormal'.

Treatment of secondary morbidity

Whatever the specific secondary condition, we begin by providing patients with an outline of a cognitively-oriented model. The assessment process is in a sense therapeutic, serving the dual function of developing an assessment map of their 'secondary condition' but, importantly, helping clients see that they can exert some control over the phenomena, thereby increasing the person's self-efficacy. Although daily recording of events, actions and cognitive activity is desirable in the recovery context, it would be accurate to state that a majority of clients are not consistent in doing this task. We have found that the use of role-plays, reverse role-plays, and guided imagery, together with simply requesting that the person recalls past events, is more likely to be successful in eliciting relevant information.

Besides the fundamental technique of teaching cognitive disputation to the patient, a library of techniques are used by us on a rational and empirical basis, including role-plays, guided imagery, graded task assignments, time-projection, psychoeducation, imaginal and *in vivo* exposure, self-instructions, and empty chair techniques (see Beck et al., 1979; Beck & Emery, 1985). The following vignette is intended to illuminate our approach.

Lucas, a 22-year-old unemployed man, was living at home with his parents. He came to the attention of EPPIC after several atypical conflicts including one in which he accused workmates of trying to get him sacked. He did subsequently lose his job, and also his place on the soccer team – a sport in which he had apparently excelled. His positive psychotic symptoms remitted with outpatient neuroleptic treatment. He remained amotivational and somewhat depressed, spending vast amounts of time either at his parents' home or that of his older brother. This led to criticism from his parents who possessed a strong work ethic. COPE assessment revealed extensive self-blaming concerning both his verbal pugnacity during the time he was psychotic and for the twin losses of his job and spot in the soccer team. It also seemed relevant that he was very perfectionistic premorbidly. He believed that he was a great disappointment to his father and felt hopeless about the future given that he had surrendered his previously-held goals and aspirations which centred around his career and sport (hoped-for selves). He was reluctant to contact his friends, fearing he would be rebuffed. The COPE therapist's approach involved psychoeducation about his psychosis, behavioural strategies for his subthreshold depressive disorder such as planning pleasant events, e.g. outings with his brother. He would not complete monitoring of his mood as a homework task and all cognitive work had to be undertaken within therapy sessions. Lucas experienced some initial difficulty in identifying his emotions and thoughts but he persisted to good effect. He learnt to identify his negative self-perceptions as a major obstacle to his progress. Cognitive challenges, graded task assignments and role-plays were used to assist him to re-contact his friends, develop new hobbies and, with the help of his friends, subsequently to contact his coach and return to his soccer team. In the latter stage of treatment, he participated in planning for retraining and return to employment.

The actual therapy techniques we employ are those used in the treatment of primary anxiety, affective and substance abuse disorders (see Cotton & Jackson, 1996) but they may need to be simplified and be 'taught' at a slower pace. Therapist expectations with regard to completion of homework exercises need to be modified. These changes are necessary because of a number of factors such as: the younger age of the patient population, their fluctuating mental state, a number of them being of lower IQ, and the possibility that their cognitive functioning may be further hampered due to the residual effects of the psychosis. There are other important factors to be considered in this young population. Some suggested by Zarb (1992) include their tendency to drop out and only present in crises, their lack of long-range perspective, and their reduced capacity for introspection. Fuller details are to be found in EPPIC (1988) and McGorry & Edwards (1997).

In COPE, the assault on the client's psychosocial development and personality is explicitly acknowledged. Although there is insufficient time in a shorter-term therapy to conduct longer-term work on personality issues, attempts should be made to prevent axis 1 psychopathologies becoming 'concretized' and enmeshed with the emergent personality structure. Therapists need to be flexible in their approach to treatment; an issue may be put aside or on hold because of an acute crisis or because some other issue is raised by the patient at the commencement of a session. Finally, in some cases, the therapist may decide not to proceed with the psychological treatment of a condition such as social anxiety, because it becomes more apparent that the social withdrawal and anxiety serves a defensive function for a patient who still retains strong paranoid ideas about other persons in their social network. It is important to recognize that the social anxiety is not the sole problem and is here trumped by the psychosis and therefore needs a different approach. Clinically, the correct path of action may be: examine and perhaps change the medication regimen (type and dose of neuroleptic); support the defensive strategy of avoidance, albeit temporarily; and use cognitive techniques to focus on, and subtly help the client to challenge the persecutory belief.

Research progress in COPE

In researching COPE we have implemented two studies to test in a preliminary way the efficacy of COPE therapy. The first is a pilot study which includes a total of 80 first-episode psychotic individuals (Jackson et al., 1996). They formed three groups: clients who attended the Early Psychosis Prevention and Intervention Centre (EPPIC; Edwards & McGorry, 1998), and were offered and accepted COPE (i.e. COPE acceptors); those who attended EPPIC, were offered but refused COPE (refusers), but continued to receive the usual range of continuing services from EPPIC; and those clients who belonged to another geographical region, received inpatient treatment from EPPIC, were never offered COPE, and did not receive any continuing outpatient services from EPPIC after the inpatient treatment period (control group). Clients were assessed on two measures of psychological functioning (the Integration/Sealing Over measure (I/SO: McGlashan et al., 1977) and the Explanatory Model (EM: Kleinman, 1980)), two 'primary' symptom measures (Brief Psychiatric Rating Scale (BPRS: Overall & Gorham, 1962) and the Schedule for the Assessment of Negative Symptoms (SANS: Andreasen, 1983)), two measures of 'secondary morbidity' ((Beck Depression Inventory, Beck & Beck, 1972) and SCL-90–R, Derogatis, 1977, 1983)), and a measure of adjustment (Quality of Life (QLS:

Heinrichs, Hanlon & Carpenter, 1984)). Relapses were also recorded. Results have been reported elsewhere (Jackson et al., 1998) but, to summarize, we found that at the end of treatment the COPE group obtained significantly superior scores to the control group on the I/SO, EM, SANS and QLS. The COPE group only significantly outperformed the refuser group on the I/SO measure, although results were in the expected direction on the EM, SANS, and QLS. Sub-analyses demonstrated that at the end of treatment bipolar clients who received COPE did better than bipolar clients who did not receive COPE on measures of psychopathology, quality of life and psychological 'integration' (Henry et al., 1997b). A one-year follow-up of the pilot study is now completed and data are currently being analysed. A second trial using a randomized controlled design is nearing completion.

Treatment for delusions and hallucinations

> Cognitive behavioural techniques used in schizophrenia have generally been developed pragmatically in clinical settings. Despite the effectiveness of antipsychotic drugs in acute schizophrenia and in preventing relapse, many patients continue to have persistent positive and negative symptoms. Even drugs such as clozapine for resistant symptoms only appear effective in up to a third of those for whom they are indicated. Side-effects also present major problems. Poor compliance occurs in up to 75% with first-episode schizophrenia ... and up to 50% of patients discharged from hospital fail to take even 75% of medication prescribed.
>
> Kingdon, Turkington & John, 1994, p. 581

Psychological interventions for persistent positive symptoms

In recent times, psychotherapists have steered away from focusing on the positive symptoms of psychosis and, indeed, since the 1960s the psychoses have fallen more firmly within the bailiwick of organically oriented psychiatry, with the symptoms expected to be responsive only to medication. What is especially interesting about the new corpus of cognitive interventions for positive symptoms is their direct challenge to the 'received wisdom' that psychological interventions have no role in the treatment of the core symptoms of psychosis. Although these approaches may manifest differences, they do share the following core commonalities: (*a*) that psychotic experiences are multidimensional in nature (Fowler & Morley, 1989), rather than being dichotomous, i.e. that they are not merely present or absent, but exist on continua, and can be described more fully by various parameters such as degree of preoccupation, frequency, intensity, and so on (Strauss, 1969) – factors not considered in official nosologies such as DSM (APA, 1980, 1987, 1994); (b) that the tenacity with which patients hold a delusion or experience hallucinatory phenomena may fluctuate over time (Fowler, Garety & Kuipers, 1995) – a view which challenges the notion of stable treatment resistance; (c) that one needs to access the ability of individuals to monitor their own behaviour, which includes the hallucinatory and delusional experiences (here the implicit assumption is that humans possess the capacity to self-influence their behaviour no matter how disturbed they appear or act); and (d) that the cognitive content (specific beliefs) and cognitive processes (cognitive distortions) which underpin delusions *and* hallucinations should be the focus of interventions.

To date, the literature on psychological interventions has focused largely on auditory hallucinations and delusions, with few papers having been written on approaches with thought disorder. The treatment of persistent hallucinations in other modalities has been virtually neglected. Methods of psychological treatments can be categorized into four groups: behavioural techniques (e.g. distraction, anxiety reduction, focusing); coping strategies (Falloon & Talbot, 1981; Breier & Strauss, 1983, 1984; Tarrier, 1992; Tarrier et al., 1993); cognitive interventions (Beck, 1952; Chadwick & Birchwood, 1994; Chadwick & Lowe, 1990; Hole, Rush & Beck, 1979); and psychodynamic approaches (Arieti, 1962; Jacobs, 1980). Most of the individuals involved in these studies have long-standing schizophrenic illness or carry diagnoses of delusional disorder. A number of readily available expositionary texts provide details of how to approach the treatment of positive symptoms. Books by Fowler et al. (1995), Chadwick et al. (1996), Haddock & Slade (1996) and Kingdon & Turkington (1994) contain useful information.

Two groups of researchers describe integrated approaches to working psychotherapeutically with people with persistent psychotic symptoms and have been particularly influential in the development of our own model which we have labelled Systematic Treatment for Persistent Positive Symptoms (STOPP). Kingdon and colleagues (Kingdon & Turkington, 1994; Kingdon, Turkington & John, 1994) describe the stages of their 'normalizing approach' as: engaging and rapport building; explaining psychosis using a normalizing rationale; examining the antecedents of psychotic symptoms; treating any co-existing anxiety and depression; reality testing; tackling entrenched psychotic symptoms; tackling negative symptoms; and relapse prevention. Garety, Fowler and their colleagues (Fowler et al., 1995; Garety et al., 1994) draw on the work of a number of researchers and include: cognitive behavioural coping strategies (Tarrier, 1992); relabelling and psychoeducation (Kingdon & Turkington, 1991); modification of delusional beliefs

(Chadwick & Birchwood, 1994); goal setting and efforts directed toward overcoming helplessness; and modification of dysfunctional assumptions about self-worth and illness (see Chadwick et al., 1996).

Methodologically, in general, the empirical studies are somewhat flawed or elementary, with sample sizes being frequently small (typically 4–6 persons); the archetypal or normative report being a single case study, or a case studies series, with and without repeated measures (e.g. Bentall, Haddock, & Slade, 1994; Fowler & Morley, 1989; Kingdon & Turkington, 1994). There are some well executed multiple baseline designs (Chadwick & Lowe, 1990; Chadwick et al., 1994; Sharp et al., 1996) but few between-group studies (Drury et al., 1996; Garety et al., 1994; Tarrier et al., 1993). Diagnoses are rarely confirmed or established via structured or semi-structured instruments and studies report no control over the effects of medication changes, or possible demand characteristics. Again, in general, there has been little or no follow-up of clients over time and follow-ups rarely exceed six months (Chadwick & Lowe, 1990; Chadwick et al., 1994); however, very recently, more convincing data has come to hand. Drawn from three randomized controlled trials, outcomes favour CBT-type treatments for chronic treatment-resistant schizophrenic-spectrum (mostly schizophrenic) clients, both at the end of treatment and at 9- or 12-months follow-up (Garety et al., 1997; Kingdon, 1997; Tarrier, 1997).

Nevertheless, treatment has not been consistently effective with *all* clients, although a mitigating factor may be that the focus has been on individuals with long-standing illness, usually with 6–20 year histories (e.g, Chadwick & Lowe, 1990). As noted by Haddock et al. (1994, p. 209) 'It is unclear what impact psychological treatments would have if these treatments were offered when individuals first presented to services...' Currently, Haddock et al. (1998) are in the process of undertaking a multi-site randomized controlled trial with first- or second-episode schizophrenic clients. This study known as SOCRATES (Study of Cognitive Re-alignment Therapy for Early Schizophrenia) is a multi-site trial of cognitive behaviour therapy (CBT) compared to supportive counselling, both in addition to routine care, and to routine care alone. The aim of the trial is to assess whether CBT is superior to the two control treatments in speeding recovery of acute psychosis and in preventing or delaying subsequent relapse in recent-onset schizophrenic clients. The trial aims to recruit 354 patients and currently has recruited 182 into the trial. When completed, it will be possible to infer whether CBT is an effective adjunct treatment in early acute schizophrenia on a range of clinical and social outcome measures, and whether a health economics analysis indicates it is cost-effective (Nick Tarrier, personal communication).

Our approach: first-episode considerations

The argument for applying psychological interventions to positive symptoms early in the course of the disorder is inherently appealing (e.g. Drury et al., 1996). Nevertheless, we have decided to implement such treatment with those individuals with first-episode psychosis who are suffering from *enduring* positive symptoms or with prolonged recovery (see Chapter 11) (Edwards et al., 1998). Certainly, it is our experience that the opportunities to shift delusional explanations using psychoeducation are more apparent in the early psychosis client. However, assessment and definition issues are often more complex.

The Systematic Treatment of Persistent Psychosis (STOPP) is a psychological therapy we have developed within EPPIC which draws on a number of perspectives. Its prime aim is to provide an integrated psychotherapy for the person experiencing *enduring* positive symptoms early in the course of a psychotic illness. In our group of clients we have found that those with *enduring* symptoms frequently present with multiple problems; drug and alcohol abuse, anxiety and depression, and dependent personality traits are common. Low self-esteem is a major feature and it is debatable whether the self-concept distortions pre-dated the onset of illness or are a consequence of slow recovery. In addition, this group seems to hold extremely negative views about mental illness. Developmental issues, common in this age group, may be particularly prominent; clients frequently describe feeling as though they have 'missed out' on aspects of growing up due to prolonged illness, or a long duration of untreated psychosis. Sometimes, developmental issues are entangled within psychotic beliefs (e.g. sexual identity, independence from parents).

The STOPP model   STOPP begins with an extensive assessment of psychopathology, specific dimensions of persistent symptoms, coping style, comorbidity, and contributing factors. Interventions draw on all four methods of psychological treatments for treatment-resistant clients mentioned earlier, notably behavioural, coping, cognitive, and psychodynamic approaches. STOPP subsumes COPE (i.e. there is a focus on the therapeutic relationship, adaptation and secondary morbidity with the aim of separating self from illness) in relation to self-esteem and stigma. There is an explicit focus on comorbidity. The therapy consists of four phases labelled assessment and rationale, psychoeducation and coping strategies, belief modification, and core beliefs. Therapy usually occurs on a weekly basis, with a six-week period of twice-weekly sessions occurring early in treatment to assist the individual in defining the issues and setting the agenda. Sessions are usually of 45 minutes' duration, but there is some flexibility with regard to the duration of the sessions. The number of therapy sessions needs to be established early in treatment. Sometimes brief therapy is indicated (e.g. if a person has a fairly focussed problem, good insight, and previous psychoeducation), and in those circumstances a coping skills approach may be most appropriate. More complex problems usually require longer periods of intervention.

Some case examples using the STOPP approach are set out below. In the first two of the following set of three vignettes we illustrate the STOPP approach to belief modification (see also phase three in Table 10.1 on page 296) with the third vignette describing the STOPP approach to exploring the meaning of symptoms (see also phase four in Table 10.1 – 'core beliefs').

A 26-year-old professional made a good recovery from a second psychotic manic episode with regard to affective symptoms. However, distressing delusions of reference remained. Behavioural analysis established television shows as instrumental in triggering these experiences. The client and therapist conjointly examined the video satellite link-up equipment located on the EPPIC site. It seemed clear that equipment that allowed one to 'be watched' was quite complex, large in size, and very expensive. The following session was conducted at the client's home and discussion centred on the television. The client and family were asked about the purchasing of their television set and whether there was any possibility of their television set being in any way 'extra special'. The client's experiences were discussed with the client's brother and the brother was asked to discuss the client's television experiences with him as they occurred later on during the evening. This was a time when particular shows that bothered the client were scheduled. The brother was asked to offer the client his interpretation of events as the shows were transmitted. On returning to the clinic the client reported that he had been watching the usual shows but was no longer receiving messages from them.

A 20-year-old university student was making a slow recovery from a protracted psychotic episode. He was still hearing voices three or four times a day. The client and therapist identified the nature of the voices – who they were, what they said, when they occurred, and so on. The client was also asked to report what made the voices better or worse. A specific trigger was identified consisting of the client seeing particular politicians on the television. The client was asked to watch the news during the week to see if he could activate the voices. The therapist agreed to tape such a program independently to watch with the client during the following therapy session. It was explained to the client that the therapist wanted him to have practice in 'bringing on the voices', and later 'in making them go away'. By the next session the voices had gone and a few weeks later the triggering and underpinning delusion of reference had disappeared completely.

Usually, individuals who are experiencing ongoing psychotic symptoms believe they have no control over their symptoms. The experiments reported in the two preceding vignettes communicate to the clients that they themselves may be able to exert some influence over their experiences. It is important that the therapist adopts an inquiring approach. Yet, at the same time a confident attitude must be conveyed. Therefore, the therapist might provide the client with examples of other individuals with whom he or she has worked, who have managed to reduce or eradicate their symptoms and how this has been accomplished. However, perhaps the most important component of these interventions is the concept of actually really caring about what the person is experiencing – to the point of taking notes in great detail. Frequently, the client has not previously explained the situation to this extent. This active listening component on the part of the therapist is helpful in terms of improving the client's self-esteem and identity, contributing towards the idea of their 'getting stronger' which is essential in accelerating recovery.

A 22-year-old man who was living with his widowed mother had a persistent delusion that he was going to hell. He was incredibly agitated about this – it preoccupied his thinking and severely restricted his activities. This young man had a homosexual orientation and had only told his mother of this after his father passed away. He obviously had concerns about a father who was 'unable to forgive him'. The therapist accompanied the client to a theological library together and researched the definition of 'hell'. This included conducting computer literature searches, asking the librarian's assistance and examining theological dictionaries. It emerged that 'hell' was usually conveyed as an 'intermediary step' and one dictionary actually described it as 'a place of rehabilitation'. The question was raised as to whether EPPIC could then be considered a form of 'hell'! The client and therapist subsequently visited the hospital pastor to obtain his opinion about the nature of 'hell'. The pastor pointed out that 'God' was forgiving and raised the question as to who was 'God' – was it possible that some of his treating clinicians had 'God' in them? Subsequently, over several sessions the underpinning belief reduced in intensity. Shortly afterwards, the client resumed attending dance parties – an activity he enjoyed immensely.

Sometimes it is possible for the therapist to 'arrive at a story' or formulation (Kingdon & Turkington, 1994) regarding a psychological understanding of the presentation (Roberts, 1991, 1992). However, this must be regarded only as a hypothesis. In working with clients with prolonged recovery it may or may not be helpful to share such interpretations with clients – they are sometimes resistant to these (as in this case where the young man described in the third vignette would have denied any concerns about what others thought about his sexual orientation) and/or where the conveying of the therapist's understanding has no impact in terms of behaviour change. It is helpful for the therapist to use these hypotheses to guide interventions, with a gradual approach to the core issues – building rapport, and developing a shared understanding and trust. The therapist must be very active in pursuing the data (e.g. in this third case visiting the library or the pastor's office) and this is helpful in conveying the therapist's desire to understand and assist. The building of self-esteem through the client and therapist having shared experiences is an essential platform for the acceptance of meaning-related comments to the client from the therapist.

Current developments with STOPP   A study is underway within EPPIC which investigates the efficacy of the atypical neuroleptic, clozapine, and STOPP, in the treatment of early enduring positive symptoms in first-onset psychosis (Maude et al., 1997). Individuals not achieving a predefined level of remission after 12 weeks of treatment are entered into one of four experimental groups for a further 12–week period: (1) thioridazine and case management; (2) thioridazine and case management plus STOPP therapy; (3) clozapine and case management; (4) clozapine and case management plus STOPP therapy. Outcome measures include severity of both positive psychotic and negative symptoms, level of depression, degree of insight, global level of functioning, and quality of life. Efficacy is determined by the degree of response and the number of patients who achieve full remission in each group.

Clients receiving STOPP are offered twice-weekly sessions for 12 weeks (24 sessions) and each session is held for approximately 45 minutes. STOPP subjects are withdrawn from the study if they miss greater than six STOPP sessions over the 12-week period. Clients in the no-STOPP conditions can be withdrawn from the study if they miss greater than six weekly case management sessions over the 12-week study period. Table 10.1 sets out the content elements of the STOPP therapy in this ongoing protocol which is delivered in a phase-like fashion (Maude et al., 1997) and is a modification of the earlier STOPP procedure reported on by Edwards et al. (1998) (see their Table 5).

Clozapine was chosen as the drug of choice in this efficacy trial because it has been shown to have differential clinical efficacy for positive symptoms in treatment-resistant patients with a psychotic disorder, and it is one of the few medications with a qualitatively lower risk of akathisia, parkinsonism, dystonia, and tardive dyskinesia (Meltzer, 1993). There are no studies to our knowledge where either psychological strategies such as STOPP and clozapine have been applied exclusively in first-episode persons experiencing prolonged recovery at three months into treatment. This is also the first study to examine the relative contribution, and combined effectiveness of these two treatments in this very early phase of the disorder.

Conclusions and future directions

The emergence of both psychological treatments like COPE developed for clients recovering from their first psychotic episode, and psychological treatments developed for positive symptoms, form one of the most important growth areas in psychosis research. This work needs to be extended and further developed; more studies need to be conducted in a variety of settings to ascertain the optimum number of treatment sessions in the hands of a diversity of researcher-clinicians. Other critical questions relate to the sequencing of treatment, the number and spacing of sessions, and comparisons of cognitive treatment (like STOPP) with and without a range of psychopharmacological agents. In this regard, the intriguing and important study of Drury et al. (1996) demands replication with acutely disturbed psychotic persons in other centres.

If the generally positive results continue to hold up and prove

Table 10.1. *The STOPP treatment outline for the 'recovery plus' treatment protocol*

Phase 1: Assessment phase:
- Assessment of explanatory model; behavioural analysis; onset of the psychotic symptoms; phenomenology of positive symptoms; drug and alcohol use; levels of anxiety and depression; personality features; and developmental issues
- Development of a psychological formulation whereby the therapist outlines his or her understanding of the aetiology and maintenance of the problem and supplies a rationale for intervention

Phase 2: Coping and psychoeducation phase:
- Teaching and initiation of coping strategies to manage positive symptoms
- Specific interventions for co-morbid anxiety and depression
- Psychoeducation and harm-minimization approach to concurrent drug and alcohol use
- Psychoeducation and interventions around medication compliance
- Introduction of normalizing models of psychosis
- Exploration of beliefs about mental illness

Phase 3: Belief modification and exploration of meaning of symptoms:
- Cognitive restructuring and belief modification around the positive symptoms. [The patient's beliefs about voices (i. e. their identity, meaning, the control they exert, the patient's compliance with them) and the evidence for those delusions are explored. Beliefs are verbally challenged and experiments to test those beliefs are pursued]
- Assessment of, and interventions around, *core* beliefs, with a particular focus on self-esteem and identity issues
- Exploration of possible meanings of the symptoms

Phase 4: Termination, review and relapse prevention

economically viable, cognitive therapeutic approaches will afford a powerful and revolutionary therapeutic possibility in the treatment of psychosis and will increase our armamentarium for improving the quality of care for early psychosis clients. Techniques such as COPE and STOPP may be used, not as second-line treatments, but as a front-line treatment concomitantly with neuroleptic therapy as reported by Drury et al. (1996).

Ultimately, the critical and as yet empirically untested question, is whether the findings obtained in settings where the techniques were developed and where expertise exists, can be 'conveyed' to other settings and taught and used by a variety of clinicians in their everyday practice to produce similarly positive results (Clarke, 1995; Seligman, 1995; Weisz et al., 1995). Right now, nevertheless, there is *some* evidence that these new approaches are potentially beneficial to our clients with psychosis. We believe that these approaches offer a counter to the overwhelmingly nihilistic ambience which usually clouds discussions of the treatment of the psychoses. Without wishing to appear wildly unrealistic, we believe that the best approach researchers and therapists can adopt to these new developments in psychological treatments for first-episode clients, is one of 'guarded optimism'.

Acknowledgments

The Early Psychosis Research Program is funded by an extensive programme grant from the Victorian Health Promotion Foundation. The authors would like to acknowledge the invaluable contributions of the following therapists for their input into the development of COPE: Lisa Henry, Shona Francey, Dana Maude, Paddy Power and John Cocks. The contributions of Dana Maude, Simone Pica and Richard Bell in the development and description of STOPP are gratefully acknowledged.

Notes

1. Liberman, Kopelowicz and Young (1994) provide an excellent overview of these biobehavioural treatments and their role in the rehabilitation of schizophrenia.
2. Interestingly, the cognitive revolution eventually began to lap on the shore of 'serious mental illness' (SMI) only after a couple of decades of focusing on the treatment of anxiety and depressive disorders. This is particularly ironic given that the major pioneer of cognitive therapy – Aaron Beck – published a paper on the treatment of a psychotic patient in 1952 (Beck, 1952).
3. Cognitive remediation appears to accept both the cybernetic metaphor for cognitive activity or processing and a disease or neural dysfunction as the prime mover in causing schizophrenia. For both a discussion of contrasting aetiological models of schizophrenia and for the proposal of a contrarian approach the reader is referred to Harrop, Trower and Mitchell (1996).
4. The biological factors include genetic factors but also more general and 'glacial' evolutionary processes (Gould, 1996a,b).
5. However, it is unlikely that development occurs in a steady linear or curvilinear progression. It is more likely that it occurs in fits and starts, akin to the evolutionary concept of 'punctuated equilibrium' described by Gould (1996a,b).

References

Amador, X. F., Strauss, D. H., Yale, S. A. & Gorman, J. M. (1991). Awareness of illness. *Schizophrenia Bulletin*, **17**, 113–32.

American Psychiatric Association (1980). *Diagnostic and Statistical Manual of Mental Disorders*, 3rd ed., DSM-III. Washington, DC: American Psychiatric Association.

American Psychiatric Association (1987). *Diagnostic and Statistical Manual of Mental Disorders*, 3rd. rev., DSM-III-R. Washington, DC: American Psychiatric Association.

American Psychiatric Association. (1994). *Diagnostic and Statistical Manual of Mental Disorders*, 4th ed., DSM-IV. Washington, DC: American Psychiatric Association.

Andreasen, N. C. (1983). *Schedule for the Assessment of Negative Symptoms.* Iowa City, Iowa: University of Iowa.

Andreasen, N. C. (1984). *The Broken Brain: The Biological Revolution in Psychiatry.* New York: Harper & Row.

Arieti, S. (1962). Hallucinations, delusions, and ideas of reference treated with psychotherapy. *American Journal of Psychotherapy*, **16**, 52–60.

Bandura, A. (1977). Self-efficacy: toward a unifying theory of behavioral change. *Psychological Review*, **84**, 191–215.

Bandura, A. (1986). *Social Foundations of Thought and Action: A Social Cognitive Theory.* Englewood Cliffs, New Jersey: Prentice-Hall.

Beck, A. T. (1952). Successful outpatient psychotherapy of a chronic schizophrenic with a delusion based on borrowed guilt. *Psychiatry*, **15**, 305–12.

Beck, A. T. & Beck, R. W. (1972). Screening depressed patients in family practice: a rapid technique. *Postgraduate Medicine*, **52**, 81–5.

Beck, A. T. & Emery, G. (1985). *Anxiety Disorders and Phobias: A Cognitive Perspective.* New York: Basic Books.

Beck, A. T., Rush, A. J., Shaw, B. F. & Emery, G. (1979). *Cognitive Therapy of Depression.* New York: Guilford Press.

Beck, A. T., Freeman, A. & Associates (1990). *Cognitive Therapy of Personality Disorders.* New York: Guilford Press.

Bellack, A. S. & Hersen, M. (eds.) (1979). *Research and Practice in Social Skills Training.* New York: Plenum Press.

Bentall, R. P. (1990). The syndromes and symptoms of psychosis. Or why you can't play 'twenty questions' with the concept of schizophrenia and hope to win. In *Reconstructing Schizophrenia*, ed. R. P. Bentall, pp. 23–60. London: Routledge.

Bentall, R. P., Haddock, G. & Slade, P. D. (1994). Cognitive behavior therapy for persistent auditory hallucinations: from theory to therapy. *Behavior Therapy*, **25**, 51–66.

Bermanzohn, P. C., Porto, L. & Siris, S. G. (1997). Associated psychiatric syndromes (APS) in chronic schizophrenia: possible clinical significance. *Paper presented at the XXVIII Congress of the European Association for the Behavioural and Cognitive Therapies*, Venice, Italy, 24–27 September, 1997.

Binder, J. L. & Strupp, H. H. (1997). 'Negative process': a recurrently discovered and underestimated facet of therapeutic process and outcome in the individual psychotherapy of adults. *Clinical Psychology: Science and Practice*, **4**, 121–39.

Birchwood, M. & Iqbal, Z. (in press). Depression and suicidal thinking in psychosis. In *Outcome and Innovation in Psychological Treatment of Schizophrenia*, ed. T Wykes, N. Tarrier & S. Lewis. Chichester, UK: Wiley

Birchwood, M. & Macmillan, F. (1993). Early intervention in schizophrenia. *Australian and New Zealand Journal of Psychiatry*, **27**, 374–8.

Birchwood, M., McGorry, P. & Jackson, H. (1997). Early intervention in schizophrenia. *British Journal of Psychiatry*, **170**, 2–5.

Bland, R. C., Newman, S. C. & Orn, H. (1987). Schizophrenia: lifetime co-morbidity in a community sample. *Acta Psychiatrica Scandinavica*, **75**, 383–91.

Blatt, S. J. (1995). The destructiveness of perfectionism: implications for the treatment of depression. *American Psychologist*, **50**, 1003–20.

Breier, A. & Strauss, J. S. (1983). Self-control in psychotic disorders. *Archives of General Psychiatry*, **40**, 1141–5.

Breier, A. & Strauss, J. S. (1984). The role of social relationships in the recovery from psychotic disorders. *American Journal of Psychiatry*, **141**, 949–55.

Bruner, J. (1986). *Actual Minds, Possible Worlds*. Cambridge, Mass. : Harvard University Press.

Chadwick, P. & Birchwood, M. (1994). The omnipotence of voices. A cognitive approach to auditory hallucinations. *British Journal of Psychiatry*, **164**, 190–201.

Chadwick, P. D. J. & Lowe, C. F. (1990). Measurement and modification of delusional beliefs. *Journal of Consulting and Clinical Psychology*, **58**, 225–32.

Chadwick, P. D. J., Lowe, C. F., Horne, P. J. & Higson, P. J. (1994). Modifying delusions: the role of empirical testing. *Behavior Therapy*, **25**, 35–49.

Chadwick, P. J., Birchwood, M. & Trower, P. (1996). *Cognitive Therapy for Delusions, Voices and Paranoia*. Chichester, UK: Wiley.

Clarke, G. N. (1995). Improving the transition from basic efficacy research to effectiveness studies: methodological issues and procedures. *Journal of Consulting and Clinical Psychology*, **63**, 718–25.

Cloninger, C. R., Dragan, M., Svrakic, D. & Pryzbeck, T. R. (1993). A psychobiological model of temperament and character. *Archives of General Psychiatry*, **50**, 975–90.

Cotton, P. & Jackson, H. (eds.) (1996). *Early Intervention and Prevention in Mental Health*. Melbourne, Australia: Australian Psychological Association.

Coursey, R. D. (1989). Psychotherapy with persons suffering from schizophrenia. *Schizophrenia Bulletin*, **15**, 349–53.

Coursey, R. D., Keller, A. B. & Farrell, E. W. (1995). Individual psychotherapy and persons with serious mental illness: the clients' perspective. *Schizophrenia Bulletin*, **21**, 283–301.

Davidson, L. (1992). Developing an empirical–phenomenological approach to schizophrenia research. *Journal of Phenomenological Psychology*, **23**, 3–15.

Davidson, L. & Strauss, J. S. (1992). Sense of self in recovery from severe mental illness. *British Journal of Medical Psychology*, **65**, 131–45.

Davidson, L. & Strauss, J. S. (1995). Beyond the biopsychosocial model: integrating disorder, health, and recovery. *Psychiatry*, **58**, 44–55.

Derogatis, L. R. (1977). *SCL-90–R: Administration, Scoring and Procedures Manual*. Towson, Maryland, USA: Clinical Psychometric Research.

Derogatis, L. R. (1983). *SCL-90–R: Administration, Scoring and Procedures Manual-II for the R(evised) Version*. Towson, Maryland, USA: Clinical Psychometric Research.

Dixon, L. B. & Lehman, A. F. (1995). Family interventions for schizophrenia. *Schizophrenia Bulletin*, **21**, 631–43.

Drury, V., Birchwood, M., Cochrane, R. & Macmillan, F. (1996). Cognitive therapy and recovery from acute psychosis: a controlled trial: Impact on psychotic symptoms. *British Journal of Psychiatry*, **169**, 593–607.

EPPIC (1997). *Psychoeducation in Early Psychosis: Manual 1 in a Series of Early Psychosis Manuals*. Melbourne, Australia: EPPIC Statewide Services and the Mental Health Branch, Department of Human Services, Victoria.

EPPIC (in press). *Cognitively-oriented Psychotherapy in Early Psychosis (COPE). A Manual in a Series of Early Psychosis Manuals*. Melbourne, Australia: EPPIC Statewide Services and the Mental Health Branch, Department of Human Services, Victoria.

Edwards, J. & McGorry, P. D. (1998). Early intervention in psychotic disorders: a critical step in the prevention of psychological morbidity. In *Cognitive Psychotherapy of Psychotic and Personality Disorders*, ed. C. Perris & P. D. McGorry. Chichester, UK: Wiley.

Edwards, J., Maude, D., McGorry, P. D., Harrigan, S. M. & Cocks, J. T. (in press). Prolonged recovery in first-episode psychosis. *British Journal of Psychiatry* (Supplement).

Erickson, E. H. (1950). *Childhood and Society*. New York: Norton.

Erickson, E. H. (1968). *Identity: Youth and Crisis*. New York: Norton.

Falloon, I. R. H. (1985). *Family Management of Schizophrenia: A Study of the Clinical, Social, Family and Economic Benefits*. Baltimore, Maryland: Johns Hopkins University Press.

Falloon, I. R. H. & Talbot, R. E. (1981). Persistent auditory hallucinations: coping mechanisms and implications for management. *Psychological Medicine*, **11**, 329–39.

Fennig, S., Kovasznay, B., Rich, C., Ram, R., Pato, C., Miller, A., Rubinstein, J., Carlson, G., Schwartz, J. E., Phelan, J., Lavelle, J., Craig, T. & Bromet, E. (1994). Six-month stability of psychiatric diagnoses in first-admission patients with psychosis. *American Journal of Psychiatry*, **151**, 1200–1208.

Folkman, S. & Lazarus, R. S. (1988). *Manual: Ways of Coping Questionnaire*. Palo Alto, California: Consulting Psychologist Press.

Fowler, D. & Morley, S. (1989). The cognitive–behavioural treatment of hallucinations and delusions: a preliminary study. *Behavioural Psychotherapy*, **17**, 267–282.

Fowler, D., Garety, P. & Kuipers, E. (1995). *Cognitive Behaviour Therapy for Psychosis: Theory and Practice*. Chichester, UK: Wiley.

Frank, A. F. & Gunderson, J. G. (1990). The role of the therapeutic alliance in the treatment of schizophrenia. *Archives of General Psychiatry*, **47**, 228–36.

Fransella, F. & Bannister, D. (1977). *A Manual for Repertory Grid Techniques.* London: Academic Press.

Frydenberg, E. & Lewis, R. (1997). *Coping Scale for Adults. Practitioner's Kit.* Melbourne, Australia: The Australian Council for Educational Research.

Garety, P. A., Kuipers, L., Fowler, D., Chamberlain, F. & Dunn, G. (1994). Cognitive behavioural therapy for drug-resistant psychosis. *British Journal of Medical Psychology,* **67**, 259–71.

Garety, P., Kuipers, E., Fowler, D., Dunn, G., Bebbington, P., Freeman, D. & Hadley, C. A randomised controlled trial of cognitive behavioural therapy for psychosis. *Paper presented at the Second International Conference on Psychological Treatments for Schizophrenia.* Oxford, England, 2nd and 3rd October, 1997.

Gergen, K. J. (1994). Exploring the postmodern: perils or potentials? *American Psychologist,* **49**, 412–16.

Gleick, J. (1994). *Chaos: Making a New Science.* London: Abacus.

Gould, R. L. (1978). *Transformations: Growth and Change in Adult Life.* New York: Simon & Schuster.

Gould, S. J. (1996a). *Dinosaur in a Haystack: Reflections in Natural History.* London: Jonathan Cape.

Gould, S. J. (1996b). *Life's Grandeur: The Spread of Excellence from Plato to Darwin.* London: Jonathan Cape.

Green, M. F. (1993). Cognitive remediation in schizophrenia: is it time yet? *American Journal of Psychiatry,* **150**, 178–87.

Greenfeld, D., Strauss, J. S., Bowers, M. B. & Mandelkern, M. (1989). Insight and interpretation of illness in recovery from psychosis. *Schizophrenia Bulletin,* **15**, 245–52.

Guidano, V. F. (1987). *Complexity of the Self.* New York: Guilford Press.

Gunderson, J. G., Frank, A. F., Katz, H. M., Vannicelli, M. L., Frosch, J. P. & Knapp, P. H. (1984). Effects of psychotherapy in schizophrenia. II. Comparative outcome of two forms of treatment. *Schizophrenia Bulletin,* **10**, 564–98.

Haddock, G. & Slade, P. D. (eds.) (1996). *Cognitive–Behavioural Interventions with Psychotic Disorders.* London: Routledge.

Haddock, G., Sellwood, W., Tarrier, N. & Yusupoff, L. (1994). Developments in cognitive–behaviour therapy for persistent psychotic symptoms. *Behaviour Change,* **11**, 200–12.

Haddock, G., Morrison, A. P., Hopkins, R., Lewis, S. & Tarrier, N. (in press). Individual cognitive–behavioural interventions in early psychosis. *British Journal of Psychiatry* (Supplement).

Halford, W. K. & Hayes, R. (1991). Psychological rehabilitation of chronic schizophrenia patients: recent findings on social skills training and family psychoeducation. *Clinical Psychology Review,* **11**, 23–44.

Harrop, C. E., Trower, P. & Mitchell, I. J. (1996). Does the biology go around the symptoms? A Copernican shift in schizophrenia paradigms. *Clinical Psychology Review,* **16**, 641–54.

Healy, D. (1990). *The Suspended Revolution: Psychiatry and Psychotherapy Reexamined.* London: Faber and Faber.

Healy, D. (1993). *Images of Trauma: From Hysteria to Post-traumatic Stress Disorder*. London: Faber and Faber.

Heinrichs, D. W., Hanlon, T. E. & Carpenter, W. T. Jr. (1984). The Quality of Life Scale: an instrument for rating the schizophrenic deficit syndrome. *Schizophrenia Bulletin*, **10**, 388–98.

Henry, L., McGorry, P. D., Jackson, H. J., Hulbert, C. A. & Edwards, J. (1997a). Cognitive psychotherapy and the prevention of secondary morbidity in first episode psychosis. *Paper presented at the XXVIII Congress of the European Association for the Behavioural and Cognitive Therapies*, Venice, Italy, 24–27 September, 1997.

Henry, L., Edwards, J., Cocks, J., McGorry, P. & Jackson, H. (1997b). Cognitively-oriented psychotherapy and the recovery process in first episode mania with psychotic features. *Paper presented at the 12th International Symposium for the Psychotherapy of Schizophrenia*, London, England, October, 1997.

Higgins, E. T. (1987). Self-discrepancy: a theory relating self and affect. *Psychological Review*, **94**, 319–40.

Hogarty, G. E., Kornblith, S. J., Greenwald, D., DiBarry, A. L., Cooley, S., Flesher, S., Reiss, D., Carter, M. & Ulrich, R. (1995). Personal therapy: a disorder-relevant psychotherapy for schizophrenia. *Schizophrenia Bulletin*, **21**, 379–93.

Hogarty, G. E., Kornblith, S. J., Greenwald, D., DiBarry, A. L., Cooley, S., Ulrich, R. F., Carter, M. & Flesher, S. (1997a). Three-year trials of personal therapy among schizophrenic patients living with or independent of family: I. Description of study and effects on relapse rates. *American Journal of Psychiatry*, **154**, 1504–13.

Hogarty, G. E., Greenwald, D., Ulrich, R. F., Kornblith, S. J., DiBarry, A. L., Cooley, S., Carter, M. & Flesher, S. (1997b). Three-year trials of personal therapy among schizophrenic patients living with or independent of family: II. Effects on adjustment of patients. *American Journal of Psychiatry*, **154**, 1514–24.

Hole, R. W., Rush, A. J. & Beck, A. T. (1979). A cognitive investigation of schizophrenic delusions. *Psychiatry*, **42**, 312–19.

Hulbert, C. A., Jackson, H. J. & McGorry, P. D. (1996). Relationship between personality and course and outcome in early psychosis: a review of the literature. *Clinical Psychology Review*, **16**, 707–27.

Hulbert, C. A., McGorry, P. D. & Jackson, H. J. (1997). Personality as a co-morbidity factor for treatment outcome in cognitively oriented psychotherapy for early psychosis (COPE). *Paper presented at the XXVIII Congress of the European Association for the Behavioural and Cognitive Therapies*, Venice, Italy, 24–27 September, 1997.

Ioannides, T. (Producer) & Hexter, I. (Director) (1994). *A Stitch in Time [Video]*. Melbourne, Australia: Early Psychosis Prevention and Intervention Centre (EPPIC) for Psychiatric Services Branch, Victorian Government Department of Health and Community Services.

Jackson, H. J., McGorry, P. D., Edwards, J. & Hulbert, C. (1996). Cognitively oriented psychotherapy for early psychosis (COPE). In *Early Intervention and*

Prevention in Mental Health, ed. P. Cotton & H. J. Jackson, pp. 131–54. Melbourne: Australian Psychological Society.

Jackson, H. J., McGorry, P. D., Edwards, J., Hulbert, C., Henry, L., Francey, S., Maude, D., Cocks, J., Power, P., Harrigan, S. & Dudgeon, P. (in press). Cognitively- oriented psychotherapy for early psychosis (COPE): preliminary results. *British Journal of Psychiatry* (Supplement).

Jacobs, L. I. (1980). A cognitive approach to persistent delusions. *American Journal of Psychotherapy*, **34**, 556–63.

Jeffries, J. J. (1977). The trauma of being psychotic: a neglected element in the management of chronic schizophrenia. *Canadian Psychiatric Association Journal*, **22**, 199–206.

Kavanagh, D. J. (1992a). Family interventions for schizophrenia. In *Schizophrenia: An Overview and Practical Handbook*, ed. D. J. Kavanagh, pp. 407–23. London: Chapman & Hall.

Kavanagh, D. J. (1992b). Recent developments in expressed emotion and schizophrenia. *British Journal of Psychiatry*, **160**, 601–20.

Kelly, G. (1955). *The Psychology of Personal Constructs*. New York: Norton.

Kessler, R. C., Foster, C. L., Saunders, W. B. & Stang, P. E. (1995). Social consequences of psychiatric disorders. I: Educational attainment. *American Journal of Psychiatry*, **152**, 1514–24.

Kingdon, D. (1997). The Wellcome study of cognitive therapy for 'treatment resistant' schizophrenia. *Paper presented at the Second International Conference on Psychological Treatments for Schizophrenia*, Oxford, England, 2nd and 3rd October, 1997.

Kingdon, D. G. & Turkington, D. (1991). The use of cognitive therapy with a normalizing rationale in schizophrenia: preliminary report. *Journal of Nervous and Mental Disease*, **179**, 207–11.

Kingdon, D. G. & Turkington, D. (1994). *Cognitive–Behavioral Therapy of Schizophrenia*. New York: Guilford Press.

Kingdon, D., Turkington, D. & John, C. (1994). Cognitive behaviour therapy of schizophrenia: the amenability of delusions and hallucinations to reasoning. *British Journal of Psychiatry*, **164**, 581–7.

Kleinman, A. (1980). *Patients and Healers in the Context of Culture. An Exploration of the Borderline Between Anthropology, Medicine, and Psychiatry*. Berkeley, California: University of California Press.

Lazarus, R. S. & Folkman, S. (1984). *Stress, Appraisal, and Coping*. New York: Springer.

Levinson, D. J. (1986). A conception of adult development. *American Psychologist*, **41**, 3–13.

Liberman, R. P. Kopelowicz, A. & Young, A. S. (1994). Biobehavioral treatment and rehabilitation of schizophrenia. *Behavior Therapy*, **25**, 89–107.

Luborsky, L., McLellan, T., Woody, G. E., O'Brien, C. P. & Auerbach, A. (1985). Therapist success and its determinants. *Archives of General Psychiatry*, **42**, 602–11.

Luborsky, L., McLellan, A. T., Diguer, L., Woody, G. & Seligman, D. A. (1997). The psychotherapist matters: comparison of outcomes across twenty-two therapists and seven patient samples. *Clinical Psychology: Science and Practice,* **4**, 53– 65.

Lundy, M. S. (1992). Psychosis-induced posttraumatic stress disorder. *American Journal of Psychotherapy,* **46**, 485–91.

Mahoney, M. J. (1991). *Human Change Processes: The Scientific Foundations of Psychotherapy.* New York: Guilford Press.

Markus, H. & Nurius, P. (1986). Possible selves. *American Psychologist,* **41**, 954–69.

Maude, D., Edwards, J., McGorry, P. D., Cocks, J., Bennett, C., Burnett, P., Pica, S., Bell, R., Harrigan, S. & Davern, M. (1997). A randomised controlled trial using cognitive–behavioural therapy and clozapine in the early treatment of persisting positive symptoms in first-episode psychosis: preliminary results. *Paper presented at the Second International Conference on Psychological Treatments for Schizophrenia,* Oxford, England, October 2nd and 3rd.

May, R. A. (1968). *Treatment of Schizophrenia: A Comparative Study of Five Treatment Methods.* New York: Science House.

McCrae, R. R. & Costa, P. T., Jr. (1990). *Personality in Adulthood.* New York: Guilford Press.

McCrae, R. R. & Costa, P. T., Jr. (1997). Personality trait structure as a human universal. *American Psychologist,* **52**, 509–16.

McGlashan, T. H. & Johannessen, J. O. (1996). Early detection and intervention with schizophrenia: rationale. *Schizophrenia Bulletin,* **22**, 201–22.

McGlashan, T. H., Wadeson, H. S., Carpenter, W. T. & Levy, S. T. (1977). Art and recovery style from psychosis. *Journal of Nervous and Mental Disease,* **164**, 182–90.

McGorry, P. D. (1992). The concept of recovery and secondary prevention in psychotic disorders. *Australian and New Zealand Journal of Psychiatry,* **26**, 3–17.

McGorry, P. D. (1994). The influence of illness duration on syndrome clarity and stability in functional psychosis: does the diagnosis emerge and stabilise with time? *Australian and New Zealand Journal of Psychiatry,* **28**, 607–19.

McGorry, P. D. (1995). Psychoeducation in first-episode psychosis: a therapeutic process. *Psychiatry,* **58**, 329–44.

McGorry, P. D. & Edwards, J. (1997). *Early Psychosis Training Pack.* Cheshire, UK: Gardiner–Caldwell Communications.

McGorry, P. D., Goodwin, R. J. & Stuart, G. W. (1988). The development, use, and reliability of the BPRS (Nursing Modification): an assessment procedure for the nursing team in clinical and research settings. *Comprehensive Psychiatry,* **29**, 575–87.

McGorry, P. D., Chanen, A., McCarthy, E., van Riel, R., McKenzie, D. & Singh, B. S. (1991). Posttraumatic stress disorder following recent-onset psychosis. An unrecognized postpsychotic syndrome. *Journal of Nervous and Mental Disease,* **179**, 253–8.

McGorry, P. D., Edwards, J., Mihalopoulis, C., Harrigan, S. M. & Jackson, H. J. (1996). EPPIC: an evolving system of early detection and optimal management. *Schizophrenia Bulletin,* **22**, 305–26.

Meltzer, H. Y. (1993). New drugs for the treatment of schizophrenia. *Psychiatric Clinics of North America,* **16**, 365–85.

Millon, T. with Davis, R. D. (1996). *Disorders of Personality: DSM^{TM} and Beyond.* New York: Wiley.

Mohr, D. C. (1995). Negative outcome in psychotherapy: a critical review. *Clinical Psychology: Science and Practice*, **2**, 1–27.

Mooney, M. & Pica, S. (1997). Social phobia in psychosis. Detection and treatment. *Paper presented at the XXVIII Congress of the European Association for the Behavioural and Cognitive Therapies*, Venice, Italy, 24–27 September, 1997.

Mueser, K. T., Goodman, L. B., Trumbetta, S. L., Rosenberg, S. D., Osher, F. C., Vidaver, R., Auciello, P. & Foy, D. W. (1998). Trauma and posttraumatic stress disorder in severe mental illness. *Journal of Consulting and Clinical Psychology*.

Murray, H. A. (1938). *Explorations in Personality.* New York: Oxford University Press.

Neimeyer, R. A. (1993). An appraisal of constructivist psychotherapies. *Journal of Consulting and Clinical Psychology*, **61**, 221–34.

Neimeyer, R. A. & Mahoney, M. J. (eds.) (1995). *Constructivism in Psychotherapy.* Washington, DC: American Psychological Association.

Ogilvie, D. M. (1987). The undesired self: a neglected variable in personality research. *Journal of Personality and Social Psychology*, **52**, 379–85.

Overall, J. E. & Gorham, D. R. (1962). The brief psychiatric rating scale. *Psychological Reports*, **10**, 799–812.

Perris, C. (1989). *Cognitive Therapy with Schizophrenic Patients.* New York: Guilford Press.

Perris, C. (1992). Some aspects of the use of cognitive psychotherapy with patients suffering from a schizophrenic disorder. In *Psychotherapy of Schizophrenia: Facilitating and Obstructive Factors*, ed. A. Werbart & J. Cullberg, pp. 131–45. Oslo: Scandinavian University Press.

Perris, C. & Skagerlind, L. (1994). Cognitive therapy with schizophrenic patients. *Acta Psychiatrica Scandinavica*, **89** (Supplement 382), 65–70.

Rey, J. M. (1992). The Epidemiological Catchment Area (ECA) study: implications for Australia. *Medical Journal of Australia*, **156**, 200–03.

Roberts, G. (1991). Delusional belief systems and meaning in life: a preferred reality? *British Journal of Psychiatry* (Supplement 14), **159**, 19–28.

Roberts, G. (1992). The origins of delusion. *British Journal of Psychiatry*, **161**, 298–308.

Robins, E. & Guze, S. B. (1970). Establishment of diagnostic validity in psychiatric illness: its application to schizophrenia. *American Journal of Psychiatry*, **126**, 983–7.

Sandler, J., Dare, C. & Holder, A. (1970). Basic psychoanalytic concepts: II. The treatment alliance. *British Journal of Psychiatry*, **116**, 555–8.

Sass, L. A. (1992). *Madness and Modernism: Insanity in the Light of Modern Art, Literature, and Thought.* New York: Basic Books.

Sass, L. A. (1994). *The Paradoxes of Delusion: Wittgenstein, Schreber, and the Schizophrenic Mind.* New York: Cornell University Press.

Schulz, R. & Heckhausen, J. (1996). A life-span model of successful aging. *American Psychologist*, **51**, 702–14.

Scott, J. E. & Dixon, L. B. (1995). Psychological interventions for schizophrenia. *Schizophrenia Bulletin*, **21**, 621–30.

Seligman, M. E. P. (1991). *Learned Optimism*. Sydney: Random House.

Seligman, M. E. P. (1995). The effectiveness of psychotherapy: the *Consumer Reports* study. *American Psychologist*, **50**, 965–74.

Sharp, H. M., Fear, C. F., Williams, J. M. G., Healy, D., Lowe, C. F., Yeadon, H. & Holden, R. (1996). Delusional phenomenology – Dimensions of change. *Behaviour Research and Therapy*, **34**, 123–42.

Singer, J. A. & Salovey, P. (1993). *The Remembered Self: Emotion and Memory in Personality*. New York: Free Press.

Smith, T. E., Bellack, A. S. & Liberman, R. P. (1996). Social skills training for schizophrenia: Review and future directions. *Clinical Psychology Review*, **16**, 599–617.

Strakowski, S. M., Tohen, M., Stoll, A. L., Faedda, G. L., Mayer, P. V., Kolbrener, M. L. & Goodwin, D. C. (1993). Comorbidity in psychosis at first hospitalization. *American Journal of Psychiatry*, **150**, 752–7.

Strakowski, S. M., Keck, P. E., Jr., McElroy, S. L., Lonczak, H. S. & West, S. A. (1995). Chronology of comorbid and principal syndromes in first-episode psychosis. *Comprehensive Psychiatry*, **36**, 106–12.

Strauss, J. S. (1969). Hallucinations and delusions as points on continua function. *Archives of General Psychiatry*, **21**, 581–6.

Strauss, J. S. (1994). The person with schizophrenia. II. Approaches to the subjective and complex. *British Journal of Psychiatry*, **164** (Supplement 23), 103–7.

Sugarman, L. (1986). *Life-span Development: Concepts, Theories and Interventions*. London: Methuen.

Tarrier, N. (1992). Management and modification of residual positive psychotic symptoms. In *Innovations in the Psychological Management of Schizophrenia: Assessment, Treatment and Services*, ed. M. J. Birchwood & N. Tarrier, pp. 147–69. Chichester, UK: Wiley.

Tarrier, N. (1997). Coping and problem-solving in the treatment of persistent psychotic symptoms. *Paper presented at the Second International Conference on Psychological Treatments for Schizophrenia*, Oxford, England, 2nd and 3rd October, 1997.

Tarrier, N., Beckett, R., Harwood, S., Baker, A., Yusupoff, L. & Ugarteburu, I. (1993). A trial of two cognitive–behavioural methods of treating drug-resistant residual psychotic symptoms in schizophrenic patients. I. Outcome. *British Journal of Psychiatry*, **162**, 524–32.

Weinberger, J. (1995). Common factors aren't so common: the common factors dilemma. *Clinical Psychology: Science and Practice*, **2**, 45–69.

Weisz, J. R., Donenberg, G. R., Han, S. S. & Weiss, B. (1995). Bridging the gap between laboratory and clinic in child and adolescent psychotherapy. *Journal of Consulting and Clinical Psychology*, **63**, 688–701.

Williams-Keeler, L., Milliken, H. & Jones, B. (1994). Psychosis as precipitating trauma for PTSD. *American Journal of Orthopsychiatry*, **64**, 493–8.

Young, J. E. (1994). *Cognitive Therapy for Personality Disorders: A Schema-focused Approach*, revised version. Sarasota, Florida: Professional Resource Press.

Zarb, J. M. (1992). *Cognitive–Behavioural Assessment and Therapy with Adolescents.* New York: Brunner/Mazel.

Zubin, J. & Spring, B. (1977). Vulnerability – a new view on schizophrenia. *Journal of Abnormal Psychology*, **86**, 103–26.

11
Preventive case management in first-episode psychosis

JANE EDWARDS, JOHN COCKS AND JAMES BOTT

> My experience as Dale's case manager has been both interesting and challenging. His progress over the past two years can be seen as mirroring the developmental tasks of adolescence, that is, development of identity, individuation, and separation; however, it has been intensified given the impact of psychosis. Accordingly, my role as case manager has changed from a paternalistic approach to a more collaborative style as Dale's sense of self has strengthened and he has felt more able to take responsibility for life decisions. Along with these changes my skills and understanding of the role of the case manager have developed. The feelings of frustration, anxiety and despair which were once almost intolerable are now more containable as they are accompanied by a sense of confidence and hope on my part regarding the degree of recovery that is possible.
>
> EPPIC case manager

Introduction

Case management as a term was first used in psychiatry in the 1960s in the context of deinstitutionalization (Ryan, Ford & Clifford, 1991). Case management was introduced as a means of avoiding fragmentation of the available community services and of providing a point of clinical accountability for the care of patients with complex problems (Harris & Bergman, 1993). In the literature, the focus within serious mental illness has been on the case management of people with chronic and stable disability, usually with a diagnosis of schizophrenia (Holloway et al., 1995).

Over the past three decades a consensus has emerged on the general features of case management: assessment of client needs; development of a comprehensive service plan to meet these needs; arrangement of service delivery; monitoring and assessment of the services; and evaluation and follow-up (Holloway et al. 1995). However, two key issues remain unresolved in the case management literature. The first issue concerns a debate between the brokerage and therapist models of case management. In a brokerage model, the case manager acts as the co-ordinator of care which is provided by other clinicians on behalf of the client. In a therapist model, the case manager is the primary treating clinician, and uses his or her clinical skills to assess the needs of the patient and the family, whilst using the developing relationship as part of the treatment itself (Lamb, 1980). The second unresolved issue involves integrated clinical care versus models which separate biological and psychosocial aspects of management. Within a case management framework, medication issues are rarely integrated with discussions of psychological or family treatments (a problem which is not limited to case management, see Hogarty, 1998). Furthermore, the case management literature generally lacks both a theoretical basis for the provision of specific interventions, and empirical support for the same (Kline, Becker & Giese, 1992). Despite this, case management is usually promoted as the framework within which optimal treatments are provided (Falloon & Fadden, 1993; Sumich, Hunt & Andrews, 1995). In this chapter we outline an approach to the case management of individuals with early psychosis, based on a therapist model, using an integrated biopsychosocial framework.

Case management in first-episode psychosis

The Nordic investigation of psychotherapeutically orientated treatment for recently diagnosed schizophrenic patients (NIPS project: Alanen et al., 1994) is the only reference to case management in a first-episode population to be found in the literature. NIPS is a multi-centre research project focussing on the provision of long-term supportive psychotherapy within the public system to newly diagnosed schizophrenic patients. Based on psychoanalytic principles, the therapy also provides a basis for family support, monitoring of medication, social rehabilitation, and crisis intervention. Gilbert & Ugelstad (1994) report on the Oslo cohort of this collaborative study and note that the 'approach has similarities with the concept of clinical case management, but since the patients were resourceful individuals and their illness was of recent onset, they needed a dialogue-based relationship more than practical case management' (p. 87). Patients voluntarily terminated therapy within 2–4 years, which Gilbert and Ugelstad suggest implies that the attachment was based on a need for help in recovering from a mental disorder, rather than assistance in dealing with persisting illness.

In this chapter we focus on the principles of preventive case management with a first-episode population. The model is considered under five headings: the clinician–patient relationship; case management tasks in each phase of disorder; prolonged recovery; use of an integrated biopsychosocial model; and management of the case management team. It is important to emphasize that a distinguishing feature of case management of the individual experiencing a first-episode psychosis is that it presents a crucial opportunity to 'get it right' in the provision of optimal clinical care. A more satisfactory quality of life will result from comprehensive assessment, formulation of a treatment plan based on this assessment, provision of optimal needs-based treatment early in the episode, and a minimization of the risks of experiencing the negative and iatrogenic effects of treatment. As an example, failing to complete secondary school whilst psychotic will impact on a person long after the psychotic episode has resolved (Kessler et al., 1995): early treatment of the episode while continuing to attend school may avoid 'post-morbid occupational decline' (Beiser et al., 1994). The emphasis in the approach outlined in this chapter is on working with the individual patient. It is crucial that case managers consider the family in their work, and the present chapter should therefore be read in conjunction with Chapter 14. However, before we turn to the specific approach to case management which we have developed, it is important to consider the context in which this occurred, since our approach to case management evolved in attempting to serve the needs of our particular patient population.

EPPIC case management context

The Early Psychosis Prevention and Intervention Centre (EPPIC) is a multicomponent service developed in order to address the needs of young adults and adolescents in the early stages of a psychotic disorder (Edwards et al., 1994; McGorry et al., 1996). The population is young with the average age for both males and females being 22 years. Ninety-five per cent remain within the parental home or in stable accommodation. The population is diverse, with individuals possessing a variety of personality types, and developmental and intellectual levels, as well as a range of life experiences. Adolescent issues are prominent (Winnicott, 1965) and are often intertwined with illness issues. Almost none of these young people have received case management services prior to the onset of psychosis. Patients bring to the treatment setting expectations based on their experience with other health carers, and portrayals of both psychosis and psychiatric workers; the latter frequently have been influenced by the popular media. While psychosis is often devastating for the young adult, the changes which have occurred in the person's life have not become immutable. In fact, a little over 90% of our patients achieve symptomatic remission from the first psychotic episode in the first 12 months of treatment (Edwards et al., 1998), and although there is a high risk of relapse, the primary tasks of case management concern promotion of recovery and prevention of persistent disability. Substance abuse is a major clinical problem with 48.3% (total $n = 147$) of our patients having problematic use at some stage prior to stabilization (Susan Harrigan, personal communication). At initial presentation, based on a sample of 347 cases, 22.2% of the population have affective psychoses, 70.9% schizophrenia spectrum disorders (i.e. schizophrenia, schizophreniform, delusional disorder and schizoaffective disorder), and 6.9% other, often transient, psychotic disorders. Twenty-eight per cent of first-episode patients avoid admission in the first three months of treatment (Power et al., 1998).

EPPIC is a regional service covering the inner city and western suburbs of Melbourne, an area of significant socioeconomic disadvantage with very few private psychiatrists servicing the area. Almost all first-episode patients with psychosis who present to EPPIC are resident in the catchment area. The Centre carries a case load of 320 patients, with 20 to 25 new referrals each month; all patients are allocated a therapist–case manager and full-time clinicians carry case loads of approximately 35 patients. Therapist–case managers within EPPIC operate within a service which offers a number of specialist subprogrammes including an assertive outreach team, an inpatient service, family work, and a recovery-based group programme. Based on the concept of a 2–5 year 'critical period' during which patients with schizophrenia are most vulnerable to deterioration (Birchwood & Macmillan, 1993), the programme currently offers up to 18 months of intensive treatment.

Clinician–patient relationship

The clinician–patient relationship is the central axis around which all treatment revolves. The therapist–case manager needs to connect with the person who is experiencing psychosis (Strauss, 1992), respect the individual's experience, acknowledge the validity of concerns raised, and be available to reality test ideas. We have found that it is impossible to duplicate the relationship which forms between patient and clinician during a time of crisis, but we are convinced that the relationship is fostered by introducing the case manager early in treatment. Consistent with the 'integrated mental health care' model (Falloon & Fadden, 1993) a case manager should be involved in the initial assessment, or otherwise see the patient and family within two working days of admission to the service. The case manager is central to all decisions across inpatient and outpatient settings and remains involved with the patient and the family throughout their time with the service.

Patients and families identify relatively few factors as being important in their relationship with the case manager. The first important factor is accessibility; both the patient and family need to know that they can contact the case manager should a crisis arise. The second is flexibility; the clinician needs to be responsive to the changing needs of the patient and the family, rather than dogmatically adhering to a particular theory or practice. The third essential factor is the maintenance of optimism on the part of the case manager; in short, the clinician needs to promote recovery, whilst expecting the patient to be actively involved in the recovery process (Anthony, 1993). Finally, the patient and family are more likely to attend to, and implement, the suggestions of clinicians whom they believe possess the relevant expertise.

The problems of a psychotic patient can draw the unwary into a morass of intra-psychic and reality-based problems. Too often case managers are left with the feeling that the patient would benefit if only the case manager could offer more. Conversely, a helpless approach can develop as a response to the seemingly overwhelming and intractable nature of problems not quickly resolved. Any intervention needs to be accompanied by careful consideration of the patient's experience of the intervention. 'Case management requirements to be human and caring do not obviate the need to monitor one's own involvement in the process and to try to make sense of the ongoing interactions ... the salient aspect of therapeutic neutrality is the willingness to observe and attempt to understand all of one's interactions with one's patients' (Kline et al., 1992, p. 372). Understanding the attachment issues for both patients and therapists may be extremely useful in tailoring interventions to individual needs (Dozier, 1993).

For example, a likeable but immature young man recovered well from a first manic episode but remained at risk of relapse and wanted to discontinue contact with the clinic. The case manager had to consider whether the difficulties that she experienced in 'letting go' reflected an anxious attachment.

A case manager may need to accept a patient's resistance to his or her awareness of the risk of relapse, in the hope that this will allow the option of further contact, rather than confronting the issue; this may lead to an explosive rejection of contact. This means that the therapist has to carry the anxiety of relapse and respond to issues of risk based on a realistic assessment.

Case managers can use their developing understanding of the patient to inform their decision making regarding the nature of interventions and style of delivery. This includes an intuitive appreciation of the patient and an examination of one's counter-transference responses.

> For example, a paranoid person may interpret attempts at frequent sessions as a threatening intrusion, and respond better to briefer and less frequent sessions. Feeling the struggle around control and domination elicited by such a patient allows one to appreciate the difficulty the patient has with these issues in the relationship, and the case manager may then give the patient more control.

This is essentially a supportive approach which aims to validate the patient's experience and, within reason, accommodate to it rather than confronting and interpreting.

Case management tasks in each phase of disorder

The division of case management tasks by phases is useful for discussion and serves to remind the clinician that recovery is to be expected (Lieberman et al., 1993; McGorry, 1992). Throughout the phases of disorder – acute, early recovery, and late recovery – case managers need to maintain both recovery and preventive foci. Typically, case managers meet with patients and families two to three times per week in the acute phase, once or twice per week in the early recovery phase, and weekly or fortnightly in later recovery, thereafter up to monthly, to continue the work of relapse prevention and monitoring. The acute phase typically refers to the initial weeks, early recovery refers to one to three months, and late recovery may extend to one year, although this pattern is highly variable, particularly in the presence of personality disorder or substance abuse. The overall tasks of the case manager include: minimizing the duration of active psychosis; preventing the toxic effects of medication using low-dose drug strategies; avoiding inpatient admission where possible, and humanizing admission when it is necessary; and actively seeking and treating secondary problems.

Acute phase

During the initial weeks of treatment, the tasks of the case manager include: engaging and developing a working therapeutic relationship with the patient and his or her family, conducting a comprehensive assessment of the individual (including undertaking risk assessment), and developing a formulation (Jackson, 1993), as well as providing symptomatic relief and containment. Engagement can be particularly difficult with the patient who attends under duress. Strategies such as asking the patient why the referring person believes him or her to be unwell, can promote discussion. It is important to let the patient recognize that the case manager takes their experiences seriously, whilst not necessarily accepting the patient's explanations. Medication forms a central component of management, and prevention and early intervention in relation to side effects are important with regard to later compliance. Strategies to manage the inevitable distress and anxiety include providing: personal support, factual information about psychosis, and reassurance. Even at this early stage it is important to start evolving a useful understanding of psychosis with the patient and family. A gentle exchange of explanatory models is useful, particularly with regard to the early planting of doubt about morbid beliefs.

> For example, a young man presented, fearing that he was being poisoned by his workmates because his thinking was confused. The case manager commented: 'I understand you believe you have been poisoned as you find that your thinking is jumbled. While I don't believe that such a poison exists I do believe that these thinking problems could be the result of a toxin from within.' The patient accepted medication to treat the effects of a 'toxin'. Over the next few sessions the case manager explored the patient's explanatory model which progressed from a 'toxin' to a 'release of an inner toxin at times of stress', to a recognition of personal vulnerability accompanied by a belief in an ability to influence positively the course of the disorder through the use of medication and stress management techniques.

Negotiations about methods of treatment in the acute phase in the first-episode patient may be very difficult, and at times impossible, as often the patient and clinician have not been able to achieve a shared understanding of the nature of the problem. The negotiation approach places emphasis on an open relationship in which the clinician strives to elicit and hear the request of the patient and then uses this request as a central part of negotiation over treatment (Eisenthal et al., 1979). 'The purpose of the negotiation is not only to have the patient accept that the clinician's definitions of the problem, goals, and methods are 'correct' ... but to have the clinician accept the possibility that the patient's definitions of the problem, desired goals, and methods are appropriate' (Lazare, Eisenthal & Frank, 1989, p. 144).

Refusal to accept treatment places the case manager in a difficult position. How much latitude the clinician should allow the patient depends on factors relating to the degree of disturbance exhibited by the patient. The clinician needs to take into account the patient's state of shock or disorganization, denial, distress, dependency, and recovery, as well as the degrees of insight and suicide risk. It is important not to be any more authoritarian than necessary. 'We must recognize that the patient has the inalienable right to determine the degree of his participation, and summary interference with his freedom of action in this regard can only be sanctioned when clear dangerousness to himself or others is evident' (Munice, 1959, p. 1320). However, there are times when this may conflict with a preventive imperative.

> At his second appointment, after a protracted inpatient admission, an 18-year-old youth who had been placed on an involuntary treatment order informed his case manager that he would no longer be taking lithium. Rather than return the patient to the inpatient facility, as the Mental Health Act allowed, the case manager suggested that they could examine the admission notes together to see if they could determine why he had been placed on lithium. By not forcing the issue, and by adopting both a collaborative and investigative approach, the young man was given an opportunity to consider the rationale for taking lithium, rather than feeling he was being controlled.

Clinical decisions in this area are often complex and, as the consequences are potentially serious, it is helpful to discuss strategies and tactics within a team structure.

Towards the end of the acute phase the young person is often eager to return to school or work. While return to normal activities should be encouraged, it may be helpful to raise with the patient and family the notion that, as with major physical illnesses, a variable period of convalescence is often required (Strauss, 1989).

> A young woman who had always been a hard worker was given a two-week sickness certificate early in the context of re-emergence of psychotic symptoms. This action alleviated her distress over her current incapacity, whilst also indicating that the case manager thought she would soon be able to return to work.

Early recovery

Ongoing involvement of the case manager during the acute phase, and extending into the recovery phase, allows a monitoring of progress and an opportunity both to understand the patient's experience of illness and to facilitate recovery. Premorbid issues tend to emerge over time, and a gradual approach to understanding the patient's life overall is most helpful. With an acute onset of illness especially, there is often an idealization of the pre-illness self and it may take a long time, perhaps up to a year, before a patient will allow himself a more realistic appraisal of what life was like before the illness developed.

> A young man recovering from a manic episode kept deferring discussion of a return to work saying that he wanted to wait until he got better. Exploration of his premorbid functioning revealed long-standing difficulties finding direction in life in association with a marked lack of self-confidence.

This distortion of the premorbid self is not uncommon; it has been suggested that awareness of impending failure may contribute to the vulnerability to psychosis in adolescence or young adult life (Arieti, 1974. Also, it is important not to close prematurely on premorbid assessment.

> A young woman used cannabis and stole regularly in the year prior to her first admission. Dismissed as being antisocial, it later emerged that she had become distressed with prodromal symptoms during that year and had self-medicated with cannabis.

11 PREVENTIVE CASE MANAGEMENT

The development of a psychotic episode involves more than the experience of symptoms. It may well be experienced as a struggle with something quite disturbing and overwhelming which arises from within. The differentiation of self from psychosis is critical in a young person struggling to establish an identity. This differentiation can be promoted in the interview through the careful use of language, e.g. 'you have experienced a psychotic episode' rather than 'you are psychotic'. It is helpful to develop the notion of a non-psychotic area of functioning within the personality. Exploring recreational and occupational skills, as well as other strengths, can assist this process.

> For example, a 20-year-old with a treatment-resistant psychosis, who viewed himself as a complete failure, was encouraged to resume golf, an activity which he had previously enjoyed and in which his skills remained.

It takes time and effort to discover such areas of able functioning and then to assist the patient in overcoming the financial and social barriers to undertaking identified activities. Resuming golf involves borrowing clubs, budgeting for green fees, telephoning the clubhouse of a local course to enquire about public hours, and establishing whether the patient is prepared to undertake the activity unaccompanied.

During this phase the patient is reintegrating a sense of self, which may include family, school, and work relationships. Case managers typically focus actively on recovery and secondary morbidity (see Chapter 10), whilst encouraging medication adherence (Falloon, 1984). The provision of support for patient and family continues. Coping strategies which increase the patient's sense of mastery, such as distraction and relaxation techniques, may be taught, and explanatory models further explored. The approach of the case manager becomes less directive and more collaborative.

During the acute phase, case managers should incorporate psychoeducation in their work with patients and families in a dynamic and creative manner. The process of psychoeducation involves an exchange of ideas about psychosis, and includes the rationale for the use of medication, the nature of psychosis – including further exploration of explanatory models, information about the course of the disorder, reassurance that recovery will occur, the challenging of negative stereotypes about illness, and an explanation of the stress–vulnerability model. The idea of potential relapse is introduced to the patient and family through the identification of possible early warning signs of relapse which were experienced or perceived during the initial prodrome. Clinicians must carefully consider the support material to be used, as much of the self-help literature is designed for patients with established and chronic illnesses. In the first-episode patient the diagnosis and prognosis is frequently unclear (McGorry, 1991), and the outcome better than has often been anticipated (Lieberman et al., 1993). Use of material which has been specifically tailored to psychosis in the first episode (e.g. Ioannides & Hexter, 1994; Schizophrenia Fellowship of Victoria, 1994) avoids misinformation. Additionally, the young patient may not be interested in reading and the use of videos and interactive computer programs may be more appealing.

Late recovery

Most patients with a first episode of psychosis will recover; however, at least with regard to non-affective psychoses, 70% will relapse within 2–3 years, 50% within ten months of stopping medication, and up to 40% will relapse whilst receiving ongoing antipsychotic medication (Gilbert et al., 1995). Lieberman et al. (1993) suggest that most patients who remit from a first episode of a schizophrenic illness relapse in the following four years. Kissling (1994) has argued that the main cause of high relapse rates is undertreatment, particularly with regard to 'doctors' non-compliance' regarding adequate duration of antipsychotic treatment. The logical extension of this, with regard to relapse and first-episode psychosis, is that one might be more optimistic about illness course if best practice is explicated, adhered to, and monitored through quality assurance mechanisms.

Relapse itself need not always impact on long-term outcome, although it is known that, in schizophrenia, each relapse brings with it an increased probability of future relapse, residual symptoms, and accompanying social disability (World Health Organization, 1979). 'We recommend treating most patients with the minimally effective dose to avoid more serious adverse effects, even at the cost of a few more relapses, provided this strategy does not lead to rehospitalisation or produce serious impairment in functioning' (Janick et al., 1993, p. 129).

Janick et al. (1993) argue that long-term maintenance medication should not be instituted in a first-episode population, and in practice very few first-episode patients would countenance such an approach. Indeed, one of the most important tasks of late recovery is the consideration of medication cessation. Non-medical case managers, in collaboration with patient and family involvement, play a major role in this decision. The stress–vulnerability model can be helpful in framing discussions which lead to the final decision. The patient's vulnerability

Table 11.1. *Guidelines for the cessation of medication in first-episode psychosis*

Non-affective psychosis	Brief episode – good prognosis	Antipsychotics 6–9* months
	Longer episode – less favourable prognosis	Antipsychotics 12–24 months
Affective psychosis	Manic – treated with lithium and antipsychotics	Lithium – 9 months, antipsychotics only until positive symptoms abate (4–6 weeks)
	Manic – treated without lithium	Antipsychotics for 6–9 months
	Depressive	Antidepressants 6–12 months, Antipsychotics short term (4–6 weeks)

* If symptoms persist these time frames will need to be lengthened correspondingly.

can be predicted with some accuracy by considering premorbid functioning and personality, duration and nature of psychopathology, and family history. By this time the case manager will have gathered further information about response to treatment, and risk factors for prolonged recovery such as family atmosphere. As a guide, we suggest that in non-affective first-episode psychosis, medication is continued for six months in the briefest and best prognosis cases, to between one and two years if the prognosis appears not so favourable. It seems sensible to maintain treatment for a period of some months after good recovery to allow for consolidation (Gilbert et al., 1995), and to taper withdrawal over several months (Jeste et al., 1995), at a time when stress for the patient is at a minimum. In the manic psychoses, debate continues about the use of lithium as treatment and/or as an adjunct to antipsychotic medication (Goodwin, 1995; Price & Heninger, 1994). If lithium is used then six to nine months of continued treatment at therapeutic levels is indicated before a tapered withdrawal (Thase, 1993). Should psychotic symptoms persist, then the time scale needs to be adjusted accordingly. Transient psychotic states present the case manager with the dilemma of targeting the stressor (e.g. grief) in a psychosocial or biomedical manner. Ideally, support should be provided and may be supplemented with the use of antianxiety agents and/or antipsychotics for brief periods. Table 11.1 summarizes guidelines for cessation of medication in first-episode psychosis.

The case manager needs to be able confidently to navigate both the service and transition periods in a manner analogous to an experienced 'tour guide' (Rosen, 1994). A major issue which demands careful planning and preparation is termination. The possible reactions of a patient to termination need to be carefully considered by the case manager. The clinician should have some understanding of attachment issues (Della Selva, 1993).

> A distant young man became psychotic within a week of being told that he was soon to finish with his case manager. In retrospect, his case manager realized that the patient's indifferent, monthly appointments indicated the firmest degree of attachment this man could achieve with his case manager.

Preparatory discharge strategies may include implementation of a 'Users Guide' (EPPIC Statewide Services, 1996); this consists of a written service orientation document which is supplied to patients and families during the engagement process and contains information about discharge planning. Regular review of progress with an explicit foreshadowing of discharge (e.g. back to the general practitioner or transfer to another mental health service or professional) is useful for a variety of reasons. First, it conveys the idea that people tend to recover. Secondly, it means that termination issues, whether they arise because the patient has completed the therapeutic contact, or has been transferred to another professional, can be addressed appropriately. Termination, notwithstanding efforts to maximize continuity of care, is a fact of life in many mental health services, and it is better if it is a planned process linked to phase of illness and the needs of the patient, rather than being a random event.

Additional tasks in late recovery focus on the individual's vulnerability to psychosis (Zubin & Spring, 1977). The work includes exploration of risk factors for relapse; identification, if possible, of an individualized relapse prodrome; and early intervention strategies based upon these, which may include guidance about appropriate help-seeking behaviour (Macmillan, Birchwood & Smith, 1992). Unfortunately, the earliest signs and symptoms of impending relapse in both affective and non-affective psychoses, including brief changes in affect, cognition and behaviour such as depression or anxiety, poor concentration, and altered sleep patterns, are non-specific (Macmillan et al., 1992), and do not always indicate early relapse. Yet, in many cases the pattern is recog-

11 PREVENTIVE CASE MANAGEMENT

nized by the patient or family members and becomes more reliably discernible with experience (Marder et al., 1994).

> A 26-year-old fitter and turner was not willing to attend the clinic following his first psychotic episode. He returned to outpatient treatment after a major relapse which resulted in his first hospitalization. The case manager spent considerable time trying to identify both his prodromal symptoms, with the assistance of tables generated through research on bipolar prodromes (Fava & Kellner, 1991; Molnar, Feeney & Fava, 1988; Smith & Tarrier, 1992), and his pathway into treatment. It was identified that both the initial episode and relapse had occurred during holiday periods. Much effort was expended on examining work issues, stress management, use of recreation, and planning ahead for vacation time. The family were seen, including the patient's sisters and brothers-in-law, and photocopies of the patient's personal early warning signs and a six-step emergency plan were distributed to each member of the family.

Patient responses to changes in mental state can, in turn, alter risk.

> One individual would become anxious at exam times, try to study harder and longer to prevent failing, go without sleep, and then use cannabis to relax, before relapsing into mania. Recognizing this pattern allowed her to consider the costs of overworking, and the injurious nature of sleep deprivation and cannabis use.

On the other hand, there can be a danger of pathologizing normal behaviour and emotions. Commonly, with relapse there is a marked increase in the sense of personal vulnerability when compared to the initial episode which can be associated with risk of suicide.

At times a case manager can model problem solving in relation to hurdles.

> Phone calls attempting to engage a young man with employment support services were made in the case manager's office. The patient located telephone numbers in the telephone book while the case manager made the calls. In this way the patient learnt how to

> navigate the telephone book, obtained 'first hand' information as to why he was not accepted in particular programmes, and watched the case manager persist in the face of unhelpful third parties.

Comorbid or premorbid problems such as substance abuse, anxiety disorders, sexual abuse or personality difficulties often become clearer in late recovery, and should be treated when appropriate.

> A 16-year-old woman began to settle after months of acute psychosis. She avoided touching numerous household objects because she believed that her grandmother, with whom she lived, was unhygienic. She felt compelled to wash her hands whenever she thought about her grandmother. As the psychosis resolved and the assessment continued, it emerged that the obsessive behaviours were longstanding and, at times, debilitating. Psychological treatment for the comorbid obsessive compulsive disorder was then accepted with good effect.

The interaction of personality and psychosis has long been a matter of debate (Hulbert, Jackson & McGorry, 1996; Smith et al., 1995). It is important to formulate a more precise diagnosis, if difficulties arise within treatment which the clinician considers reflective of possible personality issues. Consideration of several possibilities is warranted: the possibility of premorbid personality disorder; exacerbation of personality traits under the stress of the psychotic episode; the confusion of the effects of persisting psychotic and affective symptoms with personality; and the impact of unrecognized comorbid disorders on the presentation. It often takes time for the diagnoses to become clear. Borderline personality disorder is one of the more frequent comorbid diagnoses in this population (Hogg et al., 1990; Pica et al., 1990). Models of intervention suitable for non-psychotic individuals (e.g. Beck, Freeman & Associates, 1990; Benjamin, 1993; Linehan, 1993) may need to be modified under these circumstances.

Substance abuse is one of the most common comorbid problems in first-episode psychosis (Strakowski et al., 1993; 1995). While the literature about the co-existence of severe mental illness and substance abuse indicates that there is a substantial overlap of problems, particularly in adolescents and young adults, adequate data are lacking and treatment is therefore retarded (Selzer & Lieberman, 1993). However, there is little doubt that substance abuse, particularly if severe, is associated with a significantly worse outcome (Linszen, Dingemans & Lenior, 1994). In first-episode schizophrenia the temporal sequence of the onsets of psychosis and substance abuse vary (Hambrecht & Häfner, 1996; Silver & Abboud, 1994). The pattern of use is rarely fixed; patients seem to drift in and out of substance use, the substance use frequently seeming not to correlate with psychotic symptoms. For those patients with premorbid problematic substance use, the manifestation of psychotic symptoms can serve as a powerful motivator to change substance use habits. The case manager needs to assess carefully the pattern of substance use and abuse, the reasons for it in the individual case, and the perceived benefits (on the part of the patient) and likely hazards and risks for the person. An educational approach with an emphasis on health promotion can be useful. Thereafter, focussing on harm minimization within a health promotion framework (e.g. Ely et al., 1995) and applying cognitive–behavioural strategies (e.g. Kavanagh, 1995) can be effective in changing behaviour. Research on reasons and patterns of substance use and possible intervention stategies, particularly in regard to cannabis and 'hard core' polydrug users, is sorely needed in this area.

It is not always possible to follow clearly a phase-orientated approach, nor provide all the interventions outlined. It is helpful to consider levels of intervention, paralleling the concept of basic needs. Figure 11.1 outlines the ten levels of intervention which should be provided within preventive case management, moving from basic or essential interventions to more complex and supplementary, or ideal treatments. Many factors will impinge on decisions regarding the level of interventions which will be possible and/or suitable. For example, a patient with low intellectual level and a schizoid personality predisposition may not be amenable to therapy addressing recovery issues. Clearly 'treatment-reluctant' patients and/or families challenge the model, hence the separation of levels 4 and 5. In those instances a case manager may not be able to provide more than crisis interventions (level 2); the case manager should make it clear to both the individual and family that they will be available for further assistance, should it be required, thus 'leaving the door open' for further contact, and the possible institution of 'higher level' interventions.

Prolonged recovery: persistent positive symptoms

Treatment resistance is a major contributor to prolonged and persistent disability in psychosis (McGorry & Singh, 1995). The burgeoning

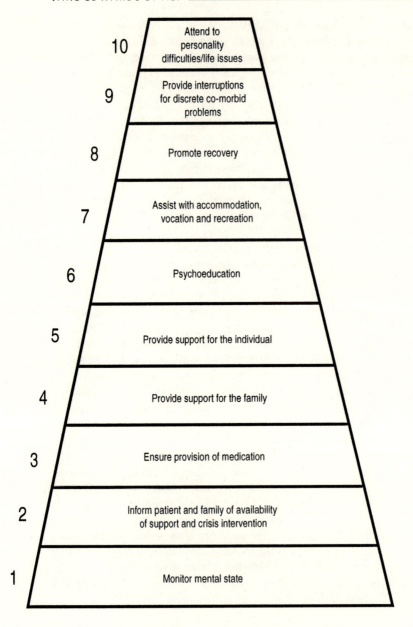

Figure 11.1. Levels of intervention in preventive case management.

literature on the psychological treatment of persistent positive symptoms focusses on patients with established diagnoses and chronic illnesses, and does not attempt to integrate psychological approaches with medication issues (e.g., Bentall, Haddock & Slade, 1994; Garety et al., 1994; Kingdon & Turkington, 1991). In developing interventions for persistent positive symptoms in the first episode (see the description of STOPP in Chapter 10) there was a need to identify patients experiencing ongoing symptoms early in the course of the disorder. Deciding at what phase of the recovery process to define 'persistent' psychotic symptoms involves consideration of appropriate passages of recovery time, given the personal and psychiatric histories of individual patients. Frequently, that endeavour also necessitates attempts to disentangle the positive symptoms indicative of acute relapse from ongoing stable symptoms. There is a need for adequate medication trials, thorough physical and neurological investigations, and the introduction of basic psychosocial interventions, to ensure that a patient is actually experiencing 'treatment resistance' rather than under-treatment, inadequate treatment, or misdiagnosis of the problem(s). Minimizing stress in the patient's social environment is an important consideration, and may include provision of adequate housing, attention to supporting relationships, and securing financial resources. Shifting the focus to the interaction between the patient and the treatments being provided at an early stage in recovery is useful. The term 'prolonged recovery' rather than 'treatment resistance' may be more accurate in a first-episode population.

Remission and the first episode

Approximately 30% of individuals with schizophrenia have a less than adequate response to neuroleptic treatment of acute symptoms (Kane, 1989). However, it is not clear how many of these patients are treatment refractory at the beginning of their illness and how many become so at a subsequent point (Lieberman et al., 1993). Lieberman et al. (1993) treated 70 first-episode schizophrenia and schizoaffective patients with a standardized antipsychotic drug protocol until recovery. Using a conservative definition of remission, a minimum of 83% of the sample recovered from their first-episode of illness after one year of treatment. Information on the degree of remission was available for 66 patients. Forty-nine patients (74%) were considered to be fully remitted (recovery with no residual symptoms), eight (12%) partially remitted, and nine (14%) had not remitted. Mean and median times to remission were 35.7 weeks and 11 weeks, respectively. It is notable that in this same sample only two patients met the criteria for the deficit syndrome

(Mayerhoff et al., 1994), using the modified criteria of Carpenter, Heinrichs & Wagman (1988) applied over a six-month period, suggesting that the prevalence of the deficit syndrome is substantially lower than that used for more chronic patients. Of the 227 individuals with first-episode psychosis who were followed up at both 3–6 months and 12 months after initial stabilization (from a total sample of 347) 6.6% experienced enduring positive psychotic symptoms (Edwards et al., 1998). When the analysis is restricted to patients with DSM-III-R diagnoses of schizophrenia, schizophreniform or schizoaffective disorders ($n = 158$), the percentage of prolonged recovery patients at 12 months rises to 8.9%. This latter figure is substantially lower than that reported by Lieberman et al. There were differences in methods between the two studies: our procedure for defining prolonged recovery was based on three follow-up points only, and may have captured some individuals who were relapsing rather than experiencing prolonged positive symptoms. Also, it did not reflect adoption of a standardized pharmacological treatment protocol – all factors which could be expected to overestimate the prevalence of prolonged recovery in our group. It is possible that our lower figures reflect the incorporation of specialized psychosocial interventions early in the treatment of the first-episode patient; comparisons with other first-episode cohorts which share a similar socio-cultural profile are required to shed light on this.

Clinical imperative

It has been observed that much of the occupational and social decline in psychosis occurs before treatment is initiated (Jones et al., 1993). It has been suggested that it is the duration of untreated frank psychosis which is an important predictor of outcome in first-episode schizophrenia (Wyatt, 1991) (see Chapters 1, 3 and 9). 'An active morbid process might occur during periods of acute symptoms or decompensation which, if not ameliorated by neuroleptic drug treatment, may result in lasting morbidity. It is possible that an extended period of dopaminergic neural dysfunction may result in a more severe, or less reversible, pathophysiologic condition' (Loebel et al., 1992, p. 1187). If this is so, it is critical, in addition to reducing the duration of untreated psychosis, i.e., prior to first effective treatment contact, to reduce the period from onset of drug therapy to remission of psychotic symptoms. That is, there is a need to accelerate recovery and remission, and reduce the percentage of treatment resistance. To prevent cases from 'slipping by' into chronicity, a consultancy service may need to be established within the clinical programme to enable case managers and psychiatrists to discuss assessment and treatment options for patients whose symptoms persist after three months of treatment. In assessing persistent positive symptoms, the clinician needs to take into account medication compliance and side effects, depression, alcohol and other substance use, and the patient's environment, including the family situation. Treatment principles include: active pursuit of effective treatment using relatively low dose strategies for adequate periods of time but with a preparedness to increase the dose or change the drug if response is delayed beyond six weeks; an expectation of at least two adequate drug trials (i.e. equivalent up to 10 milligrams of haloperidol if side-effects permit) within a three-month period; augmentation with lithium over a four-week period (Kane & Marder, 1993); use of novel antipsychotics such as risperidone and clozapine; and the addition of structured psychological and family approaches early in prolonged recovery.

Integrated biopsychosocial treatment

Preventive case management best operates within a biopsychosocial framework (Engel, 1977). Most psychotic states have a biological side and it is useful to consider biological, psychological, and social factors all impacting to shape the timing and presentation of symptoms. This model also applies to physical conditions such as asthma and dermatitis which can provide useful analogies when presenting information about psychosis. Case managers, regardless of discipline background, should be able to assess and make simple interventions across those three domains. It is also important for case managers to distinguish between the competence to prescribe a treatment, and competence to carry it out (Wooff, 1992). Where difficult problems exist, the case manager must recognize that the problem is beyond their professional or personal ability and, in line with professional and ethical guidelines, consult or make a specialist referral. Figure 11.2 outlines the skills expected of case managers in each domain and signifies the scope for individual differences in skill development.

The knowledge and skills required of a case manager are complex and broad: it includes an ability to undertake mental state assessments, make formulations on multiple levels, and provide family and psychological interventions using psychoeducation and cognitive–behavioural frameworks (Birchwood & Tarrier, 1992). The model requires 'experienced, highly trained (and well supervised) clinicians' (Shepherd, 1990, p. 60). Case managers require weekly staff development sessions, case conferences, together with individual and peer supervision, and supplemented by short courses and workshops, if their edu-

	Assessment	Simple Intervention	Complex Intervention
Social	Yes	Yes	?
Psychological	Yes	Yes	?
Biological	Yes	Yes	?

Figure 11.2. Skills required of case managers within a biopsychosocial model.

cational needs are to be met. The Thorn project (Lancashire et al., 1997) in England and the Graduate Diploma in Adolescent Health (Early Psychosis; University of Melbourne, 1995) in Melbourne have arisen from a recognition regarding the extent of training needs of case managers. Viewing case management as a task for able and skilled clinicians increases status and the possibility of attracting talented staff to case manager positions.

The biopsychosocial model does not inform a clinician as to the specific level at which to intervene, nor does it advise the clinician as to how to intervene in any particular circumstance: 'Viewing illness in the context of people's lives will enable us to retain a more realistic complexity in our descriptions of patients, and avoid simplistic reductions which sacrifice key data' (Davidson & Strauss, 1995, p. 53). For example, non-compliance with medication is often accepted as an intrinsic feature of a psychotic disorder, and often leads to an uncritical use of depot medications. Yet upon inquiring about non-compliance, a variety of reasons may be forthcoming, such as the experience of unpleasant side effects, beliefs about becoming dependent on drugs, or fears about the medication changing the patient's personality (McGorry & Kulkarni, 1994), and simple interventions may become apparent. Further, the clinician is often faced with competing needs and goals. For example, there are often times when the patient's developmental needs

11 PREVENTIVE CASE MANAGEMENT

for increasing independence and the treatment goals of the clinician conflict. One can think of a young person who wishes to discontinue any follow-up and the clinician faced with the knowledge of a high risk of relapse in an individual who seems to be experiencing deterioration in mental state. It requires fine judgement in those circumstances as to how to proceed.

> An 18-year-old man with a diagnosis of schizophrenia and with residual positive symptoms, but who was not deemed to pose an immediate risk to himself or others, angrily discontinued treatment and refused to talk to the case manager on the telephone. The case manager made it clear to the patient that the door was open and maintained contact with his mother on a monthly basis. Four months later the patient re-contacted, articulately described a two-month period of psychotic symptoms, and requested help. The case manager asked the young man for advice about which medication would be most useful and enquired as to how frequently he wished to be seen.

This case fragment illustrates that there is often tension between fostering illness self-management on the one hand, and assertive preventive intervention to avoid serious relapse on the other.

Use of the biopsychosocial model indicates that an integrated approach to management should be adopted. Integrating biochemical and psychosocial treatment can enhance recovery and result in the use of lower doses of medication (McGorry et al., 1996).

> A young woman presented at her last session with a ten-day history of depression and re-emergence of psychotic symptoms. On discussion it emerged that she had experienced influenza, was taking excessive sleeping tablets, and was experiencing difficulties at work. The case manager wanted to avoid a premature increase in antipsychotics so, after consultation with the treating psychiatrist, decided to focus on stress management. Practical suggestions included ceasing the sleeping tablets, taking a few days off work, and spending time with her sister. Within a few days the patient was greatly improved and had re-engaged in her usual activities.

The case management team

A team structure should be adopted to support case managers, with a senior clinician as a team leader who represents case managers within and outside of the service. Duties of the team co-ordinator should include: attending to the information systems required; resource management; liaising with other sub-programme co-ordinators; monitoring case loads; facilitating throughput; ensuring adequate supervision arrangements; encouraging staff development activities; co-ordinating responses to critical incidents; and identifying quality assurance activities. The co-ordinator should carry a significant clinical load as a case manager, not only to maintain skills and credibility, but also to provide formal and informal secondary consultation to colleagues and act as a general standards monitor.

Mini case conferences held on a regular basis can help case managers review progress and reasons for treatment delay, as well as assist in the co-ordination of other services the patient might be receiving. Individual supervision and small case conferences should be used to plan day-to-day management. Full team meetings are used for broad management planning with multidisciplinary input. Team reviews of patients allow both a discussion of issues which arise in treatment and a collective approach to important issues to develop.

In addition to their case management role, case managers could have a specialist role within the team, whether by profession or skill area (e.g. family worker, substance use, prolonged recovery, borderline personality disorders, anxiety disorders, vocation, suicide prevention, forensic issues, and accommodation). Additional supervision and training will be required to develop and maintain these specialist skills. Such interests can help to maintain enthusiasm, and provide the clinician with a variety of work.

There are many stresses and strains in attempting to treat patients with psychotic disorders. Patients are inevitably severely disturbed, often with marked accompanying anxiety and depression; some are suicidal or aggressive and lack insight, and their repudiation of attempts to assist can be very frustrating. Reactions to patients can include feelings of omnipotence or helplessness, despair, incompetence and self-criticism. Case managers are often presented with very difficult clinical dilemmas and need supervision; however, the relationship with the supervisor can mirror the same processes. The case manager–supervisor relationship also needs to be collaborative rather than directive. Debriefing after major incidents, such as the death of a patient or an aggressive incident, needs adequate attention, as does the need for communication between staff.

'For case management to be more than just a patchwork attempt to address systems failures and inconsistencies, clarity about task, accountability, responsibility, and authority is necessary' (Sledge et al., 1995, p. 1264). A service document, clearly specifying procedural details given the allocated resources, and which is updated by the case managers of a team on a regular basis (e.g. Early Psychosis Prevention and Intervention Centre, 1996), can facilitate understanding and ownership of organizational issues involved in case management activities.

Conflict between staff can be considered both inevitable and healthy, and is best raised and discussed. Case managers must be prepared to present their views on their own patients as well as engage in debate and exchange perspectives on the patients of other case managers. An ethos of being able to consider multiple perspectives should be actively encouraged. Case managers need to be able to refer and discharge patients as required, and liaise with new case managers, such as general practitioners, in such a way that the ongoing needs of the patient are met and the philosophy of early intervention and prevention is disseminated.

Conclusion

One of the basic tenets of preventive case management of the first-episode patient is the requirement that case managers possess the flexibility and training to respond well to the wide variety of problems as they are presented. Therefore, it becomes essential that case management skills specific to this population are developed and nurtured, and these include assessment skills and treatment skills ranging from the biological, through to the increasingly sophisticated use of psychotherapeutic interventions.

Case management of the early psychosis patient necessitates a preparedness to assess and reassess comprehensively on a continual basis. These patients are initially unknown to the psychiatric system and have illnesses which are, at least initially, unpredictable in nature. With time, the case manager gets to know the patient better and, in collaboration with the patient, develops an increased awareness of treatment response, an understanding of relapse issues, and individual challenges for recovery. Patients have diverse needs and often provoke very powerful feelings within the case manager, particularly with regard to the estimation of risk. A case manager is constantly balancing competing objectives; for example, the needs of the family versus the patient, the desire for independence and assistance. It cannot be forgotten that many of the dilemmas faced by the case manager in working with an early psychosis patient relate to adolescent issues for which the passage of time and gradual maturation processes are the only real 'cure' (Winnicott, 1965). However, at the same time, there is a need to protect the developmental processes from the possible derailment caused by a psychotic illness and its associated treatments.

Acknowledgments

Aspects of this chapter were presented by the authors at the following meetings: Case Management Making it Work – an Australian and International Review of the State of Play, Melbourne, July 1995; Early Intervention in Functional Psychosis Seminar, Stavanger, Norway, April, 1995; and 30th Congress of the Royal Australian and New Zealand College of Psychiatrists, Cairns, May, 1995. We wish to thank Annmarie Wright for permission to quote her comment on case management and her contribution to the development of Figure 11.1.

References

Alanen, Y. O., Ugelstad, E., Armelius, B., Lehtinen, K., Rosenbaum, B. & Sjostrom, R. (Eds.) (1994). *Early Treatment for Schizophrenic Patients: Scandinavian Psychotherapeutic Approaches.* Stockholm: Scandanavian University Press.

Anthony, W. A. (1993). Recovery from mental illness: the guiding vision of the mental health service system in the 1990s. *Psychosocial Rehabilitation Journal,* 16, 11–23.

Arieti, S. (1974). *Interpretation of Schizophrenia,* 2nd edn. New York: Basic Books.

Beck, A. T., Freeman, A. & Associates (1990). *Cognitive Therapy of Personality Disorders.* New York: Guilford Press.

Beiser, M., Bean, G., Erickson, D., Zhang, J., Iacano, W. G. & Rector, N. A. (1994). Biological and psychosocial predictors of job performance following a first episode of psychosis. *American Journal of Psychiatry,* **151**, 857–63.

Benjamin, L. S. (1993). *Interpersonal Diagnosis and Treatment of Personality Disorders.* New York: Guilford Press.

Bentall, R. P., Haddock, G. & Slade, P. D. (1994). Cognitive behavior therapy for persistent auditory hallucinations: from theory to therapy. *Behavior Therapy,* **25**, 51–66.

Birchwood, M. & Macmillan, F. (1993). Early intervention in schizophrenia. *Australian and New Zealand Journal of Psychiatry,* **27**, 374–8.

Birchwood, M. & Tarrier, N. (Eds.) (1992). *Innovations in the Psychological Management of Schizophrenia.* New York: Wiley.

Carpenter, W. T., Heinrichs, D. W. & Wagman, A. M. I. (1988). Deficit and nondeficit forms of schizophrenia: the concept. *American Journal of Psychiatry,* **145,** 578–83.

Davidson, L. & Strauss, J. S. (1995). Beyond the biopsychosocial model: integrating disorder, health, and recovery. *Psychiatry,* **58,** 44–55.

Della Selva, P. C. (1993). The significance of attachment theory for the practice of intensive short-term dynamic psychotherapy. *International Journal of Short-Term Psychotherapy,* **8,** 189–206.

Dozier, M. (1993). Tailoring clinical case management: the role of attachment. In *Case Management for Mentally Ill Patients: Theory and Practice,* ed. M. Harris & H. C. Bergman, pp. 41–58. Washington: Harwood Academic Publishers.

Early Psychosis Prevention and Intervention Centre (1996). *Outpatient Case Management (OCM): Principles of Practice.* Melbourne, Australia: Early Psychosis Prevention and Intervention Centre.

Edwards J., Francey, S. M., McGorry, P. D. & Jackson, H. J. (1994). Early Psychosis Prevention and Intervention: evolution of a comprehensive community-based service. *Behaviour Change,* **11,** 223–33.

Edwards, J., Maude, D., McGorry, P. D., Harrigan, S. & Cocks, J. (in press). Prolonged recovery in first-episode psychosis. *British Journal of Psychiatry* (Supplement).

Eisenthal, S., Emery, R., Lazare, A. & Udin, H. (1979). 'Adherence' and the negotiated approach to patienthood. *Archives of General Psychiatry,* **36,** 393–8.

Ely, K., Bellhouse, R., Rodrigues, A. & Roberts, P. (1995). *Get Real: A Harm-minimisation Approach to Drug Education.* Victoria, Australia: Directorate of School Education.

Engel, G. L. (1977). The need for a new medical model: a challenge for biomedicine. *Science,* **196,** 129–36.

EPPIC Statewide Services (1996). *User's Guide: Everything You'll Need to Know About EPPIC.* Melbourne, Australia: Early Psychosis Prevention and Intervention Centre.

Falloon, I. R. H. (1984). Developing and maintaining adherence to long-term drug-taking regimens. *Schizophrenia Bulletin,* **10,** 412–17.

Falloon, I. R. H. & Fadden, G. (1993). *Integrated Mental Health Care.* Cambridge, UK: Cambridge University Press.

Fava, G. A. & Kellner, R. (1991). Prodromal symptoms in affective disorders. *American Journal of Psychiatry,* **148,** 823–30.

Garety, P. A., Kuipers, E., Fowler, D., Chamberlain, F. & Dunn, G. (1994). Cognitive behavioural therapy for drug-resistant psychosis. *British Journal of Medical Psychology,* **67,** 259–71.

Gilbert, P. L., Harris, J., McAdams, L. A. & Jeste, D. V. (1995). Neuroleptic withdrawal in schizophrenic patients: a review. *Archives of General Psychiatry,* **52,** 173–86.

Gilbert, S. & Ugelstad, E. (1994). Patient's own contributions to long-term supportive psychotherapy in schizophrenic disorders. *British Journal of Psychiatry*, **164**, 84–8.

Goodwin, G. M. (1995). Recurrence of mania after lithium withdrawal: implications for the use of lithium in the treatment of bipolar affective disorder. *British Journal of Psychiatry*, **164**, 149–52.

Hambrecht, M. & Häfner, H. (1996). Substance abuse and the onset of schizophrenia. *Biological Psychiatry*, **40**, 1155–63.

Harris, M. & Bergman, H. C. (Eds.) (1993). *Case Management for Mentally Ill Patients: Theory and Practice.* Washington: Harwood Academic Publishers.

Hogarty, G. E. (in press). Integration of psychopharmacologic and psychosocial therapies in schizophrenia. *Italian Journal of Psychiatry and Behavioural Science.*

Hogg, B., Jackson, H. J., Rudd, R. P. & Edwards, J. (1990). Diagnosing personality disorders in recent-onset schizophrenia. *Journal of Nervous and Mental Disease*, **178**, 194–9.

Holloway, F., Oliver, N., Collins, E. & Carson, J. (1995). Case management: A critical review of the outcome literature. *European Psychiatry*, **10**, 113–28.

Hulbert, C. A., Jackson, H. J. & McGorry, P. D. (1996). The relationship between personality and course and outcome in early psychosis: a review of the literature. *Clinical Psychology Review*, **16**, 707–27.

Ioannides, T. (Producer) & Hexter, I. (Director) (1994). *A Stitch in Time: Psychosis ... Get Help Early* (Video). Melbourne, Australia: Published by the Early Psychosis Prevention and Intervention Centre (EPPIC) for the Psychiatric Services Branch, Victorian Government Department of Health and Community Services.

Jackson, H. J. (1993). The case formulation. *Bulletin of the Australian Psychological Society*, **15**, 7–9.

Janick, P. G., Davis, J. M., Preskorn, S. H. & Ayd, F. J., Jr. (1993). *Principles and Practice of Psychopharmacotherapy.* Baltimore, Maryland: Williams & Wilkins.

Jeste, D. V., Gilbert, P. L., McAdams, L. A. & Harris, J. (1995). Considering neuroleptic maintenance and taper on a continuum: need for an individual rather than dogmatic approach. *Archives of General Psychiatry*, **52**, 209–12.

Jones, P. B., Bebbington, P., Foerster, A., Lewis, S. W., Murray, R. N., Russell, A., Sham, P. C., Toone, B. K. & Wilkins, S. (1993). Premorbid social underachievement in schizophrenia: results from the Camberwell Collaborative Psychosis Study. *British Journal of Psychiatry*, **162**, 65–71.

Kane, J. (1989). The current status of neuroleptics. *Journal of Clinical Psychiatry*, **50**, 322–8.

Kane, J. M. & Marder, S. R. (1993). Psychopharmacologic treatment of schizophrenia. *Schizophrenia Bulletin*, **19**, 287–302.

Kavanagh, D. (1995). An intervention for substance abuse in schizophrenia. *Behaviour Change*, **12**, 20–30.

Kessler, R. C., Foster, C. L., Saunders, W. B. & Stang, P. E. (1995). Social consequences of psychiatric disorders. I: Educational attainment. *American Journal of Psychiatry*, **152**, 1026–32.

Kingdon, D. G. & Turkington, D. (1991). The use of cognitive therapy with a normalizing rationale in schizophrenia. *Journal of Nervous and Mental Disease*, **179**, 207–11.

Kissling, W. (1994). Compliance, quality assurance and standards for relapse prevention in schizophrenia. *Acta Psychiatrica Scandinavica*, **89** (Supplement 382), 16–24.

Kline, J., Becker, J. & Giese, C. (1992). Psychodynamic interventions revisited: options for the treatment of schizophrenia. *Psychotherapy*, **29**, 366–77.

Lamb, H. R. (1980). Therapist-case managers: more than brokers of services. *Hospital and Community Psychiatry*, **31**, 762–4.

Lancashire, S., Haddock, G., Tarrier N., Baguley, I., Butterworth, C. A. & Brooker, C. (1997). Effects of training in psychosocial interventions for community psychiatric nurses in England. *Psychiatric Services*, **48**, 39–41.

Lazare, A., Eisenthal, S. & Frank, A. (1989). Clinician/patient relations II: Conflict and negotiation. In *Outpatient Psychiatry: Diagnosis and Treatment*, 2nd edn, ed. A. Lazare, pp. 137–52. Baltimore, Maryland: Williams and Wilkins.

Lieberman, J., Jody, D., Geisler, S., Alvir, J., Loebel, A., Szymanski, S., Woerner, M. & Borenstein, M. (1993). Time course and biological correlates of treatment response in first-episode schizophrenia. *Archives of General Psychiatry*, **50**, 369–76.

Linehan, M. M. (1993). *Cognitive–Behavioral Therapy for Borderline Personality Disorder*. New York: Guilford Press.

Linszen, D., Dingemans, P. & Lenior, M. (1994). Cannabis abuse and the course of recent-onset schizophrenic disorders. *Archives of General Psychiatry*, **51**, 273–9.

Loebel, A. D., Lieberman, J. A., Alvir, J. M. J., Mayerhoff, D. I., Geisler, S. H. & Szymanski, S. R. (1992). Duration of psychosis and outcome in first-episode schizophrenia. *American Journal of Psychiatry*, **149**, 1183–8.

Macmillan, F., Birchwood, M. & Smith, J. (1992). Predicting and controlling relapse in schizophrenia: early signs monitoring. In *Schizophrenia: An Overview and Practical Handbook*, ed. D. Kavanagh, pp. 293–308. London: Chapman & Hall.

Marder, S. R., Wirshing, W. C., Van-Putten, T., Mintz, J., McKenzie, J., Johnston-Cronk, K., Lebell, M. & Liberman, R. P. (1994). Fluphenazine vs placebo supplementation for prodromal signs of relapse in schizophrenia. *Archives of General Psychiatry*, **51**, 280–7.

Mayerhoff, D. I., Loebel, A. D., Jose, M. J., Alvir, P. H., Szymanski, S. R., Geisler, S. H., Borenstein, M. & Lieberman, J. A. (1994). The deficit state in first-episode schizophrenia. *American Journal of Psychiatry*, **151**, 1417–22.

McGorry, P. D. (1991). The schizophrenia concept in first episode psychosis: does it fit and is it harmful? *Dulwich Centre Newsletter*, **4**, 40–4.

McGorry, P. D. (1992). The concept of recovery and secondary prevention in psychotic disorders. *Australian and New Zealand Journal of Psychiatry*, **26**, 3–17.

McGorry, P. D., Edwards, J., Mihalopoulos, C., Harrigan, S. & Jackson, H. J. (1996). EPPIC: an evolving system of early detection and optimal management. *Schizophrenia Bulletin*, **22**, 305–26.

McGorry, P. D. & Kulkarni, J. (1994). Prevention and preventively orientated clinical care in psychotic disorders. *Australian Journal of Psychopharmacology*, **7**, 62–9.

McGorry, P. D. & Singh, B. S. (1995). Schizophrenia: risk and possibility. In *Handbook of Studies on Preventative Psychiatry*, ed. B. Raphael & G. Burrows, pp. 491–514. Melbourne, Australia: Elsevier Science.

Molnar, G., Feeney, M. G. & Fava, G. A. (1988). Duration and symptoms of bipolar prodromes. *American Journal of Psychiatry*, **145**, 1576–8.

Munice, W. S. (1959). The psychobiological approach. In *American Handbook of Psychiatry*, ed. S. Arieti, pp. 1317–32. New York: Basic Books.

Pica, S., Edwards, J., Jackson, H. J., Bell, R. C., Bates, G. W. & Rudd, R. P. (1990). Personality disorders in recent-onset bipolar disorder. *Comprehensive Psychiatry*, **31**, 499–510.

Power, P., Elkins, K., Adlard, S., Curry, C. & McGorry, P. D. (in press). An analysis of the initial treatment phase in first episode psychosis. *British Journal of Psychiatry* (Supplement).

Price, L. H. & Heninger, G. R. (1994). Lithium in the treatment of mood disorders. *The New England Journal of Medicine*, **331**, 591–8.

Rosen, A. (1994). Case management: shaping services to meet individual needs. In *Mental Health – Future Directions*, ed. Australian Hospital Association, pp. 47–63. Canberra: Australian Hospital Association.

Ryan, P., Ford, R. & Clifford, P. (1991). *Case Management and Community Care*. London: Research and Development for Psychiatry.

Schizophrenia Fellowship of Victoria. (1994). *Psychosis: What is It?* North Fitzroy, Victoria, Australia: Schizophrenia Fellowship of Victoria.

Selzer J. A. & Lieberman J. A. (1993). Schizophrenia and substance abuse. *Psychiatric Clinics of North America*, **16**, 401–12.

Shepherd, G. (1990). Case management. *Health Trends*, **22**, 59–61.

Silver, H. & Abboud, E. (1994). Drug abuse in schizophrenia: comparison of patients who began drug abuse before their first admission with those who began abusing drugs after their first admission. *Schizophrenia Research*, **13**, 57–63.

Sledge, W. H., Astrachan, B., Thompson, K., Rakfeldt, J. & Leaf, P. (1995). Case management in psychiatry: an analysis of tasks. *American Journal of Psychiatry*, **152**, 1259–65.

Smith, J. A. & Tarrier, N. (1992). Prodromal symptoms in manic depressive psychosis. *Social Psychiatry and Psychiatric Epidemiology*, **27**, 245–8.

Smith, T. E., Shea, T., Schooler, N. R., Levin, H., Deutsch, A. & Grabstein, H. (1995). Studies of schizophrenia: personality traits in schizophrenia. *Psychiatry*, **58**, 99–112.

Strakowski, S. M., Tohen, M., Stoll, A. L., Faedda, G. L., Mayer, P. V., Kolbrener, B. A. & Goodwin, B. S. (1993). Comorbidity in psychosis at first hospitalisation. *American Journal of Psychiatry*, **150**, 752–7.

Strakowski, S. M., Keck, P. E., McElroy, S. L., Lonczak, H. S. & West, S. A. (1995). Chronology of comorbid and principal syndromes in first-episode psychosis. *Comprehensive Psychiatry*, **36**, 106–12.

Strauss, J. (1989). Mediating processes in schizophrenia: towards a new dynamic psychiatry. *British Journal of Psychiatry*, **155**, 22–8.

Strauss, J. (1992). The person – key to understanding mental illness: towards a new dynamic psychiatry, III. *British Journal of Psychiatry*, **161** (Supplement 18), 19–26.

Sumich, H. J., Hunt, C. & Andrews, G. (1995). *The Management of Mental Disorders: Handbook for the Schizophrenic Disorders*, Vol. 2. Sydney, Australia: World Health Organisation Training and Reference Centre for CIDI.

Thase, M. E. (1993). Maintenance treatment of recurrent affective disorders. *Current Opinion in Psychiatry*, **6**, 16–9.

University of Melbourne (1995). *Graduate Diploma in Adolescent Health (Early Psychosis)*. Faculty of Medicine, Dentistry, and Health Sciences, University of Melbourne.

Winnicott, D. W. (1965). *The Family and Individual Development*. London: Tavistock Publications.

Wooff, K. (1992). Service organisation and planning. In *Innovations in the Psychological Management of Schizophrenia*, ed. M. Birchwood & N. Tarrier, pp. 277–304. New York: Wiley.

World Health Organization (1979). *The International Pilot Study of Schizophrenia*. Chichester, UK: Wiley.

Wyatt, R. J. (1991). Neuroleptics and the natural course of schizophrenia. *Schizophrenia Bulletin*, **17**, 325–51.

Zubin, J. & Spring, B. (1977). Vulnerability – a new view of schizophrenia. *Journal of Abnormal Psychology*, **36**, 103–26.

12

Suicide and early psychosis

PADDY POWER

Introduction

The tragedy of suicide is all the more poignant when it is potentially preventable. In recent years, the incidence of suicide among young people in developed countries has been increasing at an alarming rate to become the second or third most common cause of death for 15–34-year-olds (Diekstra, 1995). Suicide rates among young males have trebled over the last 30 years in a number of industrialized countries, e.g. Australia and the USA (Australian Bureau of Statistics, 1994; Buda & Tsuang, 1990). In 1994, Australia recorded the highest rate of youth suicide among all industrialized nations with an annual incidence of 16.4 suicides per 100,000 for Australian 15–24-year-olds ('News: Suicide', 1994). It is at this particular age that major psychiatric disorders, such as affective disorders and psychosis, demonstrate their peak onset (Häfner et al., 1995; Lewinsohn et al., 1994). Among adolescents who suicide, serious mental illnesses such as the above are among the most common associated factors (Blumenthal, 1990). Surprisingly, only a small percentage of these young people who suicide are actually being treated for their mental illness at the time of their suicide (Isometsa et al., 1994; Shafii et al., 1985).

Suicide in those with serious mental illness

Retrospectively conducted psychological autopsies consistently report that between 90% and 98% of adolescent suicide victims had suffered from a psychiatric disorder either before, or at the time of, their suicide (Brent et al., 1988a; Marttunen et al., 1991; Rich, Sherman & Fowler, 1990; Runeson, 1989). Shafii et al. (1985) concluded that 95% had a diagnosable major psychiatric disorder and 81% had two or more comorbid mental disorders, compared with 29% of the controls. The

Table 12.1. *Suicide rates (percentages) among those with psychiatric disorders*

Psychiatric disorder	Suicide rate
Major affective disorders	15%
Schizophrenia	10–20%
Alcohol and drug abuse	15%
Borderline personality	5–10%

From figures quoted in Blumenthal (1990).

research by Shafii et al. suggested that 76% of those adolescents who committed suicide, suffered a major affective disorder or dysthymia, 70% had an associated substance abuse disorder, 70% had a history of antisocial behaviours, 65% had 'inhibited' personality traits, and 50% had made a previous suicide attempt.

Among those already identified as suffering from serious mental illness, lifetime rates for suicide are high (see Table 12.1), especially amongst those with psychotic disorders. Krausz, Muller-Thomsen & Maasen (1995) reported rates of suicide in 13.1% of those with adolescent-onset schizophrenia, with higher rates occurring amongst males (21.5%).

Suicide in affective disorder

Psychotic depression appears to carry a five times greater risk of suicide compared with non-psychotic depressive disorders (Roose et al., 1983). Similarly, bipolar disorders have a particularly high risk of suicide, especially around the time of switch of mood (Jamison, 1986). Mixed states of mania and depression also appear to constitute high risk periods, this possibly being due to the combination of dysphoria and impulsivity. However, suicide rarely occurs during a pure manic episode (Robins et al., 1959). Rates of suicide appear to be similar in both unipolar and bipolar disorders but are possibly higher in bipolar type II disorder (Goodwin & Jamison, 1990). Overall, suicide rates are similar in males and females with mood disorders, although female suicides tend to occur in the first 15 years of illness, while male suicides appear to be bimodally distributed between the early and late phases of illness (Goodwin & Jamison, 1990). Comorbidity with substance abuse disorders (Fawcett et al., 1990) appears to enhance the risk of suicide in affective disorders.

Suicide in schizophrenia

Among patients with schizophrenia who die by suicide, males outweigh females by a ratio of 4:1. The victims are usually single, unemployed, in the first ten years of onset of a severe chronic form of the illness (Roy, 1982), and less than 45 years old, with males usually committing suicide before 30 years of age and females before 40 years of age (Black, Winokur & Nasrallah, 1988). Fifty per cent of suicide patients with schizophrenia have made previous suicide attempts (Caldwell & Gottesman, 1990; Roy, 1986). Other studies confirm some of these risk factors and identify additional risk factors for patients, such as having: the paranoid subtype of the disorder (Fenton & McGlashan, 1991, 1996); suspiciousness in the absence of negative symptoms (Fenton et al., 1997); relatively higher intelligence (Westermeyer, Harrow & Marengo, 1991); relatively better psychosocial functioning premorbidly and higher self expectations of performance (Drake & Cotton, 1986) complicated by more severe morbidity following the illness onset; early disturbed psychosocial adjustment (Modestin, Zarro & Waldvogel, 1992); greater levels of depression (Roy, 1982); greater awareness of their pathology (Drake & Cotton, 1986); and complicating substance abuse (Runeson, 1989).

There are few available data describing rates of suicide amongst those with first-episode schizophrenia. However, Drake et al. (1984) reported that suicide rarely occurs in the acute psychotic phase of schizophrenia. Many patients show improvement clinically before the suicide, and agitation, rather than psychosis, appears to be the predominant feature at the time of suicide. 'Self-reported subjective distress', 'awareness of illness and disintegration', and 'hopelessness' all appear to be associated features. The peri-discharge period from hospital appears to be a time of very high risk for completed suicide, particularly among males (Roy, 1982), with speculation about contributing factors such as: shorter lengths of hospitalization, loss of support, reduced supervision, non-compliance with treatment, treatment resistance, and renewed exposure to stressors in the post-discharge period. Common associated stresses include family conflict and 'ejection' by the family (Breier & Astrachan, 1984).

Suicide in those with complicating alcohol and drug abuse disorders

Alcohol and drug abuse disorders are seen in 30–70% of youth suicide victims, either occurring alone as a primary disorder or in combination with other major psychiatric disorders (Shafii et al., 1988). Although alcohol and drugs may be a form of self medication in those with psychosis, it is likely that they aggravate the course of these illnesses (Brent et al., 1988a; Schuckit, 1979). Chronic alcohol abuse may induce biological effects which increase the risk of suicide through serotonergic depletion and depression (Frances, Franklin & Flavin, 1986). Many drugs of abuse, including cannabis, have psychotomimetic effects (Poole & Brabbins, 1996). In addition, alcohol and drugs of abuse potentiate the risk of other methods of suicide, such as drug overdose, through their direct metabolic effects and the indirect effects of psychological impairment (Ohberg et al., 1996).

Model of suicidality and suicide behaviours in psychosis

Figure 12.1 provides a model for suicide behaviour in psychosis. As with any model, it is limited by its attempt to simplify the complexity of the factors involved. In addition, there are a number of important points to discuss, before describing the model. Most suicides associated with psychosis appear to occur after an acute psychotic episode, and may occur as a result of the patient's depressed state, or constitute a patient's psychological reaction to the impact of their psychotic illness. However, for suicides which occur during the acute phase of psychosis, this explanation may only hold true for a proportion of victims. Although some suicide behaviours appear to be a reaction to the distressing nature of psychotic experiences, other suicides may occur as a direct response to psychotic experiences such as command hallucinations or bizarre delusions. These latter suicides may not be intentionally suicidal in nature, and may be better identified as psychotic self-destructive behaviours directly influenced by the severity of the person's psychosis (see Figure 12.1). Nonetheless, whether due to a direct or indirect effect, the experience of psychosis must significantly increase the risk of either form of suicide, and may interact in a synergistic manner with various other background and general suicide risk factors.

The model (see Figure 12.1) suggests that a dynamic state of suicidality may be manifested by the intensity of suicide ideation. It has been observed in adolescent populations that suicide ideation almost invariably precedes an attempt, and suicide behaviour appears to increase with the frequency of suicide ideation (Lewinsohn, Rhode & Seeley, 1996). Suicide ideation is best viewed as a dimensional construct (Lewinsohn, Rhode & Seeley, 1996) and, in its mild form, is a very common, though fleeting, experience in normal population samples (Zubrick et al., 1995). Psychotic experiences (including those which might directly influence behaviours which are lethal towards self) also may be best viewed as dimensional in nature (Kingdon & Turkington, 1994; Strauss, 1969). From our own clinical experience, the frequency of these psychotic suicidal behaviours appears to have a linear relationship with the corresponding psychotic-induced suicidal ideations.

This dynamic state of suicidality (vulnerability to suicide ideation) (see Figure 12.1) is created by the accumulative, modulating and interactive influences of the dimensional effects of both suicide risk factors and competing protective factors. Impacting on this state of suicidality are the final triggers or stressors (Brent et al., 1993) which mediate and influence the choice of suicide behaviour. These will determine the degree of acute lethality of the behaviour. Finally, the outcome of the suicide attempt will depend on whether detection or intervention by others is likely, or will be successful in averting death. This may depend on chance occurrences, the choice of suicide behaviour, and the setting selected by the patient.

In practice, a person may gradually reach a state of intense suicidality through the accumulation of a high level of suicide risk factors against a corresponding low level of protective factors. This state may be experienced as an intense preoccupation with cognitions of hopelessness or death, or psychotic phenomena reflecting themes of death or self-harm behaviours. When exposed to a final mediating stressor/cognition/cue/trigger, e.g. availability of means to suicide, the person is prompted to respond with a particular form of suicidal behaviour in a manner which limits access to detection or treatment. It is important to recognize that this model is a heuristic one – one developed on the basis of literature drawn from research into suicidality, depression and more chronic forms of psychosis. Whether it is applicable to the early psychosis patient must remain a question to be empirically determined.

Suicide risk factors

A number of the suicide risk factors that have been specifically associated with psychotic disorders, have been described already in the preceding sections of this chapter. The next section below, suggests some additional, though as yet unproven, possible risk factors specific to early psychosis. More non-specific risk factors for suicide, i.e. risk factors for suicide in the general population, may interact in a synergistic manner with the above specific suicide risk factors. This section discusses some of these non-specific and general risk factors for suicide.

Blumenthal (1990) suggested five overlapping and interacting domains of risk factors (referred to as the 'overlap model') which could be broadly defined as vulnerability factors for suicide in the general popu-

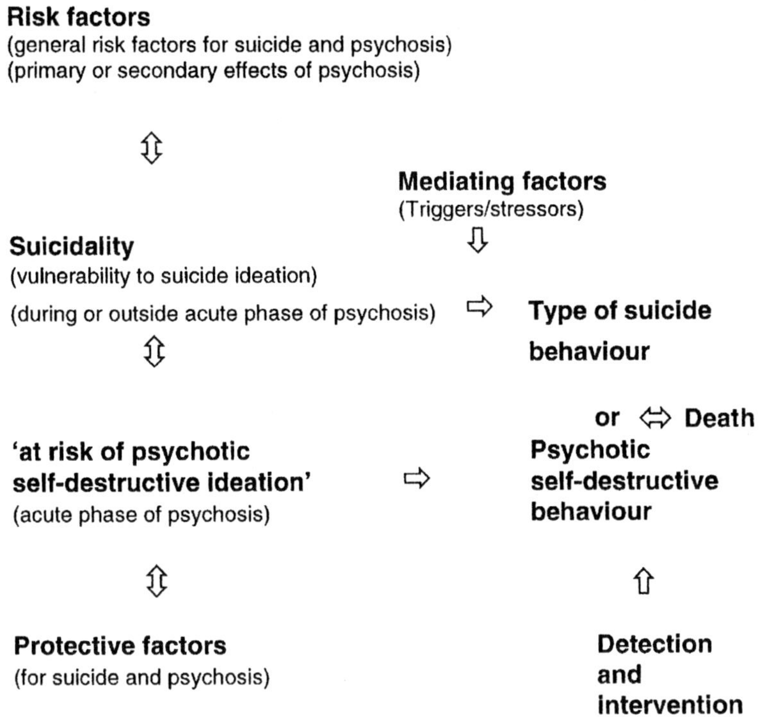

Risk factors
(general risk factors for suicide and psychosis)
(primary or secondary effects of psychosis)

⇕

Mediating factors
(Triggers/stressors)

⇓

Suicidality
(vulnerability to suicide ideation)
(during or outside acute phase of psychosis) ⇨ **Type of suicide behaviour**

⇕

or ⇔ Death

'at risk of psychotic self-destructive ideation'
(acute phase of psychosis) ⇨ **Psychotic self-destructive behaviour**

⇕ ⇧

Protective factors
(for suicide and psychosis)

Detection and intervention

Figure 12.1. A heuristic model of suicidality and suicidal behaviours.

lation. These risk factors are: genetic factors (family history of suicide); biological factors (e.g. serotonergic functioning); personality traits and cognitive style (impulsivity, cognitive rigidity, hopelessness); psychosocial milieu (e.g. life events, medical illness, and sociodemographic factors); and psychiatric disorders.

The particular cognitive styles which have been identified as risk factors for suicide in general populations have arisen from research concentrating on the relationship between suicide ideation and factors such as hopelessness and problem-solving deficits (Weishaar & Beck, 1992). However, the relationship between these factors appears to be complex and may be concomitant rather than causal (Schotte, Cools & Payvar, 1990). Beck (1987) suggested that in depressed patients with suicide ideation, these cognitive features may be *state* dependent, improving when the depression resolved. Beck also demonstrated, however, that in a contrasting group of suicide ideators, i.e. patients with alcoholism and personality disorders, suicide crises occurred in response to recent life events. These patients were characterized by *trait*-

dependent cognitive factors which persisted between suicidal episodes and included traits such as negative self-concept, cognitive rigidity, impulsivity, and problem-solving deficits. For patients with psychotic disorders there is a long tradition of research identifying a range of associated cognitive deficits. It appears that these cognitive deficits may develop before, and persist after, the onset of first-episode psychosis in a proportion of patients (Brewer et al., 1996). The association between these deficits in psychosis, and the cognitive style associated with suicide behaviours, has not yet been studied, but it is possible that these cognitive deficits in psychosis may likewise predispose psychosis patients to suicide ideation when exposed to stressful life events.

In attempting to predict future suicide, Lewinsohn, Rhode & Seeley (1996) conducted a multivariate analysis of suicide risk factors (including a number of the above) in the general adolescent population. They reported that concurrent psychopathology is the strongest determinant of suicidal behaviour. Factors other than serious mental illness include indicators of suicidality as manifested by either a history of suicide attempts (Blumenthal, 1990; Lewinsohn, Rhode & Seeley, 1996), and/or severity of hopelessness and suicide ideation (Beck, Kovacs & Weissman, 1979; Weishaar & Beck, 1992). Other additional indicators of suicide risk, but of less predictive value, include: 'poor self-concept' (Beck & Stewart, 1989; Lewinsohn, Rhode & Seeley, 1996); complicating drug (de Moore & Robertson, 1996) and alcohol abuse; a family history of suicide (Roy et al., 1991); a history of family discord (Rich, Sherman & Fowler, 1990); a suicide attempt by a friend (Lewinsohn, Rhode & Seeley, 1996); medical illness (Brent, 1986); and biological indicators, e.g. low CSF HIAA (Korn et al., 1995).

Protective factors

The importance of protective factors tends to be overlooked in reviews of suicide. However, a number of studies have identified factors which are negatively correlated with suicide risk, although in themselves they may not be of predictive value. These factors include manic states (Shaffer et al., 1988), and the presence of thought disorder in adolescents with schizophrenia (Apter et al., 1988). It might be argued on logical grounds that complicating personality traits such as obsessional traits may be associated with a reduced risk of suicide, compared with other traits such as borderline and antisocial features. Other premorbid protective factors may include certain cultural and religious beliefs, good social supports (Kerkhof & Diekstra, 1995), and good psychosocial functioning. Finally, Fenton & McGlashan (1996) and Fenton et al. (1997) have found empirical support for the notion that the deficit syndrome and prominent negative symptoms are associated with low risk of suicidality.

Clinical application of the model for suicidality and suicide behaviour in first-episode psychosis

At EPPIC and in dealing with patients with early psychosis, we have found suicide ideation and behaviours to be common, but transient, phenomena. Suicidality in early psychosis appears to be influenced by multiple interacting factors (both aggravating and protective) which wax and wane during the course of the illness. Important interactive influences appear to be those of subjective distress caused by acute psychotic or persistent negative symptoms, emerging insight into the illness, and pessimism about one's prognosis. Among the patients attending EPPIC, suicidal behaviours appear to occur most frequently during the phases of emerging psychosis, early recovery, and early relapse/prolonged recovery, but particularly during the early recovery phase.

Suicide ideation in the early phase appears particularly common during the transition from prodrome to psychosis, and usually before contact has been made with health services. Our clinical observation is that suicide ideation appears to be dependent on factors such as the degree of subjective awareness of prodrome deterioration, the speed of onset and fluctuating nature of the psychotic process, the degree of instability of mood (mixed affective features), levels of anxiety, command hallucinations, positive symptoms which represent prominent depressogenic themes, positive symptoms associated with particularly severe subjective distress, the patient's subjective impression of entrapment and hopelessness induced by psychotic experiences (see Chapters 9 and 10), the patient's impressions of significant others' responses, and the associated subjective impression of rejection or shame.

Suicide ideation during the early recovery phase appears to be more common as insight emerges during the resolution of the symptoms of psychosis. In our current practice at EPPIC, it appears to occur earlier if the patient's understanding of psychosis is coloured by expectations of poor prognosis or distress with treatment, or later, when the patient's initial relief (gained by resolving psychotic symptoms, discharge from hospital, and escape from the intense level of clinical involvement) is superseded by distress due to the experience of persistent negative symptoms, postpsychotic depression or enduring psychosocial stressors. In our experience, the period one to three months post-discharge from hospital is when suicide ideation and intent appears to peak in first-episode psychosis patients. This is often a time when follow-up services gradually reduce their involvement, either as the psychosis resolves or as the patient disengages; or conversely, the patients begin to experience difficulties attempting to reintegrate with their social network and developmental trajectory.

During the last phase, suicidal ideation appears to occur when distressing psychotic symptoms fail to resolve, or re-emerge in the context of maintained insight, or when negative symptoms persist in the context of high personal, family, or staff, expectations. This is illustrated in the following case vignette.

> A 20-year-old single, unemployed and socially isolated man, whose father had suffered from schizophrenia and had committed suicide when the patient was 10 years old, was referred to the EPPIC 'prodrome clinic' (PACE: see Chapter 4). He had no history of psychosis and presented with emerging depressive symptoms in the context of psychosocial deterioration and intermittent cannabis use. After attending the 'prodrome clinic' for a year, he precipitously developed his first-episode of acute psychosis which was complicated by very distressing paranoid delusions and hallucinations. He required several weeks of inpatient treatment before his symptoms settled. Although denying suicide ideation during the prodrome and acute psychosis phases, he was considered by inpatient and outpatient staff to be at very high risk of committing suicide. During his early recovery phase it was noted that he identified closely with his father's experience and, although he quickly developed insight into his illness, he was quite ambivalent about treatment. Three weeks after discharge from hospital, and while still attending follow-up outpatient services, he committed suicide by jumping in front of a train. The day before his death, when assessed as an outpatient by his case manager, his mental state had presented as relatively improved, there being no evidence of suicidal ideation or intent at that time. The final trigger on the day of his death remains unknown.

In hindsight, one can understand how a complex interplay of influences might conspire to cause a person to suicide. However, despite the wealth of statistics on suicide risk factors, their *predictive value* remains poor (Roy, Schreiber & Mazonson, 1988) probably because of the individual, variable and transient nature of suicidality, the large number of false positives each factor would predict, and the low base rate of suicide. Studies attempting to identify predictors of suicide are also limited by problems with methodology, e.g. definitions of suicide behaviour (Lewinsohn, Rhode & Seeley, 1996) and the lack of comprehensive models of suicide. One notable exception is a recent study by Lewinsohn, Rhode & Seeley (1996), which attempts to establish a useful clinical model which weighs the various suicide risk factors through the use of sophisticated causal modelling techniques. For early psychosis, a similar approach is required, one which involves a more comprehensive analysis of risk factors (including those which are protective), and how they relate to phase of illness or treatment. However, whilst it is difficult enough to predict suicide on a statistical basis, the problem is further compounded by the frequent inaccessibility of early psychosis patients and their inability, or unwillingness, to identify issues, cognitions or other risk factors which place them at risk of suicide. This would be consistent with the broader prevailing belief, which so far lacks empirical support, that suicide in schizophrenia is *even* less predictable than in other serious mental disorders.

Prevention and management of suicide risk in early psychosis

The prevention of suicide risk in early psychosis must first include the general principles of ensuring the prompt and effective treatment of the underlying psychotic disorder. For the subgroup identified to be at higher risk of suicide, more specific primary and secondary suicide prevention and intervention strategies are outlined below. However, as yet there is little evidence to support the efficacy of these interventions (Zubrick & Silburn, 1996), with one exception: limiting the availability of means to suicide (Gunnell & Frankel, 1994). Despite new and more effective pharmacological treatments for psychotic disorders, the suicide rate remains high among young people with psychotic disorders such as schizophrenia. Clearly, suicide prevention strategies need to be further developed.

Suicide prevention strategies should include: public education, service models, staff training, post-vention strategies to prevent 'contagion', early accurate and accessible detection strategies for those at high risk, and prompt effective treatments with easy access to intensive interventions at times of especially high risk.

Primary prevention

Service models
Service models which effectively reduce the suicide rates in those with early psychosis might be those which develop strategies to

enhance the early detection of psychosis; improved mechanisms for access to psychiatric services; 'user friendly' non-stigmatizing psychiatric services for young people; adequate supports for carers of those with psychosis; effective treatments for those either already suffering from, or at risk of developing, early psychosis; and specific suicide prevention forums or structures within health services. McGorry et al. (1996), in a review of the effect of introducing improved models of management of early psychosis, reported a sizable reduction in suicide rates with the introduction of a more comprehensive model of service delivery – the Early Psychosis Prevention and Intervention Centre (EPPIC) model. McGorry et al. (1996) reported that, within two years of entry into treatment, six cases of suicide occurred in the pre-EPPIC sample ($n = 140$) compared with seven cases in the EPPIC sample ($n = 750$).

Government social services
Effective government social policies might be those which negate the marginalization of young people with psychotic disorders, provide safety net services, e.g. youth housing which does not exclude those with psychosis or complicating substance abuse disorders, and provision of social and financial support for family and carer organizations to ensure adequate support for those with psychosis.

Education and training programmes
Despite education and training in the detection and management of those at risk of suicide being fundamental to any suicide prevention strategy, many clinicians lack adequate skills and expertise in suicide prevention techniques. Training and education programmes have been shown to provide a significant reduction in suicide rates in the regions which those 'trained' practitioners served (Rihmer, Rutz & Pihlgren, 1995). Interactive workshops and seminars in suicidology have been reported to be more effective than handing out written material (Michel & Valach, 1992) in helping clinicians to become more sensitive in assessing suicide risk, and more confident in their interventions.

Media control and prevention of contagion
Recognized preventive strategies include educational campaigns to both minimize alcohol/drug abuse and increase awareness of suicide and available services. Other factors include the minimization of the effect of 'contagion' through the control of media reports and depictions of suicide, and by the debriefing of those exposed to a suicide (Brent et al., 1988b).

12 SUICIDE AND EARLY PSYCHOSIS

Removal of lethal methods

For suicide rates in general, Lester (1995) highlights the importance of suicide prevention strategies which remove access to suicide methods. Lester suggests a number of measures which may limit access to lethal methods of suicide. These include car exhaust modifications, domestic gas modifications, restrictions and fencing around potential jumping points, limited access to household poisons, gun control legislation, and regulations to reduce the availability of 'lethal' prescriptions of medications.

Secondary and tertiary preventions in psychosis

For those at high risk of suicide generally, the detection and provision of prompt access to treatment remain poor. Studies of suicide victims' history of contact with mental health services reveal that about 50% have had no history of contact, although half of the victims had recent contact with their family doctor. Of the 50% who have had contact with mental health services, 25% had dropped out of treatment and another 25% were receiving 'inadequate care' when they committed suicide (Isometsa et al., 1994).

Because of the frequently transient nature of suicidality in psychosis, detection and treatment relies heavily on early, close, and regular monitoring of a patient's level of suicidality with prompt interventions for those identified as manifesting an immediate suicide risk.

Detection and assessment of suicide risk in early psychosis

Previous chapters have outlined mechanisms which aid in the sensitive, accurate and early detection of psychosis, and thereby identify a group of young people who carry a substantially higher risk of suicide. However, accurately detecting the subgroup (among those with early psychosis) who present an exceptionally high risk of suicide remains a problem. Assessment of the strongest predictive indicators of suicidality are: (*a*) history of suicide attempts; and (*b*) current level of suicide ideation (degree of hopelessness and entrapment (see Chapter 9) would be of most value). Other additional factors are described in the section on the model for suicide behaviour (see Figure 12.1).

There are a wide range of assessment schedules now available to rate indicators of suicidality. Although very useful as an aid to a comprehensive clinical suicide risk assessment, they cannot be relied upon on their own, and to date no schedules exist specifically designed to assess suicide risk in psychosis. Some schedules include direct measures of suicide intent (Suicide Intent Scale, Beck, Schuyler & Herman, 1974; Adolescent Suicide Questionnaire, Pearce & Martin, 1994), while others assess indirect measures which can be broadly divided into either state

(Hopelessness Scale, Beck et al., 1974; Beck et al., 1990), or trait measures of suicide risk (Risk Estimator for Suicide, Motto, 1985). Other scales include: Youth Assessment Checklist (Martin, 1995); Kienhorst's Assessment Checklist (Kienhorst et al., 1990); Scale for Suicide Ideation (Beck, Kovacs & Weissman, 1979); Lethality of Suicide Attempts Rating Scale (Smith, Conroy & Ehler, 1984); the suicidality subscale of the K-SADS (Orvaschel et al., 1982); and, finally, the suicidality subscale of the Health of the Nation Outcome Scales (HoNOS: Wing, 1994).

Given the transient nature of suicidality, regular monitoring of suicide ideation and intent is essential during the various phases of first-episode psychosis, particularly during: the transition from prodrome to psychosis; the early phase of recovery; early relapse if it occurs; and during phases when there are rapid fluctuations in mental state. Ideally, a comprehensive suicide risk assessment should be made after any behaviour suggestive of a suicide attempt. Included in this should be a exploration of the cognitions, themes (e.g. entrapment), and experiences (particularly those of psychosis) which lead the patient to choose suicide as an option, as well as the potential deterrents and factors which may aid in instilling hope in recovery. A sensitive exploration of any suicide plan is essential.

In addition to assessing suicidality itself, one needs to consider the level of stress to which the patient is currently exposed, the availability of practical and emotional support/supervision, access to means of self harm, and potential negative responses to any interventions proposed.

Specific suicide prevention interventions in early psychosis
For those with early psychosis and identified as carrying a high risk of suicide, specific treatment interventions which might be effective in reducing the high risk of suicide may mediate their effect via mechanisms which: (*a*) ensure effective treatment, e.g. for depressive features, for side effects (akathisia), for those whose psychopathology is undetected, under-treated, or resistant to standard treatments, e.g. early use of clozapine (Meltzer & Okayli, 1995); (*b*) ensure that secondary morbidity factors are being addressed, e.g. adjustment difficulties and hopelessness in the context of losses sustained (loss of relationships, employment, accommodation and, importantly, loss of self-esteem); and (*c*) address comorbid factors, e.g. substance abuse disorders, and premorbid factors, e.g. personality disorders or impaired social supports. Comorbid conditions may be quite long standing or entrenched, and may respond poorly to interventions.

Psychological interventions   Specific cognitive therapies have already been developed for suicide ideation and behaviours in general clinical population groups (Freeman & Reinecke, 1993; Perris, 1994; Rotheram-Borus et al., 1994; Salkovskis, Atha & Storer, 1990; Shearin & Linehan, 1994). Group CBT, provided in addition to individual therapy, has been demonstrated by Linehan and her colleagues (1991,1994) to be efficacious in reducing suicide behaviours in young women with borderline personality disorder. However, as yet these therapies have not been adapted for the specific needs of those with major axis I psychiatric illnesses, such as the psychotic disorders.

Both clinical experience and research suggest that patients who have suffered an acute psychotic episode are particularly vulnerable to depression and suicide ideation (Birchwood, 1996), post-traumatic stress symptoms (McGorry et al., 1991), anxiety disorders, demoralization and low self-esteem (McGorry & Kulkarni, 1994). Individually based CBT approaches which have demonstrated efficacy in psychosis (Drury et al., 1996; Jackson et al., 1996; Kemp et al., 1995) may have indirect effects on reducing suicide risk in early psychosis through their effects on the primary/secondary symptoms of psychosis, adaptation issues, insight, treatment compliance, and by maximizing protective influences against suicide through the instillation of hope in recovery. This is illustrated in the following case vignette.

> A 19-year-old single student living at home with his employed parents, presented with a three-year history of progressive severe social withdrawal, amotivation, affective blunting, increasing difficulties attending his course and tensions within the family (both parents had suffered brief episodes of psychosis in early adulthood). He was hospitalized for assessment following an unsuccessful attempt to jump off a building and repeated ingestion of poisons. Fleeting paranoid psychotic features, which included hallucinations and passivity phenomena, were noted within the setting of a rich fantasy life complicated by depressive and morbid themes. Antipsychotics provided improvement for the acute psychotic symptoms but a profound negative syndrome state persisted. This was complicated by fluctuating levels of suicidality with further serious suicide attempts requiring two re-hospitalizations within three months. Two courses of ECT and the addition of an SSRI antidepressant appeared to provide only a limited and temporary benefit in reducing his suicidality. Engagement in a rehabilitative group programme was unsuccessful. Finally, intensive individual cognitive therapy, combined with regular family counselling, began slowly to provide results in engaging the young man and understanding the nature of his suicidality, which seemed to

arise from a sense of loss of self-esteem, perceived rejection by others, social anxiety, and loss of hope in recovery. This therapy (in combination with the above pharmacotherapy) focussed directly on the issues of his suicidality in the context of psychoeducation, self-esteem, social anxiety, adjustment and recovery. Eventually, after nine months of treatment he successfully returned to his course with a resolution of his suicidality, a gradually improving level of psychosocial functioning, and resolution of family tensions.

A specific individual CBT intervention to address suicidality in psychosis is currently being developed and trialled at EPPIC as part of a federally-funded national mental health initiative to introduce suicide prevention strategies for young people with serious mental illnesses (National Mental Health Strategy, 1995). This suicide prevention CBT-based intervention draws on elements in a number of the above CBT interventions, but is applied within the context of a crisis intervention model (given the urgent and transient nature of suicidality) and supplements standard case management. The therapy aims not only to address state-related risk factors, but also to provide: psychoeducation about the mechanisms of suicidality; coping strategies for suicide ideation; coping strategies to assist with the desensitization of the impact of triggers; strategies to access assistance, augment protective factors such as 'hope' in recovery, as well as bolster self-esteem; psychoeducation about psychosis; and assist with adjustment to losses. For those with active psychotic symptoms, a greater number of sessions may prove necessary due to the more complicated nature of suicidality in acute psychosis and the not infrequent impaired information-processing problems which may accompany active psychosis. In addition to this, an adjunctive group CBT-based intervention based on the Linehan model (Linehan et al., 1994), is being trialled at EPPIC for those with persistent high levels of suicidality which have not responded to individual CBT interventions.

Psychosocial interventions   Potential psychosocial interventions may include: psychosocial measures which reduce 'hopelessness', particularly during the early recovery phase; the provision of intensive support post-discharge; minimizing the potentially disruptive impact of an episode of mental illness on the person's social milieu; protecting the person's developmental trajectory and sense of 'self', via interventions which support peer relationships, work and vocational involvements; and introducing successful role models (Lipschitz, 1995).

Given that the social network of those with psychosis often constricts to a small network of concerned relatives, interventions such as psychoeducation and therapies which reduce critical 'expressed emotion' have been suggested by Lipschitz (1995) in order to reduce the risk of suicide in psychotic disorders.

Pharmacological and physical treatments   Meltzer & Okayli (1995) recommend that clozapine should be prescribed early in patients with 'treatment-resistant' psychosis to reduce the risk of suicide, reporting that 40% of the 88 patients treated with clozapine became less suicidal according to indicators such as the number of suicide attempts and the severity of suicide ideation. Preliminary trials of the newer antipsychotics, in particular, those with D2 and 5HT2 antagonist activity (e.g. risperidone, olanzapine, sertindole, Ziprasidone and Zotepine), show promising results with fewer side effects and greater effect on negative symptoms than traditional antipsychotics, and in a small number of trials these agents have shown improvements in anxiety and depression scores (Blin, Azorin & Bouhours, 1996; Mertens, 1991). These effects, although as yet only provisionally confirmed, may impact on factors which aggravate suicide risk in psychosis.

The efficacy of antidepressants in reducing suicide in early psychosis has yet to be demonstrated. However, the combined use of anti-depressants and antipsychotics is more efficacious than monotherapy alone in the treatment of the primary symptoms of depressive psychosis (Parker et al., 1992; Spiker et al., 1985). SSRIs in combination with antipsychotics appear to be as effective as a TCA combination but possess the benefit of lower levels of side effects (Rothschild et al., 1993). In schizophrenia and schizoaffective disorders, however, the combined use of antidepressants and antipsychotic medication has been shown to delay the resolution of, or even exacerbate, psychotic symptoms in depressed and actively psychotic patients (Kramer, Vogel & Dijohnson, 1989; Prusoff, Williams & Weissman, 1979). Nevertheless, combination treatment in postpsychotic depression does appear to be beneficial (Siris et al., 1994), in both reducing depressive symptoms and rates of psychotic relapse, particularly for those who respond early to these treatments.

Lithium has been shown to be associated with lower rates of suicide in affective disorders (Coppen, 1994), but reports of its efficacy in first-episode psychosis are lacking. ECT is the most effective treatment available in the treatment of affective psychosis (Mukherjee, Sackeim & Schur, 1994; Parker et al., 1992), the disorder which carries the highest risk of suicide (Blumenthal, 1990). In five of six studies reviewed by Tanney (1986), ECT appeared to have a preventive effect on suicide behaviours, although none focussed specifically on early psychosis. However, ECT should be reserved as a second-line treatment, except in

Table 12.2. *Guidelines for the initial clinical management of a suicidal first-episode psychosis patient*

Prompt initial assessment	Prompt initial assessment of duration and severity of suicide intent, mediating factors (both risk and protective), phase and severity of psychosis, command hallucinations, degree of subjective distress, unpredictability, level of affective disturbance, access to lethal means, supervision and support available, potential for non-compliance, and patient's initial response to clinical interventions proposed. Check that patient has not made a recent attempt, e.g. recent ingestion of poison, that might require immediate medical attention.
Ensure immediate safety	Ensure patient's immediate safety by providing constant supervision and removal of any potential means to self-harm until an appropriate intervention has been decided upon.
Decide on appropriate management plan	Determine who will be the primary clinician involved and facilitate the establishment of a therapeutic alliance between the patient and that clinician throughout the high risk period. Liaise with patient's other treating clinicians, check interventions immediately available, and consult with senior clinical staff if high suicide risk is determined. Liaise with carers regarding recent and past history of factors that might indicate heightened suicide risk. Determine degree of supervision needed to minimize likelihood of a suicide attempt, balancing degree of suicide intent, willingness to comply, variability of mental state, and reliability of the least restrictive options available. Decide on necessary treatment. Negotiate options with the patient, e.g. hospitalization.
Initiate management plan	<u>Supervision</u> Provide adequate level of supervision of the patient by staff or carers with clear instructions about risk, degree of monitoring and frequency of clinical reviews needed, responses required if a deterioration is observed, e.g. who and how to consult if problems arise.

Table 12.2. (cont.)

	Safety
	Remove access to means of self-harm, e.g. razors, knives, cords, guns, medications and poisons. Limit exposure to immediate stressors and, if necessary, provide containment within a safe setting, e.g. hospital, with clear instructions to carers about limitations on patients' freedom.
	Personal contact and counselling
	Provide initial counselling and treatments while establishing rapport, understanding and trust; explore cognitions that influence level of suicidality; encourage an understanding that suicide ideation is a transient though 'painful' phenomenon related to illness factors; attempt to reframe the patient's sense of hopelessness by instilling 'hope' in recovery through treatment or therapeutic options; and finally negotiate a suicide contract.
	Immediately inform, liaise with, and provide debriefing for carers regarding suicide risk and interventions required. Defuse potential for critical comments by providing psychoeducational strategies for carers (including staff).
	Initiate treatments
	Reduce associated distress due to psychosis or suicide ideation with anxiolytics and promptly commence, ensure compliance with, and supervision of, appropriate pharmacotherapies.
	Attempt to influence psychosocial factors that might reduce suicidality, e.g. practical assistance with homelessness, access to social milieu, etc.
Review management	Regularly review and negotiate the interventions above with the patient, carers, and other clinicians involved. Ensure clear lines of clinical accountability and decision making.

emergency situations when the patient is at very high risk. In our experience, approximately 4% of patients require ECT for their first-episode of psychosis (Power et al., 1998).

In conclusion, the application of the above preventive strategies in clinical practice requires considerable expertise and skill. Table 12.2 provides guidelines for the assessment and initial intervention of patients with early psychosis presenting with a high risk of suicide.

Summary

Suicide prevention strategies in early psychosis remain relatively underdeveloped and poorly investigated despite the obvious high risk of suicide amongst those suffering from psychosis. Relatively little research has been undertaken to analyse the course and patterns of suicide ideation or behaviours in those with psychotic disorders. Even fewer studies look at the association with illness factors, such as phase of illness. Clearly, further research is needed in these areas. In addition, improving the levels of training of clinicians in suicide risk assessment and prevention is essential. Definitive studies are required to test the relative benefits of various, as yet, controversial pharmacological or psychological therapies for suicide prevention in psychosis. However, this is becoming an area of increasing interest and research as the focus turns to how to address the rising tide of suicide among adolescents. Hopefully, this is a tide which is about to turn.

References

Apter, A., Bleich, A., Plutchik, R., Mendelsohn, S. & Tyano, S. (1988). Suicidal behavior, depression and conduct disorder in hospitalised adolescents. *Journal of the American Academy of Child and Adolescent Psychiatry*, **27**, 696–9.

Australian Bureau of Statistics (1994). *Causes of Death* (Catalogue No. 4102.0). Canberra, Australia: Australian Bureau of Statistics.

Beck, A. (1987). Cognitive approaches to hopelessness and suicide. *Paper presented at the Annual General Meeting of the Association for the Advancement of Behavior Therapy*, Boston, Massachusetts.

Beck, A. & Stewart, B. (1989). The self-concept as a risk factor in patients who kill themselves. Unpublished manuscript.

Beck, A., Schuyler, D. & Herman, I. (1974). Development of suicidal intent scales. In *The Prediction of Suicide*, ed. A. T. Beck, H. C. P. Resnik & D. Lettieri, pp. 545–56. Bowie, Maryland: The Charles Press.

Beck, A., Weissman, A., Lester, D. & Trexler, L. (1974). The measurement of pessimism: the Hopelessness Scale. *Journal of Consulting and Clinical Psychology*, **44**, 861–5.

Beck, A. T., Kovacs, M. & Weissman, A. (1979). Assessment of suicidal ideation: the Scale for Suicide Ideation. *Journal of Consulting and Clinical Psychology*, **47**, 343–52.

Beck, A., Brown, G., Berchick, R., Stewart, B. L. & Steer, R. (1990). Relationship between hopelessness and ultimate suicide: a replication with psychiatric outpatients. *American Journal of Psychiatry*, **147**, 190–5.

Birchwood, M. (1996). The Birmingham Early Psychosis Program: research and clinical experience. *Paper presented at the First International Conference on*

Strategies for Prevention in Early Psychosis, Verging on Reality, Melbourne, Australia, June, 1996.

Black, D., Winokur, G. & Nasrallah, A. (1988). Effect of psychosis on suicide risk in 1593 patients with unipolar and bipolar affective disorders. *American Journal of Psychiatry*, **145**, 849–52.

Blin, O., Azorin, J. & Bouhours, P. (1996). Antipsychotic and anxiolytic properties of risperidone, haloperidol and methotrimeprazine in schizophrenic patients. *Journal of Clinical Psychopharmacology*, **16**, 38–44.

Blumenthal, S. (1990). Youth suicide: risk factors, assessment, and treatment of adolescent and young adult suicidal patients. *Psychiatric Clinics of North America*, **13**, 511–56.

Breier, A. & Astrachan, B. (1984). Characteristics of schizophrenic patients who commit suicide. *American Journal of Psychiatry*, **141**, 206–9.

Brent, D. (1986). Overrepresentation of epileptics in a consecutive series of suicide attempters seen at a children's hospital. *Journal of the American Academy of Child Psychiatry*, **25**, 242–6.

Brent, D., Perper, J., Goldstein, C., Kolko, D., Allan, M., Allman, C. & Zelenak, J. (1988a). Risk factors for adolescent suicide: a comparison of adolescent suicide victims with suicidal inpatients. *Archives of General Psychiatry*, **45**, 581–8.

Brent, D., Kupfer, D., Bromet, E. & Dew, M. A. (1988b). The assessment and treatment of patients at risk of suicide. In *American Psychiatric Review of Psychiatry*, Vol 7, ed. A. Frances & R. Hales, pp. 353–85. Washington, DC: American Psychiatric Press.

Brent, D. A., Perper, J. A., Moritz, G., Baugher, M., Roth, C., Balach, L. & Schweers, J. (1993). Stressful life events, psychopathology, and adolescent suicide: a case control study. *Suicide and Life-threatening Behavior*, **23**, 179–87.

Brewer, W., Velakoulis, D., Anderson, V., O'Brien, M., McGorry, P., Yung, A., Francey, S., Singh, B., Copolov, D. & Pantelis, C. (1996). Cognitive and olfactory deficits: course from high risk to stabilised first episode psychosis. *Paper presented at the 1996 Annual Scientific Meeting of the Australian Society for Psychiatric Research*, Newcastle, Australia.

Buda, M. & Tsuang, M. T. (1990). The epidemiology of suicide: implications for clinical practice. In *Suicide Over the Life Cycle: Risk Factors, Assessment and Treatment of Suicidal Patients*, ed. S. Blumenthal & D. Kupfer, pp. 17–37. Washington DC: American Psychiatric Press.

Caldwell, C. & Gottesman, I. (1990). Schizophrenics kill themselves too: a review of risk factors for suicide. *Schizophrenia Bulletin*, **16**, 571–89.

Coppen, A. (1994). Depression as a lethal disease: prevention strategies. *Journal of Clinical Psychiatry*, **55** (Supplement), 37–45.

de Moore, G. M. & Robertson, A. R. (1996). Suicide in the 18 years after deliberate self-harm. A prospective study. *British Journal of Psychiatry*, **169**, 489–95.

Diekstra, R. F. W. (1995). The epidemiology of suicide and parasuicide. In *Preventative Strategies on Suicide*, ed. R. F. W. Diekstra, W. Gulbinat, L. Kienhorst & D. de Leo, pp. 1–2. Leiden, Netherlands: E. J. Brill Press.

Drake, R. & Cotton, P. (1986). Depression, hopelessness and suicide in chronic schizophrenia. *British Journal of Psychiatry*, **146**, 554–9.

Drake, R. E., Gates, C., Cotton, P. G. & Whitaker, A. (1984). Suicide among schizophrenics: who is at risk? *Journal of Nervous and Mental Disease*, **172**, 613–17.

Drury, V., Birchwood, M., Cochrane, R. & Macmillan, F. (1996). Cognitive therapy and recovery from acute psychosis: a controlled trial. *British Journal of Psychiatry*, **169**, 593–601.

Fawcett, J., Schefter, W., Fogg, I., Clarke, D., Young, M., Hedeker, D. & Gibbons, R. (1990). Time related predictors of suicide in major affective disorder. *American Journal of Psychiatry*, **147**, 1189–94.

Fenton, W. & McGlashan, T. (1991). Natural history of schizophrenia subtypes. *Archives of General Psychiatry*, **48**, 969–77.

Fenton, W. & McGlashan, T. (1996). Schizophrenic symptoms: subtype and suicidality. *Paper presented at the Annual Meeting of the American Psychiatric Association*, New York, May, 1996.

Fenton, W. S., McGlashan, T. H., Victor, B. J. & Blyler, C. R. (1997). Symptoms, subtype, and suicidality in patients with schizophrenia spectrum disorders. *American Journal of Psychiatry*, **154**, 199–204.

Frances, R., Franklin, J. & Flavin, D. (1986). Suicide and alcoholism. *Annals of the New York Academy of Science*, **487**, 316–26.

Freeman, A. & Reinecke, M. A. (1993). *Cognitive Therapy of Suicide Behavior: A Manual for Treatment*. New York: Springer.

Goodwin, F. & Jamison, K. (1990). *Manic Depressive Illness*. New York: Oxford University Press.

Gunnell, D. & Frankel, F. (1994). Prevention of suicide: aspirations and evidence. *British Medical Journal*, **308**, 1227–33.

Häfner, H., Maurer, K., Löffler, W., Bustamaine, S., Anderheiden, A. W., Reicher-Rössler, A. & Nowotny, B. (1995). Onset and early course of schizophrenia. In *Search for the Causes of Schizophrenia*, Vol III, ed. H. Häfner & W. F. Gattaz, pp. 43–6. New York: Springer.

Isometsa, E. T., Henriksson, M. M., Aro, H. M., Heikkinen, M. E., Kuoppasalmi, K. & Lonnqist, J. (1994). Suicide and major depression. *American Journal of Psychiatry*, **151**, 530–6.

Jackson, H., McGorry, P., Edwards, J. & Hulbert, C. (1996). Cognitively oriented psychotherapy for early psychosis (COPE). In *Early Intervention and Prevention in Mental Health*, ed. P. Cotton & H. Jackson. pp. 131–54. Melbourne, Australia: Australian Psychological Society.

Jamison, K. (1986). Suicide and bipolar disorders. *Annals of the New York Academy of Science*, **487**, 301–15.

Kemp, R., Hayward, P., Applewhaite, G., Everitt, B. & David, A. (1995). Compliance therapy in psychotic patients: randomised controlled trial. *British Medical Journal*, **312**, 345–9.

Kerkhof, A. J. & Diekstra, R. F. (1995). How to evaluate and deal with acute suicide risk. In *Preventive Strategies on Suicide*, ed. R. F. Diekstra, W. Gulbinat, I. Kienhorst & D. de Leo., pp. 97–119, Leiden, Netherlands: E. J. Brill Press.

Kienhorst, C., deWilde, E., Van den Bout, J., Broese van Groenou, M., Diekstra, R. & Woltus, W. (1990). Self-report suicidal behaviour in Dutch secondary education students. *Suicide and Life Threatening Behavior*, **20**, 101–12.

Kingdon, D. & Turkington, D. (1994). *Cognitive–Behaviour Therapy of Schizophrenia*. London: Guilford Press.

Korn, M. L., Brown, S. L., Kotler, M., Gordon, M. & Van Praag, H. M. (1995). Biological aspects of suicide. In *Preventive Strategies on Suicide*, ed. R. F. Diekstra, W. Gulbinat, I. Kienhorst & D. de Leo, pp. 311–37. Leiden, Netherlands: E. J. Brill Press.

Kramer, M., Vogel, W. & Dijohnson, C. (1989). Antidepressants in 'depressed' schizophrenic inpatients. A controlled trial. *Archives of General Psychiatry*, **46**, 922–8.

Krausz, M., Muller-Thomsen, T. & Maasen, C. (1995). Suicide among schizophrenic adolescents in the long-term course of illness. *Psychopathology*, **28**, 95–103.

Lester, D. (1995). Preventing suicide by restricting access to methods for suicide. In *Prevention Strategies on Suicide*, ed. R. Diekstra, W. Gulbinat, I. Kienhorst, & D. de Leo. pp. 163–71. Leiden, Netherlands: E. J. Brill Press.

Lewinsohn, P. M., Clarke, G. N., Seeley, J. R. & Rhode, P. (1994). Major depression in community adolescents: age at onset, episode duration, and time to recurrence. *Journal of the American Academy of Child and Adolescent Psychiatry*, **33**, 809–18.

Lewinsohn, P. M., Rhode, P. & Seeley, J. R. (1996). Adolescent suicidal ideation and attempts: prevalence, risk factors, and clinical implications. *Clinical Psychology: Science and Practice*, **3**, 25–46.

Linehan, M., Armstrong, H., Suarez, A. & Allmon, D. (1991). Cognitive behavioral treatment of chronically parasuicidal borderline patients. *Archives of General Psychiatry*, **48**, 1060–4.

Linehan, M., Tutek, D., Heard, H. & Armstrong, H. (1994). Interpersonal outcome of cognitive behavioral treatment for chronically suicidal borderline patients. *American Journal of Psychiatry*, **151**, 1771–6.

Lipschitz, A. (1995). Suicide prevention in young adults. *Suicide and Life-threatening Behavior*, **25**, 155–69.

Martin G. (1995). *Youth Assessment Checklist*. Flinders Medical Centre, Child and Adolescent Mental Health Service, Bedford, South Australia.

Marttunen, M. J., Aro, H. M., Henricksson, M. M. & Lonnqvist, J. K. (1991). Mental disorders in adolescent suicide: DSM-III-R axes I and II diagnoses in suicides among 13 to 19 year olds in Finland. *Archives of General Psychiatry*, **48**, 834–9.

McGorry, P. & Kulkarni, J. (1994). Prevention and preventively oriented clinical care in psychotic disorders. *Australian Journal of Psychopharmacology*, **7**, 62–9.

McGorry, P., Chanen, A., McCarthy, E., Van Riel, R., McKenzie, D. & Singh, B. (1991). Post-traumatic stress disorder following recent onset psychosis: an unrecognised post-psychotic syndrome. *Journal of Nervous and Mental Disease*, **179**, 253–8.

McGorry, P., Edwards, J., Mihalopoulos, C., Harrigan, S. & Jackson, H. (1996).

EPPIC: an evolving system of early detection and optimal management. *Schizophrenia Bulletin*, **22**, 305–26.

Meltzer, H. & Okayli, G. (1995).The reduction of suicidality during clozapine treatment in neuroleptic resistent schizophrenics. *American Journal of Psychiatry*, **152**, 183–90.

Mertens, P. (1991). Longterm treatment of chronic schizphrenic patients with risperidone. In *Risperidone, Major Progress in Antipsychotic Treatment*, ed. J. Kane, pp. 33–48. Oxford: Oxford Clinical Communications.

Michel, K. & Valach, L. (1992). Suicide prevention: spreading the gospel to general practitioners. *British Journal of Psychiatry*, **160**, 757–60.

Modestin, J., Zarro, I. & Waldvogel, D. (1992). A study of suicide in schizophrenic inpatients. *British Journal of Psychiatry*, **160**, 398–401.

Motto, J. (1985). Development of a clinical instrument to estimate suicide risk. *American Journal of Psychiatry*, **142**, 680–6.

Mukherjee, S., Sackeim, H. & Schur, D. (1994). Electroconvulsive therapy of acute manic episodes: a review of 50 years' experience. *American Journal of Psychiatry*, **151**, 169–76.

National Mental Health Strategy (1995). Canberra, Australia: Department of Health and Family Services, Commonwealth of Australia, Canberra.

News: Suicide (1994). *British Medical Journal*, **308**, 7–11.

Ohberg, A., Vuaori, I., Ojanpera, I. & Lonnqvist, J. (1996). Alcohol and drugs in suicides. *British Journal of Psychiatry*, **169**, 75–81.

Orvaschel, H., Puig-Antich, J., Chambers, W. J., Tabrizi, M. A. & Johnson, R. (1982). Retrospective assessment of pre-pubertal major depression with the Kiddie-SADS-E. *Journal of the American Academy of Child and Adolescent Psychiatry*, **21**, 392–7.

Parker, G., Roy, K., Hadzi-Pavlovic, D. & Pedic, F. (1992). Psychotic depression: a meta-analysis of physical treatments. *Journal of Affective Disorders*, **24**, 17–24.

Pearce, C. & Martin, G., (1994). Predicting suicide attempts among adolescents. *Acta Psychiatrica Scandinavica*, **90**, 324–8.

Perris, C. (1994). Cognitive therapy in the treatment of patients with borderline personality disorders. *Acta Psychiatrica Scandinavica*, **89** (379, Supplement), 69–72.

Poole, R. & Brabbins, C. (1996). Drug induced psychosis. *British Journal of Psychiatry*, **168**, 135–9.

Power, P., Elkins, K., Adlard, S. P., Curry, C., McGorry, P. & Harrigan, S. (in press). An analysis of the initial treatment phase in first episode psychosis. *British Journal of Psychiatry*.

Prusoff, B., Williams, D. & Weissman, M. (1979). Treatment of secondary depression in schizophrenia: a double blind, placebo controlled trial of amitriptyline added to perphenazine. *Archives of General Psychiatry*, **36**, 569–75.

Rich, C. L., Sherman, M. & Fowler, T. C. (1990). San Diego Suicide Study: the adolescents. *Adolescence*, **25**, 855–65.

Rihmer, Z., Rutz, W. & Pihlgren, H. (1995). Depression and suicide in Gotland. An intensive study of all suicides before and after a depression-training programme for general practitioners. *Journal of Affective Disorders*, **35**, 147–52.

Robins, E., Murphy, G., Wilkinson, R., Gasner, S. & Kayes, J. (1959). Some clinical considerations in the prevention of suicide based on a study of 134 successful suicides. *American Journal of Public Health*, **49**, 888–98.

Roose, S. P., Glassman, A. H., Walsh, T., Woodring, S. & Vital-Herne, J. (1983). Depression, delusions, and suicide. *American Journal of Psychiatry*, **140**, 1159–62.

Rotheram-Borus, M. J., Piacentini, J., Miller, S., Graae, F. & Castro-Blanco, D. (1994). Brief cognitive–behavior treatment for adolescent suicide attempters and their families. *Journal of the American Academy of Child and Adolescent Psychiatry*, **33**, 508–17.

Rothschild, A. J., Samson, J. A., Bessette, M. P. & Carter-Campbell, J. T. (1993). Efficacy of the combination of fluoxetine and perphenazine in the treatment of psychotic depression. *Journal of Clinical Psychiatry*, **54**, 338–42.

Roy, A. (1982). Suicide in chronic schizophrenia. *British Journal of Psychiatry*, **141**, 171–7.

Roy, A. (1986). Suicide in schizophrenia. In *Suicide*, ed. A. Roy, pp. 97–112. Baltimore: Williams and Wilkins.

Roy, A., Schreiber, J. & Mazonson, A. (1988). Suicidal behavior in chronic schizophrenic patients: a follow-up study. *Canadian Journal of Psychiatry*, **31**, 737–40.

Roy, A., Sega, N., Centerwall, B. & Robinette, D. (1991). Suicide in twins. *Archives of General Psychiatry*, **48**, 29–32.

Runeson, B. (1989). Mental disorder in youth suicide: DSM-III-R axes I and II. *Acta Psychiatric Scandinavica*, **79**, 490–7.

Salkovskis, P., Atha, C. & Storer, D. (1990). Cognitive behavioural problem solving in the treatment of patients who repeatedly attempt suicide: a controlled trial. *British Journal of Psychiatry*, **157**, 871–6.

Schotte, D. E., Cools, J. & Payvar, S. (1990). Problem solving deficits in suicidal patients: trait vulnerability or state phenomenon? *Journal of Consulting and Clinical Psychology*, **58**, 562–4.

Schuckit, M. (1979). Alcoholism and affective disorder: diagnostic confusion. In *Alcoholism and Affective Disorders. Clinical Genetic and Biochemical Studies*, ed. D. Goodwin & Erickson, pp. 9–20. New York: SP Medical & Scientific Books.

Shaffer, D., Garland, A., Gould, M., Fisher, P. & Trautman, P. (1988). Preventing teenage suicide: a critical review. *Journal of the American Academy of Child and Adolescent Psychiatry*, **27**, 675–87.

Shafii, M., Carrigan, S., Whittinghill, J. R. & Derrick, A. (1985). Psychological autopsy of completed suicide in children and adolescents. *American Journal of Psychiatry*, **142**, 1061–4.

Shafii, M., Steltz-Lenarsky, J., Derrick, A., Beckner, C. & Whittinghill, J. (1988). Comorbidity of mental disorders in the post-mortem diagnosis of completed suicide in children and adolescents. *Journal of Affective Disorders*, **15**, 227–33.

Shearin, E. & Linehan, M. (1994). Dialectic behaviour therapy for borderline personality disorder. *Acta Psychiatrica Scandinavica*, **89** (Supplement 379), 61–8.

Siris, S., Bermanzohn, P., Mason, S. & Shurwall, M. (1994). Maintenance imipramine therapy for secondary depression in schizophrenia. *Archives of General Psychiatry*, **51**, 109–15.

Smith, K., Conroy, R. W. & Ehler, B. D. (1984). Lethality of Suicide Attempt Rating scale. *Suicide and Life-threatening Behavior*, **14**, 215–42.

Spiker, D. G., Weiss, J. C., Dealy, R. S., Griffin, S. J., Hanin, I., Neil, J. F., Perel, J. M., Rossi, A. J. & Soloff, P. H. (1985). The pharmacological treatment of delusional depression. *American Journal of Psychiatry*, **142**, 430–5.

Strauss, J. S. (1969). Hallucinations and delusions as points on continua function. *Archives of General Psychiatry*, **21**, 581–6.

Tanney, B. L. (1986). Electroconvulsive therapy and suicide. In *Biology of Suicide*, ed. R. Maris, pp. 116–40. New York: Guilford Press.

Weishaar, M. & Beck A. (1992). Hopelessness and suicide. *International Review of Psychiatry*, **4**, 177–84.

Westermeyer, J., Harrow, M. & Marengo, J. (1991). Risk for suicide in schizophrenia and other psychotic and non-psychotic disorders. *Journal of Nervous and Mental Disease*, **179**, 259–66.

Wing, J. K. (1994). Health of the Nation Outcome Scale: HoNOS field trials. London: Royal College of Psychiatrists Research Unit.

Zubrick, S. & Silburn, S. (1996). Suicide prevention. In *Early Intervention and Prevention in Mental Health*, ed. P. Cotton & H. Jackson, pp. 193–209. Melbourne, Australia: The Australian Psychological Society.

Zubrick, S., Silburn, S., Garton, A., Dalby, R., Carlton, J., Shepherd, C., Lawrence, D. & Burton, P. (1995). Western Australian Child Health Survey: developing health and well being in the '90s. Perth: Australian Bureau of Statistics and the Institute for Child Health Research.

13

Early psychosis and substance abuse

DONALD H. LINSZEN AND MARIE E. LENIOR

Introduction

Psychoactive substance abuse and schizophrenia both have their onset in adolescence and young adulthood. North American studies have reported high prevalence rates of substance abuse amongst young patients with schizophrenia with cited figures ranging from 25 to 60% (Regier, Farmer & Rae, 1990; Test, Wallisch & Allness, 1989). Substance abuse by schizophrenic patients constitutes a common, rather than exceptional, event, with the variation in rates being explained by differences in diagnostic criteria, patient selection, geographical location, and social class, as well as by actual substance use varying over time. Nevertheless, in the rigorous Epidemiologic Catchment Area (ECA) study, young schizophrenic patients abused alcohol or drugs three times as much as the same age group in the general population (Regier, Farmer & Rae, 1990). In a large sample of schizophrenic patients presenting with a first episode of psychosis, the prevalence of substance abuse proved to be high as well (Hambrecht & Häfner, 1996). The most commonly abused psychoactive substances for patients with schizophrenia have been found to be alcohol, cannabis and stimulants such as cocaine and amphetamines (Barbee et al., 1989; Mueser et al., 1990). It has been suggested that psychostimulant drugs are preferred by schizophrenic patients (Schneier & Siris, 1987); in other studies, alcohol use (Drake, McHugo & Noordsey, 1993) and combined cannabis and alcohol use (Cuffel, Heithoff & Lawson, 1993) were found to be far more common. These discrepant findings regarding drug preferences have also been reported in a population of young schizophrenic patients (Caton, Gralnick & Bender, 1989). Two main hypotheses have been proposed to explain the frequent comorbidity of substance abuse of young patients with schizophrenia:

(1) The *vulnerability* hypothesis. Drug and alcohol abuse may contribute to the development of schizophrenia, or may precipitate signs and symptoms of the illness in individuals who later become schizophrenic (Breakey et al., 1974; Mueser et al., 1990; Richard, Liskow & Perry, 1985). Further evidence in favour of this hypothesis is that schizophrenic patients with substance abuse tend to have more psychotic relapses than non-abusers (Mueser et al., 1990; Osher & Kofoed, 1989).

(2) The *self-medication* hypothesis. Patients with schizophrenia may attempt to alleviate the distressing symptoms of the illness, or the side-effects of pharmacotherapy, through the use of alcohol and drugs (Dixon et al., 1991). Experiencing an early symptom onset in schizophrenia, may constitute a risk factor for substance abuse.

Whether substance abuse precipitates, or is a consequence of, schizophrenia is often a difficult question to answer. The main difficulty is the impossibility of proving that psychotic symptoms would not have occurred without drug use. Still, the high rates of comorbidity for schizophrenia and substance abuse highlights the importance of examining the effect of substance abuse on the onset and course of schizophrenia, and the reasons for substance abuse.

Substance abuse has been associated with a more severe course of schizophrenia (Mueser et al., 1990), whilst cannabis abuse has been associated with earlier psychotic relapses in young first-episode schizophrenic patients (Linszen, Dingemans & Lenior, 1994). This underlines the need for the development of more effective treatments for comorbid schizophrenia and substance abuse, aimed at improving the outcome of schizophrenia.

Onset of substance abuse and schizophrenia

The incidence and prevalence of substance abuse in adolescents and young adults is high. For instance, the 1985 National Household Survey revealed that 25% of the young adult population between 18 and 25 reported having ever used cocaine, and 60% reported having ever used hashish or marijuana (National Household Survey on Drug Abuse, 1985). Psychotic symptoms can occur in association with intoxication or withdrawal of substances. Although varying considerably with substances, psychotic symptoms usually disappear after a few days following discontinuation of the drug use. However, amphetamine use has been associated with persistent psychotic symptoms (McLellan, Woody & O'Brien, 1979). Cocaine and phencyclidine have also been reported to induce psychotic states which persisted for weeks despite controlled substance abstinence (APA, 1994). A Swedish epidemiological study

(Andreasson et al., 1987) and a Dutch study (Linszen et al., 1994) revealed that cannabis abuse one year prior to the illness was an independent risk factor for schizophrenia. In Germany (Hambrecht & Häfner, 1996) one-third of first-episode schizophrenic patients with a high rate of comorbid substance abuse, started their habit before the first signs of schizophrenia, whereas the rest started the substance abuse around, or after, the first signs.

When the prevalence, and more particularly the incidence, rates of schizophrenia are compared with those for substance abuse, the onset of schizophrenia turns out to be a relatively rare event. The incidence rates of schizophrenia between the ages of 15 and 24 ranged from 0.02 to 0.04% per 1000 population (World Health Organization, 1973). Therefore, the psychotic and negative symptoms associated with the diagnosis of schizophrenia are likely to be attributed to substance abuse, especially in the early phases of the disorder. The early diagnosis of schizophrenia may thus be missed and intervention directed at schizophrenia subsequently hindered for months, even years. This is important because untreated psychotic illness with a duration of more than one year is a major predictor of symptomatic deterioration in the onset phase of schizophrenia (Loebel et al., 1992). Therefore, overdiagnosing schizophrenia in the presence of substance abuse must be balanced against missing a diagnosis of schizophrenia. Consideration of the clinical evidence in association with the empirical data reveals similarities between the symptomatology of alcohol and other substance abuse, and the symptoms and symptom dimensions of schizophrenia (Liddle, 1987; Van der Does et al., 1995). This similarity in symptoms between schizophrenia and drug use, combined with the characteristics of drug use, in particular polydrug use, conspire to make it very difficult on occasion to distinguish substance abuse from schizophrenia, particularly in the prodromal stages of the latter (Jackson, McGorry & Dudgeon, 1995). The similarities are: (1) The presence of psychotic (positive) symptoms both in schizophrenia and in the intoxication and abuse phases of psychostimulants such as amphetamines (Hall & Hando, 1994) or amphetamine-like substances including 3,4–methylenedioxymethamphetamine (MDMA: 'ecstasy') (Steele, McCann & Ricaurte, 1994), phencyclidine (Wright et al., 1988) and cocaine (Satel, Southwick & Gawin, 1991); cannabis (Thornicroft, 1990) and hallucinogens (such as LSD, PCP, and psilocybin: Strassman, 1984). Psychotic episodes may also be elicited by withdrawal states from opiates, sedatives and alcohol. Brief psychotic episodes with visual and tactile hallucinations (e.g. triggered by cocaine), instead of auditory hallucinations and reasonable functioning between episodes, suggest repeated abuse. (2) The presence of negative symptoms in schizophrenia, in cannabis and opioid abuse (apathy, psychomotor retardation), as well as in amphetamine (including phencyclidine and ecstasy), and cocaine withdrawal (fatigue, psychomotor retardation) (Dixon et al., 1991). (3) The presence of disorganization symptoms both in schizophrenia (Liddle, 1987) and in cannabis abuse (disorganized speech, inappropriate affect) (Thomas, 1993). (4) The decline in social and occupational functioning in schizophrenia and the persistent problems caused by recurrent substance abuse during adolescence and young adulthood, with the person failing to perform adequately at work, school and home, inflicting harm on themselves, and suffering damaging interpersonal relations. Physical signs and symptoms of intoxication which develop within a few hours after the ingestion of substances can help to differentiate toxic psychosis from the psychotic, negative and other symptoms of schizophrenia (APA, 1994). These are described in Tables 13.1 and 13.2. Table 13.1 records symptoms and signs and the drugs with which they are associated, whilst Table 13.2 delineates the *comparative effects* of substance intoxication on *specific* physical signs and symptoms.

Initial assessment of the patient with the dual diagnoses of substance abuse and schizophrenia, involves both the taking of a history and the conducting of a physical examination. Moreover, information needs to be obtained not only from the patient but also from at least one relative, as well as from former treatment agencies. This procedure will help determine whether schizophrenia was apparent (*a*) before the onset of substance abuse, (*b*) followed a period of several weeks to months of substance abstinence, or (*c*) emerged during a period of increasing usage. One indicator of schizophrenia which is independent of substance abuse is persistent psychotic ('revealed psychosis'), negative or disorganization symptomatology, remaining after weeks. Financial problems and homelessness are also frequently associated with significant substance abuse in schizophrenic patients (Mueser et al., 1990). Last, but not least, laboratory findings are useful tools in drawing a distinction between the two conditions. Laboratory tests are particularly important, since self reports about substance abuse are often unreliable.

Substance abuse and the course of schizophrenia

Clinicians should be aware of substance abuse among schizophrenic patients, since substance abuse is associated with non-compliance and treatment resistance. Young male patients with recent onset schizophrenia may be particularly prone to use drugs in an attempt to self-

Table 13.1. *Symptoms or signs and the drugs with which they are associated*

Symptoms or signs	Drugs
Tachycardia	Cannabis, LSD, PCP, amphetamine, cocaine, MDMA, psilocybin
Hypertension	Amphetamine, cocaine, LSD, PCP, MDMA, psilocybin
Increased respiratory rate	Cocaine (in severe intoxication: depressed)
Mydriasis	Amphetamine, cocaine, LSD, PCP, MDMA, psilocybin
Tremor	Cannabis, LSD
Dry mouth	Cannabis, LSD
Increased perspiration	Amphetamine, cocaine, LSD
Conjunctival injection	Cannabis
Blurred vision	LSD
Nausea	Amphetamines, LSD, PCP, MDMA
Lost appetite	Amphetamines, cocaine

Table 13.2. *Comparative effects of substance intoxication on specific physical signs and symptoms*

		Stimulants		Hallucinogenic-related substances	
	Cannabis	Amphetamines	Cocaine	LSD	PCP
Heart rate	↑		↑	↑	↑
Blood pressure		↑	↑	↑	↑
Respiratory rate			↑	↑	↑
Pupillary dilatation	−	+	+	+	+
Tremor	+	+	+	+	+/−
Dry mouth	+	−	−	+	−
Perspiration	−	↑	↑	↑	−
Conjunctival injection	+	−	−	−	−

↑ = increased; + = symptom present; − = symptom absent.

medicate their psychotic, negative, depressive and other symptoms, or they may attempt to alleviate the consequences of the disorder, e.g. homelessness, by being admitted to a psychiatric hospital. A small group of schizophrenic patients abuse heroin and other opiates for their antipsychotic properties, although alcohol and sedatives may also reduce the intensity or discomfort of psychotic symptoms (Millman, 1982). Methadone has been used in a study with treatment-resistant patients; although there was a decrease in psychotic symptomatology in the acute phase of treatment, tolerance occurred with chronic use (Brizer et al., 1985).

Psychotic and schizophrenic patients also use cannabis and cocaine or speed, although these are psychotomimetic and are associated with marked increases in readmission due to psychotic relapse (LeDuc & Mittleman, 1995). Patients may attempt to take control of the hallucinations or delusions by using substances which create or enhance them, or distance themselves from their symptoms. We have noted that some patients want to avoid being stigmatized as 'psychotic' or 'schizophrenic' or as a 'psychiatric' patient. They may prefer to be regarded as an 'addict', instead of being considered as 'mad' or as a 'lunatic'.

Moreover, as Mueser et al. (1990) have mentioned, drug abuse seems likely to be determined by the availability of illicit drugs; patients will often use the drug available - even if it means feeling worse! Despite the subjective relief substance abuse may provide to patients with recent onset schizophrenia, it can have negative and deleterious effects on psychotic illness, such as exacerbating symptomatology, precipitating psychotic relapses and rehospitalizations, and increasing suicidality and violence (Smith & Hucker, 1994). It can also undermine psychosocial functioning, cause financial problems and homelessness, and can result in higher service utilization (Mueser et al., 1990).

Cannabis abuse and the early course of schizophrenia

In 1845 Moreau de Tours, a doctor working in the French Bicetre asylum, described the effects of the acute and chronic intoxication produced by cannabis (Moreau de Tours, 1845). He observed a great diversity of psychological phenomena such as euphoria, intensified hearing, irresistible impulses, anxiety, dissociation of ideas, avolition, disorientation in time and place and, with higher doses, delusions and hallucinations. The manifold presentations of symptoms and signs led him to develop the first 'model' for an experimental psychosis. Since then, studies examining the relationship between cannabis use and psychotic disorders, i.e. schizophrenia, have consisted of case series, in which possible relationships between cannabis abuse and psychotic symptoms were difficult to test. In a few case-control studies, psychotic symptoms were evaluated retrospectively, using hospital files (Negrete et al., 1986). Also, the observation period was typically of only one week's duration, and schizophrenic symptoms were evaluated once, on a cross-sectional basis (Peralta & Cuesta, 1992).

Since then, studies have found the following: (1) an increase of psychotic (positive) symptoms in cannabis-abusing schizophrenic patients (Chopra & Smith, 1974; Cleghorn et al., 1991; Martinez-Arevalo, Calcedo-Ordoñez & Varo-Prieto, 1994; Treffert, 1978; Weil, 1970), or no difference in psychotic symptoms in comparison to non-cannabis-abusing schizophrenic populations (Knudsen & Vilmar, 1984); (2) a decrease in negative symptoms; in cannabis-abusing patients fewer negative symptoms such as affective flattening have been found (Knudsen & Vilmar, 1984).

In the first large prospective cohort study with a relatively young sample (Linszen et al., 1994), conducted over the course of a year using monthly BPRS assessments, the relationship between cannabis abuse and the symptomatic course of recent-onset schizophrenia and related disorders was examined. Twenty-four cannabis-abusing patients were compared with 69 non-abusers. The mean age when they started abusing cannabis was 16 years and the mean duration of abuse before admission was 3.9 years. All but one of the cannabis-abusing patients commenced their habit at least one year prior to their first psychotic symptoms (mean = 3 years, range = 0–7 years). Within the group of 24 cannabis abusers, 13 heavy abusing patients (54%) could be identified, this group being defined in terms of using more than one cigarette per day. The mild abusing group ($n = 11$) consumed between one cigarette a week and one a day. Hard drug abuse was rare (two patients used cocaine and ecstasy; one of these patients used hard drugs sporadically in combination with heavy cannabis abuse). The most relevant finding of this prospective study in patients with recent-onset schizophrenia and schizophrenia-related disorders, was the occurrence of significantly more, and earlier, psychotic relapses or exacerbations in the total group of cannabis-abusing patients ($n = 24$) over a 12-month period. When a distinction was made with respect to the intensity of abuse, it appeared that it was the particularly heavy cannabis-abusing patients who relapsed more frequently and earlier. This finding was not confounded by exposure to alcohol and/or any other (psychoactive) drugs, nor by differences in antipsychotic medication compliance and dosage. Two additional findings indicated a possible causal relationship between cannabis and psychotic relapse. First, 14 out of 24 cannabis-abusing patients reported an immediate increase in psychotic symptoms after resuming cannabis abuse; 13 of these 14 patients were clinically in remission when they reported the increase of psychotic symptoms. Six patients noted no such increase, and only one patient reported a decrease in psychotic symptoms when abusing cannabis.

The relationship between cannabis abuse and the symptom dimensions of recent-onset schizophrenic disorders was also examined over a 12-month period. Positive, negative, disorganization and depressive symptom dimensions were analysed for the same group of cannabis-abusing patients when compared with non-abusing patients. No effect was found for the positive syndrome ($p = 0.43$), the negative syndrome ($p = 0.23$), or the depression syndrome ($p = 0.27$). However, a main effect for cannabis abuse was found for the course of the symptoms of the disorganization dimension ($p = 0.01$), with the scores tending to increase over the 12-month period ($p < 0.01$). In the mild-abusing group, symptoms of anxiety and depression tended to be less present than in the non- and heavy-abusing group. Therefore, the self-medication hypothesis was only supported for patients with mild cannabis abuse. The existence of an amotivational syndrome, with an increase of negative symptoms in the cannabis-abusing group of young schizophrenic patients, was not tenable, particularly for the heavy cannabis-abusing group.

Treatment of schizophrenia and substance abuse

Clarification of the relationship of the two disorders could help us develop practical applications for the treatment of patients with substance abuse and schizophrenia or other psychotic disorders. Although the effectiveness of a treatment programme for patients with schizophrenia and substance abuse has yet to be established, some of the ingredients of such specialized treatment programmes have been defined. First, treatment of substance abuse in schizophrenia is probably best provided by psychiatric intervention programmes, rather than by specialized drug or alcohol programmes (Minkoff, 1989; Osher & Kofoed, 1989). Potentially, the latter programmes may be too stressful for patients with schizophrenia (Ridgely, Goldman & Willenbring, 1990).

A period of inpatient care may be necessary to clarify the diagnosis and to facilitate detoxification *and* treatment of the acute psychosis (Smith & Hucker, 1994). Initial treatment should be supportive, with the patient being provided with a warm, safe environment, and with frequent reassurance that the perceptions, thoughts and feelings experienced by the patient are a function of the drug use and will pass.

Substance-abusing patients with schizophrenia may have a distinctively different response to treatment than other schizophrenic patients, because substance abuse can affect pharmacotherapy and treatment compliance (Siris, 1990). Dually diagnosed patients may be more accepting of, and responsive to, new atypical antipsychotic medication because of their reduced level of extrapyramidal side-effects. Benzodiazepines should be administered to alleviate anxiety during drug-free periods and in order to differentiate between drug-related psychotic episodes and uncomplicated functional psychotic disorders. During the initial phase, neuroleptics may exacerbate psychotic symptoms, or even cause delirium through their anticholinergic side-effects; if there are signs of intoxication or recent heavy use, neuroleptics may be reserved for the later stages of treatment. If the psychotic symptoms persist after several days to weeks of abstinence, the symptomatology should be treated as being essentially similar to functional psychotic disorders. It is likely that persistent psychotic symptoms are a function of a continuing vulnerability and will probably not resolve spontaneously.

Promising ingredients of pilot psychosocial intervention projects seem to be as follows: since patients with schizophrenia tend to deny their substance abuse, they should be persuaded that they have a drug or alcohol problem. Psychoeducation should be provided for patients and families about the course and complications of both schizophrenia and substance abuse disorders and the detrimental effects of substance abuse. Abstinence from alcohol and street drugs should be the goal of treatment, and techniques such as motivational interviewing may be useful. Comorbid patients should be actively engaged, with assertive and continuous case management being given even more emphasis than with the non-abusing schizophrenic patient. This is because substance-abusing schizophrenic patients often fail to comply with inpatient or outpatient treatment (Fariello & Scheidt, 1989). Structured treatment programmes should include a combination of group and individual work (Smith & Hucker, 1994); the latter should include training in relaxation, social skills, assertiveness and problem-solving. The development of appropriate attitudes and avoidance skills towards drug abuse should be an additional focus of case work. Practical advice should be provided along with assistance to overcome social problems such as homelessness, financial difficulties and law breaking.

Conclusion

Further studies are needed to continue the systematic study of the relationship between substance abuse and schizophrenia. Questions such as 'How does cannabis use influence the onset of psychotic disorder?', 'Do variable amounts of substance consumption exert differential effects on the symptoms of schizophrenic patients?', or 'Do positive consequences such as the relief of psychotic or negative symptoms, occur with some level of substance use?' need to be answered.

Clarification of the relationship between schizophrenia and substance abuse would have both the theoretical benefits of elucidating the mechanisms of onset and relapse of psychotic and negative symptoms, as well as having practical import for the treatment of substance abusers with schizophrenia or related psychotic disorders. These studies should include quantitative estimations of substance abuse repeated over time, laboratory confirmation of single- or poly-substance abuse, along with repeated assessments of dose–response effects as soon as possible after abuse in substance-abusing patients.

In Amsterdam, a specific in- and outpatient treatment programme which involves peer-based support seems effective in preventing patients from dropping out of treatment. Some of these young cannabis-abusing patients manage to stop their habit once they are able to relate increases in their psychotic symptomatology as being directly due to their cannabis abuse. Atypical antipsychotic medication may reduce the need for patients to abuse substances in order to alleviate the side-effects of typical antipsychotic medication. Integrated psychosocial treatment programmes for substance abuse and schizophrenia need to be developed and evaluated as a matter of urgency.

Acknowledgments

The cannabis study was funded in part by Grant 28–1241 from the 'Praeventiefonds'. The authors thank J. Verhoeff MD, J. B. van Borssum Waalkes MD and Professor B. Gersons MD, PhD, for their support of the study. The authors are also grateful to Professor Henry Jackson PhD, of the University of Melbourne, for his motivational support.

References

American Psychiatric Association (1994). *Diagnostic and Statistical Manual of Mental Disorders*, 4th edn Rev. (DSM-IV-R). Washington, DC: American Psychiatric Association.

Andreasson, S., Allebeck, P., Engström, A. & Rydberg, U. (1987). Cannabis and schizophrenia. A longitudinal study of Swedish conscripts. *Lancet*, **2**, 1483–6.

Barbee, J. G., Clark, P. D., Crapanzano, M. S., Heintz, G. C. & Kehoe, C. E. (1989). Alcohol and substance abuse among schizophrenic patients presenting to an emergency psychiatric service. *Journal of Nervous and Mental Diseases*, **177**, 400–7.

Breakey, W. R., Goodell, H., Lorenz, P. C. & McHugh, P. R. (1974). Hallucinogenic drugs as precipitants of schizophrenia. *Psychological Medicine*, **4**, 255–61.

Brizer, D. A., Hartman, N., Sweeney, J. & Millman, R. B. (1985). Effects of methadone plus neuroleptics in treatment-resistant chronic paranoid schizophrenia. *American Journal of Psychiatry*, **142**, 1106–7.

Caton, C. L. M., Gralnick, A. & Bender, S. (1989). Young chronic patients and substance abuse. *Hospital and Community Psychiatry*, **40**, 1037–40.
Chopra, G. S. & Smith, J. W. (1974). Psychotic reactions following cannabis use in East Indians. *Archives of General Psychiatry*, **30**, 24–7.
Cleghorn, J. M., Kaplan, R. D., Szechtman, B., Szechtman, H., Brown, G. M. & Franco, S. (1991). Cannabis abuse and schizophrenia: effect on symptoms but not on neurocognitive function. *Journal of Clinical Psychiatry*, **52**, 26–30.
Cuffel, B. J., Heithoff, K. A. & Lawson, W. (1993). Correlates of patterns of substance abuse among patients with schizophrenia. *Hospital and Community Psychiatry*, **44**, 247–51.
Dixon, L., Haas, G., Weiden, P. J., Sweeney, J. & Frances A. J. (1991). Drug abuse in schizophrenic patients: clinical correlates and reasons for use. *American Journal of Psychiatry*, **148**, 224–30.
Drake, R. E., McHugo, G. J. & Noordsey, D. L. (1993). Treatment of alcoholism among schizophrenic outpatients: 4 year outcomes. *American Journal of Psychiatry*, **150**, 328–9.
Fariello, D. & Scheidt, S. (1989). Clinical case management of the dually diagnosed patient. *Hospital and Community Psychiatry*, **40**, 1065–7.
Hall, W. & Hando, J. (1994). Route of administration and adverse effects of amphetamine use in young adults in Sydney, Australia. *Drug and Alcohol Review*, **13**, 277–84.
Hambrecht, M. & Häfner, H. (1996). Substance abuse and the onset of schizophrenia. *Biological Psychiatry*, **5**, 56–62.
Jackson, H. J., McGorry, P. D. & Dudgeon, P. (1995). Prodromal symptoms of schizophrenia in first-episode psychosis: prevalence and specificity. *Comprehensive Psychiatry*, **36**, 241–50.
Knudsen, P. & Vilmar, T. (1984). Cannabis and neuroleptic agents in schizophrenia. *Acta Psychiatrica Scandinavica*, **69**, 162–74.
LeDuc, P. A. & Mittleman, G. (1995). Schizophrenia and psychostimulant abuse: a review and re-analysis of clinical evidence. *Psychopharmacology*, **121**, 407–27.
Liddle, P. (1987). The symptoms of chronic schizophrenia. A re-examination of the positive–negative dichotomy. *British Journal of Psychiatry*, **151**, 145–51.
Linszen, D. H., Dingemans, P. M. & Lenior, M. E. (1994). Cannabis abuse and the course of recent-onset schizophrenic disorders. *Archives of General Psychiatry*, **51**, 273–9.
Loebel, A. D., Lieberman, J. A., Alvir, J. M. J., Mayerhoff, D. I., Geisler, S. H. & Szymanski, S. R. (1992). Duration of psychosis and outcome in first episode schizophrenia. *American Journal of Psychiatry*, **149**, 1183–8.
Martinez-Arevalo, M. J., Calcedo-Ordoñez, A. & Varo-Prieto, J. R. (1994). Cannabis consumption as prognostic factor in schizophrenia. *British Journal of Psychiatry*, **164**, 679–84.
McLellan, A. T., Woody, G. E. & O'Brien, C. P. (1979). Development of psychiatric illness in drug abusers: possible role of drug preference. *New England Journal of Medicine*, **301**, 1310–4.
Millman, R. B. (1982). The provision of opioid therapy to the mentally ill:

conceptual and practical considerations. In *Opioids in Mental Illness: Theories, Clinical Observations, and Treatment Possibilities*, ed. K. Vereby, pp. 178–85. New York: The New York Academy of Sciences.

Minkoff, K. (1989). An integrated treatment model for dual diagnosis of psychosis and addiction. *Hospital and Community Psychiatry*, **40**, 1031–6.

Moreau de Tours, J. (1845). *Du Hachisch et de L'aliénation Mentale*. Paris: Collection 'Esquirol'.

Mueser, K. T., Yarnold, P. R., Levinson, D. F., Singh, H., Bellack, A. S., Kee, K., Morrison, R. L. & Yadalam, K. G. (1990). Prevalence of substance abuse in schizophrenia: demographic and clinical correlates. *Schizophrenia Bulletin*, **16**, 31–56.

Negrete, J. C., Knapp, W. P., Douglas, D. E. & Smith, B. (1986). Cannabis affects the severity of schizophrenic symptoms: results of a clinical survey. *Psychological Medicine*, **16**, 515–20.

National Household Survey on Drug Abuse (1985). *National Institute on Drug Abuse*. Rockville, Maryland: US Department of Health and Human Services.

Osher, F. C. & Kofoed, L. L. (1989). Treatment of patients with psychiatric and psychoactive substance abuse disorders. *Hospital and Community Psychiatry*, **40**, 1025–30.

Peralta, V. & Cuesta, M. J. (1992). Influence of cannabis abuse on schizophrenic psychopathology. *Acta Psychiatrica Scandinavica*, **85**, 127–30.

Regier, D. A., Farmer, M. E. & Rae, D. S. (1990). Co-morbidity of mental disorders with alcohol and other drug abuse. Results from the Epidemiological Catchment Area (ECA) study. *Journal of the American Medical Association*, **264**, 2511–18.

Richard, M. L., Liskow, B. I. & Perry, P. J. (1985). Recent psychostimulant use in hospitalized schizophrenics. *Journal of Clinical Psychiatry*, **46**, 79–83.

Ridgely, M. S., Goldman, H. H. & Willenbring, M. (1990). Barriers to the care of persons with dual diagnosis: organisational and financial issues. *Schizophrenia Bulletin*, **16**, 123–32.

Satel, S. L., Southwick, S. M. & Gawin, F. H. (1991). Clinical features of cocaine induced paranoia. *American Journal of Psychiatry*, **148**, 495–8.

Schneier, F. R. & Siris, S. G. (1987). A review of psychoactive substance use and abuse in schizophrenia: patterns of drug choice. *Journal of Nervous and Mental Disease*, **175**, 641–52.

Siris, S. G. (1990). Pharmacological treatment of substance abusing schizophrenic patients. *Schizophrenia Bulletin*, **16**, 111–22.

Smith, J. & Hucker, S. (1994). Schizophrenia and substance abuse. *British Journal of Psychiatry*, **165**, 13–21.

Steele, T. D., McCann, U. D. & Ricaurte, G. A. (1994). 3,4–Methylenedioxymethamphetamine (MDMA), 'ecstasy': pharmacology and toxicology in animals and humans. *Addiction*, **89**, 539–45.

Strassman, R. J. (1984). Adverse reactions to psychedelic drugs: a review of the literature. *Journal of Nervous and Mental Diseases*, **172**, 577–82.

Test, M. A., Wallisch, L. & Allness, D. J. (1989). Substance use in young adults with schizophrenic disorders. *Schizophrenia Bulletin*, **15**, 465–76.

Thomas, H. (1993). Psychiatric symptoms in cannabis users. *British Journal of Psychiatry*, **163**, 141–5.

Thornicroft, G. (1990). Cannabis and psychosis: is there epidemiological evidence for an association? *British Journal of Psychiatry*, **157**, 25–33.

Treffert, D. A. (1978). Marijuana use in schizophrenia: a clear hazard. *American Journal of Psychiatry*, **135**, 1213–15.

Van der Does, A. J. W., Dingemans, P. M. A. J., Linszen, D. H., Nugter, M. A. & Scholte, W. F. (1995). Dimensions and subtypes of recent-onset schizophrenia: a longitudinal analysis. *Journal of Nervous and Mental Diseases*, **183**, 681–8.

Weil, A. T. (1970). Adverse reactions to marijuana, classification and suggested treatment. *New England Journal of Medicine*, **282**, 997–1000.

World Health Organization. (1973). *Report on the International Pilot Study of Schizophrenia*. Geneva: World Health Organization.

Wright, H. H., Cole, E. A., Batey, S. R. & Hanna, K. (1988). Phencyclidine induced psychosis: eight year follow-up of ten cases. *Southern Medical Journal*, **81**, 565–8.

14

Family intervention in early psychosis

JOHN GLEESON, HENRY J. JACKSON, HEATHER STAVELY
AND PETER BURNETT

Rationale for a preventive model in family work

Young people throughout the western world are faced with increasing rates of unemployment, together with rising costs in education and accommodation (Gunn, 1997). These pressures, as reflected in higher numbers of young people delaying the move from the parental home (Gunn, 1997), have arguably prolonged the final steps towards independence. Of course, any serious illness during this period can significantly compound the challenges involved in the transition to adulthood and prolong the caregiving role for family members.

The threat to the process of individuation is clearly exacerbated with the onset of psychosis (McGorry & Singh, 1995) which has a median age of onset during the late teenage years (Kosky & Hardy, 1992; Regier et al., 1984). However, 'developmental stagnation' may precede the acute illness, since the prodromal phase has been associated with deterioration in functioning (Häfner et al., 1995; Jackson, McGorry & Dudgeon, 1995; Jones et al., 1993; McGorry et al., 1996; Yung et al., 1996). It is not surprising, therefore, that 63% of consecutive new patients to the EPPIC programme between 1992 and 1996 were residing with their parents (Early Psychosis Prevention and Intervention Centre, 1997). This figure is at the upper end of published data which suggests that the proportion of adult patients living with their relatives, ranges from 30 to 65% (Solomon & Draine, 1995).

A further line of evidence suggests that families are critical caregivers for patients suffering psychosis: Jackson and Edwards (1992), in reviewing the social network and schizophrenia literature, concluded that with increasing length of illness, social network size and support diminishes, and that it tends to shrink in a fairly predictable sequence, with friends and acquaintances dropping out first, leaving the patient increasingly reliant on the family unit for support. Ultimately, and where increasing chronicity and continuing illness occur, sometimes even the family unit is unable to tolerate the demands imposed on them, and this leaves the patient restricted to receiving support from professionals. Of more serious concern is the evidence that this deterioration commences well prior to the first episode and can happen very rapidly (Häfner et al., 1995; Jones et al., 1993). This process is more likely to accelerate if the cohesion of the family is seriously threatened by other influences, e.g. physical and sexual abuse, poverty, substance abuse, and unemployment. Another factor likely to impact on family burden is the duration of untreated psychosis (DUP) described by Loebel et al. (1992) and McGlashan and Johannessen (1996), although prospective data are required formally to confirm this relationship between deterioration in network size and support, and symptoms prior to the first episode of psychosis.

This pattern of erosion of the social network, particularly the peer group, leads to a 'developmental reversal' whereby, instead of the patient becoming less reliant on the family and more reliant on others, e.g. the peer group (Levinson, 1986), the exact reverse occurs. This puts the patient out of step developmentally with his or her peers and subject to family pressure to be 'developmentally appropriate'. Consequently, the patient may miss out on opportunities to develop generalized skills, e.g. social competency and intimacy, as well as skills in one or more specialized domains, e.g. leisure pursuits and vocational development.

It is therefore a great advantage for the family unit to remain functional in order to support the patient and prevent further deterioration, by providing the patient with a safe environment to convalesce, gain a 'breathing space', and 'woodshed' their skills (Davidson & Strauss, 1995; Strauss, 1989, 1994). To achieve this without derailing the normal developmental process of individuation and separation from the family of origin represents a major challenge. In other words, the rationale for family work in first-episode psychosis extends beyond the support of parents, siblings and partners as primary carers since it is an integral component of the preventive approach to the treatment of first-episode psychosis (McGorry & Singh, 1995). This paradigm postulates that intensive intervention which is initiated as early as possible in the course of psychosis lessens the likelihood of long-term disability and secondary morbidity, such as depression, anxiety and the symptoms of posttraumatic stress (Birchwood, McGorry & Jackson, 1997; Falloon et al., 1996; McGlashan & Johannessen, 1996; McGorry et al., 1996). Support for the model has been provided by three strands of evidence and, although they have been detailed in earlier chapters of this book, they are briefly reiterated at this juncture. First, long-term outcome studies have shown a wide variability in the level of long-term disability, which challenges the assumptions of inevitable deterioration and disability which underpin the neo-Kraepelinian 'disease' concept of schizophrenia (Carpenter & Strauss, 1991; Harding, Zubin & Strauss, 1987). Second, studies of first-episode patients have indicated that significant delays in accessing appropriate treatment, which are associated with poorer outcomes, occur commonly after the initial onset of illness (Lieberman et al., 1993; Loebel et al., 1992). Third, a range of studies, examining neurobiological, symptomatic and functional outcomes, has indicated that the rate of deterioration is most rapid during the first two years of illness (see Chapter 9) (Birchwood & Macmillan, 1993; McGlashan & Johannessen, 1996), highlighting the need for intensive intervention during this so-called 'critical period' (see Chapter 9) (Birchwood & Macmillan, 1993; Birchwood et al., 1997).

Summary

These lines of evidence converge to suggest: that the family can play an important role in providing a supportive recovery environment for the patient during, as well as following, the first episode of illness by allowing the patient 'time-out', during which to recoup and gather strength to venture back into the world; that a message of balanced optimism needs to be communicated to the parents which indicates that, even if the early course of illness is problematic, there is a good chance of improvement; and that this initial psychotic episode constitutes a critical opportunity for the family to receive support, and to support the patient.

Further points emerge if one adopts a stress–vulnerability framework and accepts that the family is the group which typically provides most support to the patient. First, family work provides an opportunity to ameliorate stress which arises from within the family context and which potentially interacts with enduring patient vulnerability to exacerbate symptoms or trigger subsequent episodes of psychosis (Nuechterlein et al., 1992; Nuechterlein, Snyder & Mintz, 1992). The second point is more tentative, namely that family interventions matched to the needs of families during the early phases of illness prevent or reduce the severity of family morbidity including depression, anxiety and complicated grief reactions. Such interventions may also reduce the risk of deterioration in the family patterns of relating evident in more chronic populations. A related notion is the need to identify carefully the treatment-resistant or frequent relapsing patient early in the illness course, because the pattern of illness erodes the family's ability to support him. It may be helpful to postulate a closed-loop system in which family pathology interacts in complex ways with the pathology of the individual, exacerbating both symptoms and burden, and generally 'raising the temperature' for all concerned. Currently, this model remains an empirically untested proposition, although it is consonant with the recursive self-sustaining systemic constructs discussed elsewhere (Kavanagh, 1996; Kelly, 1995).

Empirical research with 'first-episode families'

It is important to state clearly from the outset that the empirical work with first-episode families has been limited. One starting point can be to consider principles gleaned and extrapolated from family research conducted with more chronic patients and their relatives although, as with other aspects of treatment, this can be risky. Currently, the two largest areas comprising this body of family research have been the 'expressed emotion' (EE) and 'family burden' literatures. With regard to the EE research, this has been concerned with two topics, namely, the association of EE with relapse and more particularly the ability of EE to predict relapse; and, secondly, working with families with the twin expectations of directly reducing patient relapse or symptom exacerbations by changing the family climate, and of helping families to cope with the illness of their relative. The family burden literature has a much shorter history than the EE literature. We examine each in turn.

Expressed emotion

Expressed emotion and relapse

Studies examining levels of emotional tension in families of patients have focussed virtually exclusively on the study of EE, an empirical construct which has been defined in terms of one or more of three subcomponents – the expression of hostility, emotional overinvolvement, and the number of critical comments directed toward the patient. At the end of a nine-month period subsequent to the initial EE assessment, approximately 50% of patients in the high EE group have relapsed compared with 21% of patients in the low EE group (see Bebbington & Kuipers, 1994, for an aggregate analysis; see also Kavanagh, 1992). This finding has held up across culture and gender, with the major moderating variables being the amount of time spent with family members, and use of regular antipsychotic medication (Bebbington & Kuipers, 1994; Kavanagh, 1992).

However, the relevance of the EE construct to first-episode patients is much less clear. In particular, the insufficient attention paid to issues such as length or phase of illness and the period of untreated illness prior to first presentation means it is difficult to extrapolate from these findings to the first-episode population (see Macmillan et al., 1986). Therefore, it is necessary to examine the EE literature which deals with first-episode patients.

Predictive power of EE in first-episode families

As previously stated, both EE and intervention studies have reported on patients with established schizophrenic illnesses of varying durations, but only a small number of studies have examined the power of EE to predict relapse in first-episode patients. Stirling et al. (1991) interviewed key relatives of 33 recent-onset psychotic patients with early onset being defined as within the previous two years. The authors found no association between household EE and relapse rate at 12 months' follow-up. An examination of the EE data reveals that the authors found a much higher occurrence of 'emotional overinvolvement' (EOI) and a much lower incidence of criticism than reported in the bulk of the studies dealing with patients with established illness (see Kavanagh, 1992). It is possible that this finding reflects families' reliance upon 'emotion-focussed coping' which occurs after all available 'problem-focussed' strategies are found wanting. In short, the family are faced with a significant crisis which elicits an appropriate emotional response.

Rund et al. (1995) found no correlation between EE and relapse but the sample only comprised 12 patients. Barrelet et al. (1990) found a significant association between EE and relapse in 36 'first-admission' patients, although the results failed to reach significance when only the patients who were living with their relatives were included.

The median age of the Barrelet et al. sample was 24.5 years compared with epidemiological studies which indicate that the median age of onset is approximately 19 years (Regier et al., 1984); so there exists an issue pertaining to the representativeness of the sample.

Huguelet et al. (1995) attempted to address the issue of the relationship between EE and relapse across time by prospectively monitoring 44 first-admission patients with a diagnosis of schizophrenia. Patients living with high EE relatives presented significantly more often with a premorbid personality disorder, a slower onset, more substance abuse, and a poorer premorbid adaptation than those living with low EE relatives. EE status did not correlate with relapse until the third year of follow-up. This finding suggests that EE during the initial two-year 'critical period' is not predictive of relapse. A major weakness of the study was the 34% attrition rate, which allows for the interpretation that the sample became progressively more representative of the subset of first-episode clients who develop prolonged psychosis.

Given that the duration of untreated psychotic symptoms (DUP) was not directly assessed in the above study (Huguelet et al., 1995), it remains possible that 'slower onset' was confounded with DUP. In fact, it has been suggested (Parker, Johnston & Hayward, 1988) that high EE might reflect a response to the period of decline in functioning of the schizophrenic member. Yet almost invariably, researchers have failed to measure the duration of untreated symptoms prior to first admission, thus raising questions about the influence of pre-treatment chronicity within the sample (Barrelet et al., 1990; Rund et al., 1995). This interpretation is supported by a first-episode study (Macmillan et al., 1986) which found a positive correlation between EE and relapse, but the authors determined that this relationship was explained by the duration of untreated illness and the use of antipsychotic medication. However, Mintz et al. (1989) showed that high EE parents overestimate the duration of illness, which casts doubt on this assertion.

Nuechterlein et al. (1992) attempted to address the question of whether the relationship between EE and relapse could be accounted for by other variables in the first-admission population. They recruited a 'mixed' sample of 43 consecutive first-admission and recent-onset schizophrenic patients with a mean age of 22.7 years. Within one month of admission a significant relative was assessed for EE. Of the 31 patients from high-EE families, 39% had relapsed by 12 months according to their scores on the BPRS, while none of the 12 patients from the low-EE families had relapsed. The authors conducted a number of path analyses to test a range of possible interpretations of this outcome, concluding that the data fitted two models. The first model suggested that living with the patient during the period preceding admission, which was more likely to occur if the patient had an earlier age of onset of illness, may have partly accounted for the development of high EE. A separate analysis suggested that the severity of the illness may have accounted for the development of high EE, early onset, and living at home. Unfortunately, DUP was not measured, leaving open the possibility that DUP was the underlying latent or encrypted variable, which is consistent with other findings that DUP is related to severity of illness (Loebel et al., 1992). (See also the discussions by Halford, Schweitzer & Varghese (1991) and Rosenfarb et al. (1995), concerning the directions of causation between family environment and patient symptom level and/or adjustment).

Summary and conclusions about the EE literature

In summary, the evidence for a relationship between high EE and relapse during the critical period of first-episode psychosis is equivocal. Further studies are required to test the hypothesis that DUP may account for both the emotional response of relatives and the course of illness. High EE at first onset may be partially indicative of a short-term emotional response on the part of caregivers facing a significant crisis. Both may share a relationship with relapse because *both* factors derive at least partially from DUP. Furthermore, EE at three years may be more reflective of longer-term stress in family members which may share a more direct relationship with relapse if family members have increasing difficulty supporting their relatives emotionally as the illness progresses. In terms of the needs of first-episode families, the Macmillan et al. (1986) study supports the aforementioned interpretation highlighting that first-episode families, along with the patients themselves, require crisis support and assistance in understanding the early signs of psychosis and accessing appropriate treatment for their relative as soon as possible, so that the duration of untreated symptoms can be minimized. If and when the illness progresses into prolonged psychosis, most families will benefit from early identification of patterns of communication related to relapse, so that the efficacy of psychoeducation regarding the management of interpersonal conflict can be maximized. It also seems logical, since 'EE' has been accepted as influencing the course of a whole range of disorders, that it may be more useful to demystify it and break the problem down into more widely interpretable elements, e.g. coping, distress, burden and burnout.

In conclusion, we submit that new methodologies need to be adopted to test squarely the relevance of the EE concept to the first-episode population. Repeated measures designs need to be conducted over lengthy time periods. Using larger sample sizes than has hitherto been the case, statistical models such as latent growth models, structural equational modelling and random effect regression models, would permit the testing of various alternative models of how symptoms, functioning, and premorbid characteristics interact with one another over time, and would capture whatever data exist at each time point, pragmatically allowing for the fact that data may be missing for particular individuals at various time points. The study by Nuechterlein et al. (1992) provides some approximation of what we have in mind, although the sample size was small for this kind of model, which in all likelihood would not prove to be particularly robust. Furthermore, those authors assumed a direction of influence with their path analyses, rather than examining a larger number of competing models.

As for many fields of investigation in psychosis, significant further methodological advances can be made. Sample sizes need to be increased, and power calculations performed prior to the conduct of studies. Representative samples, not convenience samples, are needed for these studies. Also, measures assessing quality of life and functioning are needed, not just symptom and relapse measures. The course of the illness prior to first contact must be fully documented, as must the premorbid characteristics of the person and their functioning. If this were carried to its logical conclusion then, instead of being reliant on retrospective reports of pre-first contact functioning, the enlisting and assessing of prodromal patients and their families would constitute the superior methodology, permitting more rigorous mapping and documentation of the 'pre-illness' family climate (e.g. Yung et al., 1996). It would also permit the examination of an important thesis currently unfalsifiable using current designs and samples, but which perhaps covertly informs some clinicians' approach to family work; this is the view that the EE construct may represent longstanding premorbid high EE in one or both members of the parental dyad, so that if EE is not truly aetiological then it may, at least for some families, constitute a precipitant for the emergence of initial psychotic disturbance in a family member.

Family burden and first-episode psychosis

A second body of research has examined the impact or 'burden' of the psychosis upon family members. Surprisingly little research has focussed upon the distress or burden experienced by families during the early stages of illness, but it has been assumed that relatives experience shock, confusion, guilt about having caused the illness, and fear about the future (Halford, 1992; Hatfield, 1978; Hatfield & Lefley, 1993; Maurin & Boyd, 1990; Mueser et al., 1996; see also Jackson, Robinson & Pica, 1996). With regard to psychopathology, Salleh (1994) found that 23% of 210 carers developed neurotic disorders nearly half of whom had neurotic depression.

Most of the work has been undertaken with chronic populations and the data may not be extrapolated easily to the first-episode population. Generally, the findings with chronic populations suggest that poorer coping and greater objective or subjective burden for family members is associated with dual diagnoses (e.g. substance abuse), high EE, increasing negative symptoms, behaviours related to low levels of activity and poor self-care (Clarke, 1994; Gopinath & Chaturvedi, 1993; Jackson, Smith & McGorry, 1990; Smith et al., 1993; Vettro et al., 1994), more contact (Winefield & Harvey, 1994), and increasing levels of disturbance (Winefield & Harvey, 1993). By contrast, patients with greater self-care and communication skills were regarded as more enjoyable to live with (Winefield & Harvey, 1993). Other research has indicated that burden may emerge as problems with individuation become more evident following the first episode; for example, Pickett, Cook & Cohler (1994) interviewed 123 mothers and 99 fathers of 134 17–40-year-old children, most with a diagnosis of schizophrenia, and found that 'off-timedness' of development was associated with stronger burden (see the work of Hatfield & Lefley, 1993).

With regard to intervention with burden, in China, Xiong et al. (1994) provided either standard care or a family-based intervention to 63 schizophrenic patients who were living with family members. Patients were evaluated at 6-, 12-, and 18-month follow-ups. Family intervention was associated with significantly lower levels of family burden. Reinhard (1994), Loukissa (1995) and Soloman and Draine (1995), also found professional support and social support selectively reduced burden, whereas practical advice on managing disruptive behaviours reduced objective burden.

Summary of family burden research

In summary, further research is required to fully ascertain the specific nature and extent of the distress and burden experienced by first-episode families. First, there is a need for determining the emotional consequences of living with a relative experiencing a first episode of psychosis which may include acute stress disorder, symptoms of post-traumatic stress and depression. In addition, more data are required regarding the incidence of dangerous events in first-episode households and the extent of the disruption in household routines – especially in the light of shifts toward community-based services for the acute phase of illness (see Chapter 3). Finally, there is a need for prospective longitudinal studies which assess the distress and needs of families from the point of initial contact, thus enabling at-risk family members to be identified as early as possible in the course of illness.

Efficacy of family intervention in first-episode psychosis

The older corpus of studies share the goal of reducing relapse and helping families cope with the schizophrenic illness of their relative (Falloon et al., 1982, 1985; Hogarty et al., 1986; Leff et al., 1982, 1985,1989; Tarrier et al., 1988). These studies have demonstrated a consistent reduction in both the relapse rate and the level of EE (Falloon et al., 1982, 1985; Lam, 1991; Mari & Streiner, 1994). Common features of the studies include the selection of high EE families and the use of maintenance antipsychotic medication. The family interventions were sustained over a period of time, emphasized respect for the family and patient, and included an educational component and a behavioural approach involving communication and problem-solving skills. We are not clear that the results would be the same for early psychosis families and patients who may have different concerns and issues, and it would seem important that an attempt is made to ascertain the findings in early psychosis.

A search of the literature revealed five published papers which examined family-based intervention in early-onset psychosis. Goldstein et al. (1978) used a randomized four-cell design comprising high- and low-dose fluphenazine and crisis-oriented family therapy with psychosocial control of weekly individual visits. The family therapy consisted of six sessions, and the follow-up period was six months. EE status was not reported. The authors reported that 'Relapses during the six-week trial period and at six-month follow-up were least in patients who received *both* high-dose and family therapy (0%) and greatest (48%) in the low-dose-no-therapy group.' (p. 1169). On the BPRS, there was a significant result in favour of crisis-oriented therapy at six weeks, but it was sustained only for those patients who received the high drug dose.

Zhang et al. (1994) conducted a randomized controlled trial of family intervention in 78 first-episode male schizophrenic patients in China. The experimental group attained a significantly better outcome. However, the relatively long duration of illness for a first-episode group (their mean duration of illness was 33.4 months, and for the controls it was 35.7 months), combined with the lack of objective clinical outcome criteria and the idiosyncratic diagnostic criteria employed in this study, all conspire to significantly weaken the generalizability of the findings to other first-episode populations.

From Finland, Lehtinen (1993) reported a five-year follow-up study of 28 first-contact schizophrenic patients treated in a programme with a strong systemic family and crisis orientation. He compared his cohort to one recruited seven years earlier who were treated with an individually-focussed psychodynamic and therapeutic milieu approach. The readmission rate in the first year after intake was roughly equal, with 87% in the old cohort and 82% in the new. Thereafter, the readmission rate declined greatly in the family-treated cohort, down to 11–18% per year over the next four years, versus 36–47% for the old cohort. The new cohort also required considerably less outpatient treatment. Once again this study was weakened by the use of readmission as an indicator of clinical outcome rather than ratings on objective clinical instruments, thereby rendering unclear conclusions regarding the relationship between treatment and outcome. In addition, the historical nature of the comparison makes interpretation of this study difficult, but the low rate of readmission in the family-treated group after the first year is encouraging.

A more recent study by Linszen et al. (1996) included 97 recent-onset patients who entered the inpatient component of the study (although only 76 of them entered the controlled outpatient trial) and their families. Patients were aged between 15 and 26 years of age and had a DSM-III-R diagnosis of schizophrenia or related disorder. Relapse was defined according to 'Brief Psychiatric Rating Scale' criteria supplemented by clinical criteria. At entry all patients participated in an inpatient milieu treatment programme which varied according to the time to remission. Seventy-six patients and families agreed to be followed up in an outpatient treatment programme. Then the families were stratified into high and low EE subgroup using the 'Camberwell Family Interview' (CFI), and patients were assigned randomly to either patient-oriented psychosocial intervention alone, or psychosocial intervention in combination with behavioural family intervention; the latter included psychoeducation, communication training and problem-solving skills training.

The authors found evidence supporting the predictive power of EE, particularly when no effort was made to change the family environment (i.e. the group who did not receive the family intervention showed a significant correlation between relapse and EE). Overall, adding a behavioural intervention did not reduce the relapse rate. This result may have been due to the low overall relapse rate (16% in 12 months), which in turn may reflect the efficacy of the patient-oriented psychosocial intervention. Interestingly, patients from low EE families were slightly more likely to relapse when they received the behavioural family intervention. Retrospectively, the clinicians rated the ease or difficulty of implementing interventions whilst being blind to EE status. In their discussion, the authors noted that the behavioural family intervention was carried out with considerable difficulty in 60% of the low EE and 32% of the high EE families, and that many families reported that the focus of behavioural communication tasks interfered with their need to deal with emotions regarding the recent episode of illness. The authors concluded that family interventions should be more tightly linked to the stage of illness and that for first-episode families more attention should be paid to facilitating the processes of grief and mourning.

Finally, Rund et al. (1995) administered a two-year psychoeducational treatment programme for their 12 first-episode patients, which included educational sessions for relatives. Fifty-eight per cent of parents changed from high to low EE status over the two-year period.

However, the lack of a control group combined with the very small sample size does not enable an association to be established with any degree of confidence between the treatment package and the outcome.

Summary
In summary, studies which have investigated the efficacy of family interventions in first-episode psychosis have utilized varying diagnostic and relapse criteria rendering generalizations difficult. Secondly, the family interventions have varied markedly from study to study, with little attempt to isolate the efficacious components. In terms of the needs of first-episode families, there are some hints in the literature that in the initial stages of the illness families require an opportunity to express their emotions; attempting to modify these processes of coping may even be associated with worse outcomes for some patients and their families. By using interventions designed for use with more chronic populations, and imparting an excessively pessimistic attitude to patients and their families regarding course and outcome, there is the capacity for causing harm to patients.

An approach to meeting the needs of first-episode families

The process of interactions between patient and other family members can be segmented into key 'nodal' stages, which roughly map onto the early course of psychosis (McGorry et al., 1996). In terms of the course of the illness itself, the key transition points can be divided into 'prodrome to psychosis', 'first-episode to the two-year critical period', and from 'critical period to prolonged psychosis', with a proportion crossing each node (McGorry et al., 1996). However, in describing the course of psychosis in relation to the family, it may be more useful to label these nodal points as 'predetection to detection', 'detection to initial recovery', and 'initial recovery to first relapse or prolonged psychosis'. While it remains important to emphasize that family members may shift back and forth between stages and that some stages will be redundant for some families, this model of the course of psychosis provides a useful heuristic tool for generating hypotheses about the needs of first-episode families, for both research and clinical purposes.

Stage 1: Before detection: perceptions and explanations

During the prodromal phase families are faced with changes in a relative which they may deny (at first), or which may be mistaken for developmental or personality changes (Hulbert, Jackson & McGorry, 1996). This may be one of the reasons for patients taking time to access appropriate care; this can later foster guilt, anxiety and confusion for family members (see Chapter 3). There is the possibility, nonetheless, that the young adolescent's personality structure may be inextricably and pervasively changed by the insidious development of psychotic symptoms on the underlying character structure (see Hulbert et al., 1996). This pathoplastic process would result in an amalgam of symptoms and pre-existing personality traits which might now be best described as personality style (Hulbert et al., 1996). In terms of attribution theory, the ambiguous nature of the symptoms is likely to propagate varying and even contradictory explanations for the symptoms among family members (Buchanan & Seligman, 1995). The non-specificity of prodromal symptoms may interact with the diversity in explanatory styles across family members, thus prolonging the time taken to reach consensus about the problem, and lengthening the DUP. According to this notion, families with at-risk adolescents need ready access to information about the early warning signs with accessible assessment services for early detection. In addition, clinicians should be mindful of reviewing and normalizing conflicts which may have developed within first-episode families prior to contact with specialist services.

Stage 2: After detection: grief and stress

The transition to stage 2, 'after detection', may often be precipitated by a crisis which forces the family to consider an illness explanation and the need for urgent assessment. While stage 1 may be dominated by a search for explanations and appropriate help, during stage 2 families are confronted with a 'general' diagnosis (e.g. psychosis) and the commencement of treatment. Although research evidence is required, anecdotal evidence indicates that, during stage 2, family members are often at risk of developing the symptoms of acute stress disorder marked by anxiety symptoms, depressive features, and complicated grief reactions, especially when faced with repeated traumatic incidents in the home.

Clinicians need to acknowledge to families that the onset and detection of a psychotic episode, and the process of being referred to a psychiatric service, constitutes a period of great stress and upheaval. This stress may be further complicated by uncertainty in the minds of clinicians, patients and family members, regarding diagnosis and treatment efficacy. In some cases this period of diagnostic uncertainty may have to be tolerated by family members for a considerable length of time, although treatment can usually be initiated in the short term. For many families the uncertainty is accompanied by the decision to initiate treatment or organize hospital admission against the patient's will, an almost universally distressing experience often followed by feelings of regret mixed with relief. In short, the detection and initiation of treatment in first-episode psychosis is a major trauma for families.

In general, the literature gives little formal consideration to encouraging families to talk in an unstructured way about their experiences and their misgivings in obtaining psychiatric assistance. Of course, these issues are routinely explored in the early stages of most interventions, but the process is often not reported explicitly. In our view, there must be the provision of space and opportunity for the family members, particularly the parents, to ventilate and express their concerns (see Linszen et al., 1996). Failure to do so means that psychoeducational sessions are less effective and the engagement of the family in further work is less likely.

Anecdotal evidence suggests that the biggest challenge for families at this point is to process new information about the illness and its treatment while coping with symptoms of grief and acute stress disorder. This underscores the point that many family members need repeated access to information, together with opportunities for emotional support. An important compounding factor here is the tenebrous connotations of the diagnoses people receive, particularly the word 'schizophrenia', and particularly for those families with a family history of this illness. Other families without family histories of psychosis may share the community's stereotypes of patients being dangerous and intellectually impaired. This underscores the importance of clinicians identifying the family's explanatory model of the illness, and the stereotypes families hold of 'mental illness', and 'psychiatrically ill patients'.

A final issue is the extent to which individual differences within the family are addressed in the early stages of family work. There can be a tendency on the part of clinicians to assume that the needs of family members are the same. Failure to recognize differences impairs engagement and reduces the effectiveness of interventions.

Stage 3: Toward recovery: coping, competence and adaptive functioning

A 'competence paradigm', integrated with a stress and coping model, offers a schema for generating hypotheses regarding the needs of families as the young person begins to respond to treatment. The central components of this model include family life events (including the onset of the psychosis), resources available to the family (which may offset the stress of life events), the family's appraisal of their situation (which moderates the level of stress), and the ability to adapt to the changing circumstances. This paradigm offers a developmental model which views families as competent or potentially competent partners in the recovery process while recognizing that the unfamiliar nature of the illness may lead to competency deficits (Marsh, 1992; EPPIC, 1997). The paradigm suggests that those families who face a less severe psychosis, and who have a history of optimism in the face of challenges and access to a wide range of supports, may benefit from education regarding the illness without the need for ongoing input from specialist family workers. Other families, faced with a relative with severe, treatment-resistant psychosis, who have limited resources and who have a sense of hopelessness about the future, may be at risk of developing more chronic depressive and stress-related disorders. Families in this situation will require access to practical and intensive emotional support during the recovery phase in combination with more intensive treatment of the patient's psychosis. However, it is important to emphasize that patients with a severe, treatment-resistant psychosis, constitute only a small subset of first-episode patients (about 10% in our experience at EPPIC), while a larger subset have a relapsing course of illness.

Stage 4: First relapse and prolonged recovery

A relapse or deterioration in mental state following recovery often represents a pivotal event in the lives of families, forcing another reconstruction of the family's explanatory model from 'unstable' (i.e. temporary) to more 'stable' explanations, and from 'external' to 'internal' (i.e. something inherent in the client). The risk of depression, complicated grief reactions and marital conflict may be increased for parents as concerns emerge regarding long-term burden and loss of expectations for their child. Anecdotal evidence suggests that during this phase siblings may develop anxiety about their own vulnerability to psychosis, together with anxiety about feeling torn between supporting their parents and becoming more independent from the family. This all suggests that families facing relapse need access to early and intensive treatment of the relapse, together with ongoing emotional support, education and, in some cases, access to structured family therapy (e.g. see Anderson, Hogarty & Reiss, 1986).

The three foci of family intervention and prevention: a model of service delivery

The family literature in established psychotic illness reveals a predominance of studies examining the impact of family interactions upon the course of psychosis, in particular the relationship between EE and relapse. However, as emphasized above, the onset of psychosis often represents a traumatic upheaval which can also impact significantly upon the lives of individual family members and upon the life of the 'family system'. Therefore, both the design of future research endeavours and models of service delivery to first-episode families should be driven by consideration of a broader range of inter-relations between psychosis and the life of the family.

One method of construing these inter-relationships is in terms of the 'three foci' of prevention and intervention which can be matched to specific treatment goals. The first focus represents the impact of the psychosis upon the life of the 'family system' as a whole and upon key 'subsystems'. This focus has largely been ignored in the empirical research literature. From this standpoint the goals for prevention and intervention include minimizing the disruption to the life of the family throughout the prodromal and acute phases of illness and maximizing adaptive functioning in the aftermath of the acute psychosis. Specific interventions aimed at achieving these goals include: providing ongoing psychoeducation, optimizing problem solving and communication, and bolstering 'subsystems' within the family (e.g. empowering parents to maintain their 'executive functioning'). Of course, any preventive family interventions are predicated upon optimal treatment of the acute psychosis itself and early recognition of treatment-resistant psychosis (see Chapters 7, 9 and 11).

The second focus, the impact of the psychosis upon individual family members, highlights the preventive goals of minimizing the risk of long-term morbidity in all family members, facilitating an understanding of the psychosis for each individual, and minimizing the risk of the client becoming either overly dependent or alienated from their family. From this perspective clinicians may need to be mindful of 'staggering' the engagement process to match the readiness of the individuals within the family, and this may necessitate the design of separate interventions. Within this focus, interventions include prompt access to debriefing following critical events, which also permits a preliminary assessment of the impact of the psychosis and related critical events upon the functioning and well-being of each family member. At-risk family members may need monitoring and follow-up with access to crisis intervention and emotional and practical support. In terms of the impact of the psychosis upon the client's relationship to the family, the clinician can attempt to minimize the risks of alienation and long-term dependency through attempts at reconstructing the family's enduring 'internal/ stable' attributions regarding the client's behaviour. This can be achieved by supplementing a 'package' approach to psychoeducation with individual education with family members. The clinician can thereby facilitate the 'thawing' of the family's response to the client during the critical period which may develop during the acute stages of illness and become 'frozen' by anger or anxiety.

The third focus, the interaction between the family and the course of the psychosis, leads to the goals of maximizing communication and problem-solving skills in the family, maximizing the preparedness of the family to respond to relapse and crises associated with the psychosis, and minimizing the development of criticism, hostility and emotional over-involvement. Interventions are centred around overtly incorporating the family within the treatment team so that early warning signs of relapse can be identified. In some families, where there is evidence of sustained conflict, a more intensive focus upon minimizing unhelpful responses should be adopted (Anderson et al., 1986; Falloon, Boyd & McGill, 1984). McFarlane et al., (1995), as a component of a project linking Norway, Denmark and the United States, have developed a modified family intervention for this focus for first-episode families (T. H. McGlashan & J. O. Johannessen, personal communication to Patrick McGorry).

Considered as a whole, these three foci provide a schema for providing assessment, psychoeducation, support and family therapy to first-episode families across the phases of illness.

A description of the EPPIC family services

Service philosophy

The approach to family work within EPPIC is underpinned by a first assumption of 'least pathology', i.e. that first-episode families are no different from others in their ability to solve the array of problems associated with both the acute and recovery phases of psychosis. The second key assumption is that optimal delivery of services requires a collaborative approach which promotes a view of families and clients as active members of the treatment team. Thirdly, there is a recognition that services should be flexible in meeting the needs of individuals which may vary as a function of family role (i.e. parent, spouse, sibling, child), or as a function of the phase of the illness from 'detection' to 'prolonged psychosis'. Finally, rather than only being the prerogative of specialist family therapists, family work is integrated across the components of the EPPIC programme, with specialist consultation available from a consultant psychiatrist and designated family workers for more complex cases.

The engagement and assessment process

A number of obstacles confront clinicians who are attempting to engage families (see Smith, 1992). Many families suspect that they will be blamed for the psychosis; others may prefer to avoid the stigma associated with mental health services, or they may feel that family interventions will be intrusive, ineffectual, or prejudicial to their attempt to maintain the patient's trust.

Within EPPIC, in cases where families are not involved in the initial referral process, attempts are made to contact family members as soon as possible. This typically occurs in the first instance, through the 'Early Psychosis Assessment and Community Treatment Team' (EPACT), a 24-hour mobile team which provides both a single point of entry into the service and an intensive home-based treatment service during the acute phase of illness. This system inevitably focusses on the staff engaging with families, and contrasts with the tendency for families to be excluded during the inpatient stays and from involvement with case managers unless efforts are made to counter this.

Clinicians are mindful of making services as accessible and 'user-friendly' for families as possible. Initial orientation 'packages' are provided in written and video formats and by allocating sufficient time to allow families to express their own concerns. All families are given a written invitation to attend the family and friends information sessions as soon as possible (see Psychoeducation, below). The following case fragment gives some indication of an initial contact with a family.

Frank (father of 22-year-old Joe) telephoned the Early Psychosis Assessment and Community Treatment Team (EPACT) regarding his concerns about changes in his son over the previous six months. Frank explained that he and his son had lived alone since he separated from his wife five years earlier. Over the previous six months Frank had noticed that Joe was seeing less of his friends and spending more and more time at home, although Joe continued in his employment as a full-time panel beater. Frank reported that two weeks earlier, after some encouragement, Joe confided in him that a group of friends were planning to falsely implicate him in an elaborate fraud which involved the Federal and Victorian Police forces. Joe had told Frank that his suspicions were confirmed when he discovered that cars he was asked to work on were bugged so that his friends could provide information to the Police.

Frank explained that he had been highly ambivalent about contacting EPACT because, although he recognized that 'something was not quite right' with Joe, he was very anxious to maintain his son's trust, especially as Joe became increasingly suspicious of others. In addition, Frank was forthcoming regarding his concerns that medication would reduce his son's spontaneity and make it impossible for him to function in his job. The EPACT staff member responded by acknowledging Frank's mixed feelings and explained that many parents experienced the same conflict. Frank was invited to an appointment the next day with two of the EPACT staff members who discussed the risks of leaving Joe untreated and the possible outcomes if an assessment proceeded. Frank was shown an educational video, given some reading material, and introduced to some of the other treating staff.

Over the next four days EPACT continued to initiate regular telephone contact with Frank regarding the possibility of proceeding with an assessment. The team explained to Frank how he might be able to broach the issue with his son. Despite some residual ambivalence, Frank raised the issue with his son, after which an assessment interview was scheduled, with Joe's somewhat reluctant approval.

A more detailed assessment of the needs of families is more commonly conducted by the patient's outpatient case manager (OCM) or, for more complex cases, by an EPPIC family worker. This assessment process is deliberately distinguished from the procedure of obtaining collateral information from the family during the assessment of the patient. Clinicians invite families to a session 'to give them an opportunity to have questions answered', and families are encouraged to set the agenda. Families are interviewed together or separately, with an emphasis initially upon allowing the family to express concerns and ask questions. Clinicians then attempt to assess the family's knowledge about psychosis, the impact of the psychosis upon family members, concurrent stressors, family patterns of communication and problem solving and family coping resources. Finally, more detailed attention is given to more complex needs which may include extreme levels of distress, verbal or physical violence, or focusing on recent arrivals from non-English speaking countries, and the stress that surrounds that major transition. The following case fragment illustrates such a case.

Peter, a 19-year-old man, was referred to EPPIC by his 22-year-old sister, Mary. Both had left Bosnia six months previously for Melbourne where they were residing temporarily with their paternal uncle and aunt. Mary explained her reactions to Peter's deteriorating mental state with the assistance of an interpreter in a family meeting scheduled soon after Peter was diagnosed with 'first-episode psychosis' by the home treatment team.

Mary: 'Why now? We had both survived so much together, leaving our family, leaving university, leaving our friends, even being in fear of our lives at times during the war...and now, suddenly, he gets really sick! Sometimes I wonder if maybe I just didn't protect him enough from all the upheavals, and I worry that things built up inside him because he didn't want to show me that he wasn't coping, in case I didn't think he was grown up enough. Or maybe I overlooked the signs of his illness for months. But the problem is that when you hear about your cousins being killed and when you have to leave everyone behind, you expect to be frightened and you expect to have nightmares. I probably should have listened to what he was saying to me. I feel I have let him down, I should have protected him more.'

Psychoeducation

Education is provided to individual families but also delivered within a multiple family group format (known as the 'family and friends' sessions). There are several major considerations which inform our approach to education with individual families. First, the education process begins from the first point of contact. At the point of referral parents are often informed that a first episode of an unspecified mental illness may be emerging which requires urgent assessment to avoid the risk of exacerbation. The rationale and procedure for all assessments are thoroughly explained. At this point the family are usually faced with an acutely psychotic relative, so allowances must be made for their capacity to process new information being compromised at this time. This means that family members often need unambiguous messages which are repeated frequently via several modalities. Of course, most families are eager for a diagnosis and causal explanation; clinicians are careful to explain the risk of a premature diagnosis and the need for a thorough organic screen and, indeed, the nature and purpose of a psychiatric diagnosis – a shorthand description of the clinical features which guides decisions on treatment. Once the diagnosis has been confirmed it is usually described as a 'first episode of a psychosis' and relatives are informed that the cause is not associated with family processes. It is usually explained that schizophrenia is only one of a variety of subtypes which are subsumed under psychosis. As mentioned earlier, the clinician needs to recognize that family members may share many of the community's negative stereotypic pictures of psychosis, schizophrenia and psychiatric patients in general. It is the job of the family worker to help detoxify the stereotypes. Later, families may begin to raise questions concerning prognosis. At this earlier stage, diagnosis, treatment and short-term recovery are the focus of the family's concerns.

Also, at this stage many family members may be working with the acute home treatment team to enable their relative to remain at home. These families often require practical advice and coaching in managing disturbed behaviour, responding to positive psychotic symptoms, monitoring medication and recognizing side-effects (see Chapter 8). In addition, clinicians explain the association between the client's behaviours and subjective psychotic experiences, which reduces confusion for families and minimizes the risk of misinterpretations leading to conflict. In these circumstances clinicians work to minimize the uncertainties for families by providing information about what improvements and problems they can expect over the immediate short term and over the ensuing weeks.

Following the initial acute phase of treatment, families often need more detailed information about symptoms of psychosis, aetiology, course of illness and treatment. While the delivery of information must be guided by an assessment of the family's knowledge base and explanatory model of the illness, clinicians generally utilize the 'stress-vulnerability' model as an explanation which minimizes blame and which provides a rationale for a broad psychosocial approach to treatment beyond the acute phase of treatment. Clinicians need to be adaptable and flexible in their approach and they need to tailor ideographically their intervention to the individual needs of the patient and family. Furthermore, clinicians need to suspend assumptions which may underscore psychoeducational material designed for family work with more chronic populations. The general aims of psychoeducational input are displayed in shorthand in Table 14.1.

Working with first-episode families is unique in the sense that families are usually naïve to the experience of psychosis and its treatment or, in the case where the family have a history of psychosis, their experience of mental health services may have been aversive. Their participation in a treatment plan must therefore be predicated upon: the provision of knowledge, the opportunity to adjust to the crisis, and a therapeutic alliance in which they feel comfortable. By contrast, families who have faced several episodes of illness are more familiar with the issues and stressors involved in symptom exacerbations and relapses, and are more able to negotiate the health system. However, in our clinical experience, this latter group are often angry, guilt-ridden, and depressed, due to failed coping, frequently exacerbated by a failure to be appropriately supported in the optimal manner described.

Table 14.1. *General aims of psychoeducation input*

To reduce distress, burden and anxiety
To permit time to ventilate, discuss with therapist
To provide support to families and friends in their own right to reduce their own morbidity, or risk of same
To provide accurate information using both written and verbal materials
To assist families and friends in integrating the information with their particular experiences of their relative and the notion of recovery
To enable families and friends to recognize and utilize their own particular strengths and resources
To facilitate a collaborative approach with families and friends that acknowledges the importance of their role with the patients and in the treatment process
Via the medium of multi-family psychoeducation groups, to provide a safe environment to ask questions, discuss their own concerns and experiences

---

Family members may experience psychopathology in the form of depression, grief, substance abuse, presenting either *de novo*, or as an exacerbation of pre-existing, or comorbid, problems. This is an area which requires sensitivity and diplomacy from the family worker. Families often feel guilty and responsible for the occurrence of the psychosis, and interpret discussion of their own problems as confirmation that they were indeed to blame (see Jackson et al., 1996). Therefore, during the psychoeducation process, it must be made clear that family problems do not cause psychosis, but may impede the recovery process unless they can adapt successfully, and may well require some support and skilled intervention in their own right to help them to do this.

On occasion, specialist work may be required, such as specific marital work for the parents of a younger patient or for the patient and his or her partner, or family therapy and/or specific individual work with children, siblings and so on.

Multiple family group format
All families are invited to a series of evening sessions entitled 'family and friends' which are scheduled over four consecutive weeks. In addition to providing opportunities for structured learning, the group reduces the effects of social isolation and stigma. The group is open, although participants are encouraged to attend from the first session. Usually facilitated by two staff members, the format alternates between didactic presentations and general discussion, which allows participants to exchange experiences and provide support to one another.

The information provided across the four interactive sessions is outlined below in Table 14.2. We have found that families need to feel

Table 14.2. *Outline of family and friends sessions*

Session 1.	What is psychosis? This session covers the stress-vulnerability model, and the nature, signs and symptoms (positive, negative and affective) of psychosis
Session 2.	Medication. This session introduces the range of neuroleptics, mood stabilizers, antidepressants, benzodiazepines and side-effect medications, including information about effects and side-effects
Session 3.	Recovery. This session introduces the phase model of psychosis with a discussion regarding the changes that relatives may have noticed during each phase. Emphasis is given to the improvements and challenges which relatives may be faced with during the recovery phase. Recovery is defined and the psychological issues and stages of recovery described. Information is provided as to how the family may best assist in the patient's recovery process
Session 4.	The future. This session explores concerns and expectations for the future and informs participants about further available sources of information and support. Families are given information on how to maintain recovery, how to detect and cope with relapse, and the resources and services available to them if relapse occurs

supported and assisted with integrating new information via case examples. In particular, information is most helpful when it elucidates the relationship between observed changes in their relative's behaviour and symptoms, as illustrated in the following case example.

> After the facilitator provided didactic material to the group about the symptoms of psychosis, a mother explained that, although she had already been given information, she remained uncertain about how to respond to her son. She explained that she felt anxious when her son accused his sister of 'messing with his mind', and confused about whether to punish or protect him.
> The facilitator incorporated this example into an explanation of the link between psychotic experience and behavioural responses, explaining that during the active phase of illness, family members (and indeed clinicians) often had to infer this connection based on observations of the client's behaviour. The facilitator explained that the woman's son may have held a belief that his sister was controlling his thinking or reading his mind, which understandably led him to make accusations.

> Other members of the group supported this interpretation through examples of similar symptoms in their relatives. At the encouragement of the facilitator, the group was able to shift to generating strategies for responding to a relative who believed that a sibling was interfering with their mind.

Not only can such sessions help families by providing them with an understanding of their relative, but they can also aid families in realizing that they are not alone in their experience of shock, distress and confusion. This can be facilitated by outlining some of the stages families often experience in the transition from prodrome to acute illness.

A second group intervention, which provides further support and psychoeducation for families with a relative with a more persistent illness, has more recently been developed within the EPPIC programme to complement the initial four-session group. In fact, according to McFarlane et al. (1995), psychoeducational multiple-family groups (MFGs) constitute a powerful and viable treatment option, particularly where patients suffer from persistent positive symptoms. McFarlane et al. (1995) found MFGs to be more effective than individual family work in reducing relapse and promoting remission. Those authors commented that they believed that this was because MFGs extended mutual support across families and patients, and increased their problem-solving capabilities and options, thereby reducing morbidity in the form of anxiety and stress in family members. This stands in direct contrast to the more usual scenario whereby, with continuing psychosis, social networks and social support contract, and the risk of burden and morbidity in family members increases (Jackson & Edwards, 1992).

Support
During the acute phase clinicians can have a role in providing practical support to families through offering suggestions, helping family members solve problems, and offering management advice. There is also a prominent role for clinicians in providing emotional support to the family with particular emphasis upon ameliorating the impact of guilt, fear and anger, and reducing stigma for family members. It is important to encourage family members to access existing support networks as a means of buffering stress and preventing family morbidity, and to encourage family members to address their own needs in addition to the needs of the patient. A summary of the general principles for working with families with an early psychosis member are outlined in Table 14.3.

The success of this range of interventions is predicated upon a well-

Table 14.3. *General principles for working with families with an early psychosis member*

Recognize the phase nature of the patient's illness, and that family work needs to be adaptable and flexible in approach
Recognize that families will have a range of different feelings, worries and questions
Recognize that families need time and an opportunity to deal with the crisis and ensuing stressors
Recognize that the explanations that families have for what has happened to them need to be heard and understood
Recognize that families need a framework for understanding
Recognize that families also need a recovery time and may go through particular stages
Recognize that the family work may change over time, ranging from a maintenance role to dealing with longer-term, ongoing issues
Recognize that family work is a preventive intervention. It is aimed at addressing levels of distress, burden, coping, social functioning and general health for all family members

resourced outpatient programme which allows for case managers or psychiatrists to work flexibly with specialist family workers. Optimal arrangements may vary, including: the primary clinician providing both the individual and family work; the primary clinician and specialist family worker providing cotherapy; while in some cases family work may need to be separated from the individual work – especially when countertransference issues, therapeutic skills or other pressures may impede the effectiveness of family interventions provided by the case manager or psychiatrist.

Future directions

Future directions in first-episode family work should first clarify the needs and experiences of families; in particular, hypotheses regarding the stage model need to be tested empirically. Are all the components reflective of the experience of the majority of families? Do the stages unfold in a sequential building block fashion? What is the impact of psychoeducation and support when provided early in the course of illness upon the subsequent morbidity in the family? What are the outcome data for patients when this is undertaken? Secondly, we need to identify protective factors and risk factors regarding prolonged morbidity in family members. Similarly, we need more flexible assessment tools which separate out stable and temporary communication patterns in families, rather than taking for granted the assumption that the communication patterns and emotional concomitants are 'trait-like'.

However, there is already sufficient information available from clinical practice and research to suggest guidelines for family work in early psychosis. Families need to be provided with clear and accurate information about psychosis. They need reassurance about the excellent prospects for recovery from the first episode, tempered with appropriate realism about the risks of relapse. They need an opportunity to express their own feelings about their relative's illness and opportunities to ask questions. They need support to work through any anxiety, grief or despair. Finally, they need information about the kind of emotional environment which facilitates recovery, and sometimes they need specific help in working towards such an environment.

References

Anderson, C., Hogarty, G. & Reiss, D. (1986). *Schizophrenia and the Family*. New York: Guilford Press.

Barrelet, L., Ferrero, F., Szigethy, L., Giddey, C. & Pellizzer, G. (1990). Expressed emotion and first-admission schizophrenia. Nine month follow-up in a French cultural environment. *British Journal of Psychiatry*, **156**, 357–62.

Bebbington, P. & Kuipers, L. (1994). The predictive utility of expressed emotion in schizophrenia: an aggregate analysis. *Psychological Medicine*, **24**, 707–18.

Birchwood, M. & Macmillan, F. (1993). Early intervention in schizophrenia. *Australian and New Zealand Journal of Psychiatry*, **27**, 374–8.

Birchwood, M., McGorry, P. & Jackson, H. (1997). Editorial – Early intervention in schizophrenia. *British Journal of Psychiatry*, **170**, 2–5.

Buchanan, G. M. & Seligman, M. E. P. (1995). *Explanatory Style*. New Jersey: Lawrence Erlbaum.

Carpenter, W. T. & Strauss, J. S. (1991). The prediction of outcome in schizophrenia. IV: Eleven-year follow-up of the Washington IPSS cohort. *Journal of Nervous and Mental Disease*, **179**, 517–25.

Clarke, R. E. (1994). Family costs associated with severe mental illness and substance use. *Hospital and Community Psychiatry*, **45**, 808–13.

Davidson, L. & Strauss, J. S. (1995). Beyond the biopsychosocial model: integrating disorder, health and recovery. *Psychiatry*, **58**, 44–55.

Early Psychosis Prevention and Intervention Centre (1997). *Working with Families in Early Psychosis: No 2 in a Series of Early Psychosis Manuals*. Victoria, Australia: Psychiatric Services Branch, Human Services Victoria.

Falloon, I., Boyd, J. & McGill, C. (1984). *Family Care of Schizophrenia*. New York: Guilford Press.

Falloon, I. R. H., Boyd, J. L., McGill, C. W., Razani, J., Moss, H. B. & Gilderman,

A. M. (1982). Family management in the prevention of exacerbations of schizophrenia: a controlled study. *The New England Journal of Medicine*, **306**, 1437–40.

Falloon, I. R. H., Boyd, J. L., McGill, C. W., Williamson, M., Razani, J., Moss, H. B., Gilderman, A. M. & Simpson, G. M. (1985). Family management in the prevention of morbidity of schizophrenia: clinical outcome of a two-year longitudinal study. *Archives of General Psychiatry*, **42**, 887–96.

Falloon, I. R. H., Kydd, R. R., Coverdale, J. H. & Laidlaw, T. M. (1996). Early detection and intervention for initial episodes of schizophrenia. *Schizophrenia Bulletin*, **22**, 271–82.

Goldstein, M. J., Rodnick, E. H., Evans, J. R., May, P. R. & Steinberg, M. (1978). Drug and family therapy in the aftercare of acute schizophrenia. *Archives of General Psychiatry*, **35**, 1169–77.

Gopinath, P. S. & Chaturvedi, S. K. (1993). Distressing behaviour of schizophrenics at home. *Acta Psychiatrica Scandinavica*, **88**, 221–2.

Gunn, M. (1997). Youth suffers identity crisis as the rites of passage blur. *The Weekend Australian*, April 26–27, p. 7.

Häfner, H., Maurer, K., Löffler, W., Bustamante, S., an der Heiden, W., Riecher-Rössler, A. & Nowotny, B. (1995). Onset and early course of schizophrenia. In *Search for the Causes of Schizophrenia*, Vol III, ed. H. Häfner & W. F. Gattaz, pp. 43–66. Berlin: Springer-Verlag.

Halford, W. K. (1992). Assessment of family interaction with a schizophrenic member. In *Schizophrenia: An Overview and Practical Handbook*, ed. D. J. Kavanagh, pp. 254–74. London: Chapman & Hall.

Halford, W. K., Schweitzer, R. D. & Varghese, F. N. (1991). Effects of family environment on negative symptoms and quality of life of psychotic patients. *Hospital and Community Psychiatry*, **42**, 1241–7.

Harding, C. M., Zubin, J. & Strauss, J. S. (1987). Chronicity in schizophrenia: fact, partial fact, or artifact? *Hospital and Community Psychiatry*, **38**, 477–86.

Hatfield, A. B. (1978). Psychological costs of schizophrenia to the family. *Social Work*, **23**, 5–12.

Hatfield, A. B. & Lefley, H. P. (1993). *Surviving Mental Illness: Stress, Coping, and Adaptation*. New York: Guilford Press.

Hogarty, G. E., Anderson, C. M., Reiss, D. J., Kornblith, S. J., Greenwald, D. P., Javna, C. D., Madonia, M. J., and Environmental/Personal Indicators in the Course of Schizophrenia Research Group. (1986). Family psychoeducation, social skills training, and maintenance chemotherapy in the aftercare treatment of schizophrenia. 1. One-year effects of a controlled study on relapse and expressed emotion. *Archives of General Psychiatry*, **43**, 633–42.

Huguelet, Ph., Favre, S., Binyet, S., Gonzalez, Ch. & Zabala, I. (1995). The use of the Expressed Emotion Index as a predictor of outcome in first admitted schizophrenic patients in a French speaking area of Switzerland. *Acta Psychiatrica Scandinavica*, **92**, 447–52.

Hulbert, C. A., Jackson, H. J. & McGorry, P. D. (1996). Relationship between personality and course and outcome in early psychosis: a review of the literature. *Clinical Psychology Review*, **16**, 707–27.

Jackson, H. J. & Edwards, J. (1992). Social networks and social support in schizophrenia: correlates and assessment. In *Schizophrenia: An Overview and Practical Handbook*, ed. D. J. Kavanagh, pp. 275–92. London: Chapman & Hall.

Jackson, H. J., McGorry, P. D. & Dudgeon, P. (1995). Prodromal symptoms of schizophrenia in first-episode psychosis: prevalence and specificity. *Comprehensive Psychiatry*, 36, 241–50.

Jackson, H., Robinson, T. & Pica, S. (1996). State psychiatric hospitals and psychiatric wards in general hospitals. In *Clinical Psychology: Profession and Practice in Australia*, ed. P. R. Martin & J. S. Birnbrauer, pp. 103–28. Melbourne, Australia: Macmillan.

Jackson, H. J., Smith, N. & McGorry, P. (1990). Relationship between expressed emotion and family burden in psychotic disorders: an exploratory study. *Acta Psychiatricia Scandinavica*, 82, 243–9.

Jones, P. B., Bebbington, P., Foerster, A., Lewis, S. W., Murray, R. M., Russell, A., Sham, P. C., Tone, B. K. & Wilkins, S. (1993). Premorbid social underachievement in schizophrenia: results from the Camberwell Collaborative Psychosis Study. *British Journal of Psychiatry*, 162, 65–71.

Kavanagh, D. J. (1992). Recent developments in expressed emotion and schizophrenia. *British Journal of Psychiatry*, 160, 601–20.

Kavanagh, D. J. (1996). Family interventions in relapse prevention of schizophrenia. In *Early Intervention and Prevention in Mental Health*, ed. P. Cotton & H. Jackson, pp.155–72. Melbourne, Australia: Australian Psychological Society.

Kelly, K. (1995). *Out of Control: The New Biology of Control*. London: Fourth Estate.

Kosky, R. & Hardy, J. (1992). Mental health: is early intervention the key? *Medical Journal of Australia*, 256, 147–48.

Lam, D. H. (1991). Psychosocial family intervention in schizophrenia: a review of empirical studies. *Psychological Medicine*, 21, 423–41.

Leff, J. P., Kuipers, L., Berkowitz, R. & Sturgeon, D. (1982). A controlled trial of social intervention in the families of schizophrenic patients. *British Journal of Psychiatry*, 141, 121–34.

Leff, J., Kuipers, L., Berkowitz, R. & Sturgeon, D. (1985). A controlled trial of social intervention in the families of schizophrenic patients: two year follow-up. *British Journal of Psychiatry*, 146, 594–600.

Leff, J. P., Berkowitz, R., Shavit, N., Strachan, A., Glass, I. & Vaughn, C. (1989). A trial of family therapy vs. a relatives group for schizophrenia. *British Journal of Psychiatry*, 154, 58–66.

Lehtinen, K. (1993). Need-adapted treatment of schizophrenia: a five-year follow-up study from the Turku project. *Acta Psychiatrica Scandinavica*, 87, 96–101.

Levinson, D. J. (1986). A conception of adult development. *American Psychologist*, 41, 3–13.

Lieberman, J. A., Jody, D., Geisler, S. H., Alvir, J. M. J., Loebel, A. D., Szymanski, S. R., Woerner, M. & Borenstein, M. (1993). Time course and biological correlates of treatment response in first-episode schizophrenia. *Archives of General Psychiatry*, **50**, 369–76.

Linszen, D., Dingemans, P., Van Der Does, J. W., Nugter, A., Schote, P., Lenior, R. & Goldstein, M. J. (1996). Treatment, expressed emotion and relapse in recent onset schizophrenic disorders. *Psychological Medicine*, **26**, 333–42.

Loebel, A. D., Lieberman, J. A., Alvir, J. M. J., Mayerhoff, D. I., Geisler, S. H. & Szymanski, S. R. (1992). Duration of psychosis and outcome in first-episode schizophrenia. *American Journal of Psychiatry*, **149**, 1183–8.

Loukissa, D. A. (1995). Family burden in chronic mental illness. A review of research studies. *Journal of Advanced Nursing*, **21**, 248–55.

McFarlane, W. R., Lukins, E., Link, B., Dushay, R., Deakins, S. A., Newmark, M., Dunne, E. J., Horen, B. & Toran, J. (1995). Multiple-family groups and psychoeducation in the treatment of schizophrenia. *Archives of General Psychiatry*, **52**, 679–87.

McGlashan, T. H. & Johannessen, J. O. (1996). Early detection and intervention with schizophrenia: rationale. *Schizophrenia Bulletin*, **22**, 201–22.

Macmillan, J. F., Gold, A., Crow, T. J., Johnson, A. L. & Johnstone, E. C. (1986). The Northwick Park Study of first episodes of schizophrenia. IV. Expressed emotion and relapse. *British Journal of Psychiatry*, **148**, 133–43.

McGorry, P. D., Edwards, J., Mihalopoulos, C., Harrigan, S. M. & Jackson, H. J. (1996). EPPIC: an evolving system of early detection and optimal management. *Schizophrenia Bulletin*, **22**, 305–26.

McGorry, P. D. & Singh, B. S. (1995). Schizophrenia: the risk and possibility of prevention. In *Handbook of Studies on Preventive Psychiatry*, ed. B. Raphael & G. Burrows, pp. 491–514. Amsterdam: Elsevier Science.

Mari, J. J. & Streiner, D. L. (1994). An overview of family interventions and relapse on schizophrenia: meta-analysis of research findings. *Psychological Medicine*, **24**, 565–78.

Marsh, D. T. (1992). *Families and Mental Illness: New Directions in Professional Practice*. New York: Praeger.

Maurin, J. T. & Boyd, C. B. (1990). Burden of mental illness on the family: a critical review. *Archives of Psychiatric Nursing*, **4**, 99–107.

Mintz, L. I., Nuechterlein, K. H., Goldstein, M. J., Mintz, J. & Synder, K. S. (1989). The initial onset of schizophrenia and family expressed emotion: some methodological considerations. *British Journal of Psychiatry*, **154**, 212–17.

Mueser, K. T., Webb, C., Pfeiffer, M., Gladis, M. & Levinson, D. F. (1996). Family burden of schizophrenia and bipolar disorder: perceptions of relatives and professionals. *Psychiatric Services*, **47**, 507–11.

Nuechterlein, K. H., Dawson, M. E., Gitlin, M., Ventura, J., Goldstein, M. J., Snyder, K. S., Yee, C. M. & Mintz, J. (1992). Developmental processes in schizophrenic disorders: longtitudinal studies of vulnerability and stress. *Schizophrenia Bulletin*, **18**, 387–425.

Nuechterlein, K. H., Snyder, K. S. & Mintz, J. (1992). Paths to relapse: possible transactional processes connecting patient illness onset, expressed emotion, and psychotic relapse. *British Journal of Psychiatry*, **161** (Supplement 18), 88–96.

Parker, G., Johnston, P. & Hayward, L. (1988). Parental 'expressed emotion' as a predictor of schizophrenic relapse. *Archives of General Psychiatry*, **45**, 806–13.

Pickett, S. A., Cook, J. A. & Cohler, B. J. (1994). Caregiving burden experienced by parents of offspring with severe mental illness: the impact of off-timedness. *Journal of Applied Social Science*, **18**, 199–207.

Reinhard, S. C. (1994). Living with mental illness: effects of professional support and personal control of caregiver burden. *Research in Nursing Health*, **17**, 79–88.

Regier, D. A., Myers, J. K., Kramer, M., Robins, L. N., Blazer, D. G., Hough, R. L., Eaton, W. W. & Locke, B. Z. (1984). The NIMH epidemiologic catchment area program. Historical context, major objectives, and study population characteristics. *Archives of General Psychiatry*, **41**, 934–41.

Rosenfarb, I. S., Goldstein, M. J., Mintz, J. & Nuechterlein, K. H. (1995). Expressed emotion and subclinical psychopathology observable within the transactions between schizophrenic patients and their family members. *Journal of Abnormal Psychology*, **104**, 259–67.

Rund, B. R., Aeie, M., Borchgrevink, T. S. & Fjell, A. (1995). Expressed emotion, communication deviance and schizophrenia. *Psychopathology*, **28**, 220–8.

Salleh, M. R. (1994). The burden of care of schizophrenia in Malay families. *Acta Psychiatrica Scandinavica*, **89**, 180–5.

Smith, J. (1992). Family interventions: service implications. In *Innovations in the Psychological Management of Schizophrenia*, ed. M. Birchwood & N. Tarrier, pp. 235–51. Chichester, UK: John Wiley.

Smith, J., Birchwood, M., Cochrane, R. & George, S. (1993). The needs of high and low expressed emotion families. A normative approach. *Social Psychiatry and Psychiatric Epidemiology*, **28**, 11–16.

Solomon, P. & Draine, J. (1995). Subjective burden among family members of mentally ill adults: relation to stress, coping and adaptation. *American Journal of Orthopsychiatry*, **65**, 419–27.

Stirling, J., Tantam, D., Thomas, P., Newby, D., Montague, L., Ring, N. & Rowe, S. (1991). Expressed emotion and early onset schizophrenia: a one year follow-up. *Psychological Medicine*, **21**, 675–85.

Strauss, J. S. (1989). Subjective experiences of schizophrenia: toward a new dynamic psychiatry – II. *Schizophrenia Bulletin*, **15**, 179–87.

Strauss, J. S. (1994). The person with schizophrenia as a person. II: Approaches to the subjective and complex. *British Journal of Psychiatry*, **23** (Supplement), 103–7.

Tarrier, N., Barrowclough, C., Vaughn, C., Bamrah, J. S., Porceddu, K., Watts, S. & Freeman, H. (1988). The community management of schizophrenia. A controlled trial of a behavioural intervention with families to reduce relapse. *British Journal of Psychiatry*, **153**, 532–42.

Vettro, F., Magliano, L., Lobace, S., Morosini, P. L. & Maj, M. (1994). Burden on key relatives with schizophrenia vs neurotic disorders: a pilot study. *Social Psychiatry and Psychiatric Epidemiology*, **29**, 66–70.

Winefield, H. R. & Harvey, E. J. (1993). Determinants of psychological distress in relatives of people with chronic schizophrenia. *Schizophrenia Bulletin*, **19**, 619–25.

Winefield, H. R. & Harvey, E. J. (1994). Needs of family caregivers in chronic schizophrenia. *Schizophrenia Bulletin*, **20**, 557–66.

Xiong, W., Phillips, M. R., Hu, X., Wang, R., Dai, Q., Kleinman, J. & Kleinman, A. (1994). Family-based intervention for schizophrenic patients in China. A randomised controlled trial. *British Journal of Psychiatry*, **165**, 239–47.

Yung, A. R., McGorry, P. D., McFarlane, C. A., Jackson, H. J., Patton, G. C. & Rakkar, A. (1996). Monitoring and care of young people at incipient risk of psychosis. *Schizophrenia Bulletin*, **22**, 283–303.

Zhang, M., Wang, M., Li, J. & Phillips, M. R. (1994). Randomised-control trial of family intervention for 78 first-episode male schizophrenic patients. *British Journal of Psychiatry*, **165** (Supplement), 96–102.

15

The role of day programmes in recovery in early psychosis

SHONA M. FRANCEY

Introduction

The emergence of psychotic illness for the first time is a frightening and confusing experience for the individual and their friends and family. The experience threatens an individual's sense of self and identity, and has the potential to seriously disrupt developmental trajectories in vocational, educational and social domains (Jackson et al., 1996). It is during this early period following the onset of a psychotic disorder that there is the greatest opportunity to intervene to prevent the development of psychosocial disability (Birchwood & Macmillan, 1993). This idea is supported by the results of several long-term follow-up studies which indicate that a relatively stable state is achieved by people with psychotic illnesses after about five years, and that prior to this the emerging range of psychosocial interventions for serious mental illness are likely to have the greatest impact (see Chapter 9) (Birchwood & Macmillan, 1993; Carpenter & Strauss, 1991; McGlashan, 1984). Among a variety of modalities of interventions useful at this stage of illness, day programmes offer a number of features which are particularly relevant to the needs of a young person recovering from their first episode of psychosis.

However, to date, there have been no studies of the efficacy of day programmes in facilitating recovery in first-episode psychosis. When consulting the literature in order to glean directions for programme development, it has been necessary to attempt to extrapolate from, and adapt, programmes from two more general areas. Although sparse, there are studies which examine the efficacy of programmes attempting to address general adolescent mental health needs (e.g. following delinquency or substance abuse problems), and there is a small literature on day programmes set up to assist individuals with long-term psychiatric disabilities. The principles, supported by studies from these two domains, can be applied to the exploration of the role of day programmes in recovery from early psychosis, and the need for more specific studies will be highlighted.

Young people recovering from a first episode of psychosis represent a special population with particular needs, and our experience with this group suggests that the day programme modality may be especially helpful. Particular needs and goals which seem to be addressed through this group-based intervention include: the rebuilding of social networks; the establishment of a peer group; the regaining of confidence for social interaction, goal setting, and activity scheduling; learning about psychosis; building life skills and confidence; fostering independence; and interacting with people who are further along in their recovery and thus provide inspiration and hope for the future. There is also the opportunity to witness the effects of factors inhibiting recovery, e.g. drug abuse, and learn vicariously about behaviours to be avoided.

This chapter begins with an examination of the definitions and a review of the efficacy of day programmes, followed by a brief review of the literature about the needs of recovering patients in general. Also, the psychosocial rehabilitation paradigm and its applicability to recovering first-episode patients is explored briefly. The remainder of the chapter is devoted to a description and preliminary evaluation of a day programme specifically designed to facilitate recovery from first-episode psychosis.

What is a day programme?

'Day programme' is a term poorly defined in the literature on psychiatric treatment modalities, with a number of terms, e.g. partial hospitalization, day care, day treatment, and day hospital, used to describe a variety of services. These services may differ in terms of the location of service, population treated, or function of the service (Rosie, 1987). The single common defining characteristic of all the services described by these terms is that the recipients of the service do not sleep at the treatment site; unlike inpatient units, participants in day programmes return to their own accommodation at night, and this is frequently cited as a major advantage of this type of service, especially for young people. This is because of the reduced costs associated with non-residential treatment, the increased efficacy thought to result from the encouragement of involvement with community resources which enhances the generalization and maintenance of skills acquired in the programme, and the reduced restrictiveness of the treatment setting (Gabel & Finn, 1986; Kiser, 1991). Reviews and studies conducted under the heading of partial hospitalization have provided the clearest delineation of the functions of these types of programmes. However, it must be emphasized that the lack of consistency in the use of terms, the wide variety of target groups, structures of programmes and interventions used, combined with the distinct lack of outcome studies, means that there is little useful material to guide day programme development.

Rosie (1987) reviewed partial hospitalization programmes in North America and Europe and provided a definition from the American Association of Partial Hospitalization. 'Partial hospitalization is an ambulatory treatment programme that includes the major diagnostic, medical, psychiatric, psychosocial, and prevocational treatment modalities designed for patients with serious mental disorders who require co-ordinated intensive, comprehensive, and multidisciplinary treatment not provided in an outpatient setting. It allows for a more flexible and less restrictive treatment programme by offering an alternative to inpatient treatment' (p. 1291). He goes on to distinguish between day hospitals, day treatment programmes and day care centres. Day treatment programmes are designed to treat patients who have achieved some recovery and may be in transition from hospital to outpatient care. They have the goal of improved functioning for the patient and involvement is time-limited. This is in contrast to 'day hospitals' which provide diagnostic and treatment services for acutely ill patients who would otherwise be treated as inpatients, and 'day care centres' which aim to maintain stability in chronic psychiatric patients and therefore offer long-term care. In addition, day treatment programmes are often specifically designed to meet the needs of particular populations of patients.

Adolescents and young adults represent a special population because this life stage constitutes a period of rapid change and development often experienced as highly stressful (Rice, Herman & Petersen, 1993). It is a time of life when peer group influences are at their peak, and educational and social structures for young people commonly adopt group formats. Thus, young people may find it easier to engage in group programmes and this is likely to be an effective medium for the delivery of various forms of intervention. For these reasons, adolescents and young adults have been considered to be a group for whom day treatment utilizing group-based interventions may be particularly appropriate. However, there is a marked paucity of research evidence to support this idea. Kettlewell, Jones and Jones (1985) reported that there is only a sparse literature on adolescent partial hospitalization programmes and few studies attempt to evaluate such programmes. However, Kettlewell et al. (1985) note that the stresses entailed in adolescence are increasing, as indicated by escalating suicide rates, and that psychiatric problems during this period require innovative programming. They used multiple outcome measures obtained from patients, parents and therapists derived from scores on three instruments: the Child and Adolescent Behavior Checklist (Fineberg, Kettlewell & Sowards, 1982), Goal Attainment Scaling (Kiresuk & Sherman, 1968), and the Assessment of Current Functioning Scale (Lefkovitz, Morrison & Davies, 1982). Results suggested that their 12-week programme was effective for adolescents and thus provided support for the effectiveness of this treatment modality.

Kiser et al. (1986) conducted a survey of 82 child and adolescent day treatment programmes in the USA, and found huge variability in all aspects of the programmes. While beginning from the unproven assumption that this type of treatment is important for adolescents, these investigators stressed that it is largely under-utilized due to a lack of definition and standards. They argue that it is essential to gather data to support the effectiveness of this type of programme, in order to compete for health care funding. Isenberg (1983) described and evaluated a day treatment programme for young adults with chronic severe mental illness. The participants were described as having multiple deficits in independent functioning and difficulties with separation from their families of origin. This programme evaluation supported the day treatment modality as being effective in helping severely ill young people achieve greater independent functioning, but it is based on a small sample of 22 patients. The patients had a mean of 3.5 prior psychiatric hospitalizations and there were 12 with a diagnosis of chronic schizophrenia, six with personality disorder diagnoses and four were dually diagnosed with bipolar disorder and a personality disorder. Clearly, there is an urgent need for further research to demonstrate the effectiveness of day treatment for adolescents and young adults with psychiatric difficulties, to support the clinical intuitions of those who are establishing these programmes. It is important that carefully designed studies using formal methods of assessment to establish diagnoses, sufficiently lengthy periods of follow-up, including long-term follow-up after several years, accurate records of attendance, and the targetting of the particular population under consideration (i.e., young people with recent-onset psychosis as opposed to those with longstanding illnesses), be conducted in order to demonstrate the efficacy of this treatment modality. These factors have not been addressed in most of the relevant literature reviewed (Isenberg, 1983; Kettlewell et al., 1985; Kiser et al., 1986). Second generation studies are needed to determine the most efficacious and potent components of day treatment for first-episode psychosis. These would assist in the refinement of programmes.

What do day programmes do?

Hoge et al. (1987, 1988) conducted interview studies with staff and psychiatric patients of their partial hospitalization programme, in order to define the functions and the therapeutic factors believed to underpin the programme. Their findings indicated that the programme functioned to reduce symptomatology, decrease demoralization, and facilitate re-entry into the community. These investigators noted that the ability of the programme to achieve education, skill building, and the connecting of patients with community resources, was limited due to the short (one month) duration of their programme. In terms of therapeutic factors purported to facilitate the positive changes observed as programme outcomes, these have remarkable concordance with the factors thought to facilitate recovery which are outlined below. The patients in these studies were young adults with a mean age of 30 years; 50% had schizophrenia-related disorders, 35% affective disorders, 10% anxiety disorders and 5% adjustment disorders. A quarter of the patients had a dual diagnosis of substance abuse, and 60% were diagnosed with a personality disorder on axis II of DSM-III.

Structure, encompassing routine, direction, activity, and purpose or role in life, was identified by 95% of the subjects as important in their improvement. Similarly, interpersonal contact, providing acceptance, a sense of belonging, support and companionship, were cited by almost all of the study subjects as important aspects of the programme. The opportunity to contribute to the programme in some way, or to help others, was seen to be beneficial, as was the chance to ventilate strong feelings in a 'safe' environment. Other factors of the programme which were listed as therapeutic included: learning about illness, receiving feedback on behaviour, practising things at home, encouraging patient autonomy, the security of being monitored, and the feeling of mastery derived from successful completion of the programme. While it should be noted that these findings are from a small sample of 20 subjects, they suggest that this treatment modality may be useful for a population of young people recovering from psychosis. However, the sample's mean age of 30 years suggests that the majority of these subjects were unlikely to be recovering from a first-episode of psychosis and thus raises questions about the direct applicability of these results to the younger first-episode psychosis group.

Most day programmes for people who have experienced serious mental illness would be considered to be offering psychosocial rehabilitation. This is a field of endeavour which has emerged in the wake of the deinstitutionalization movement and which resulted in the discharge of large numbers of previously chronically-hospitalized mental patients into the community. The philosophy of psychosocial rehabilitation has evolved over time from beginnings which emphasized the training of patients (presumed to have permanent disabilities) in skills to help them live with, or improve, their disabilities, to the more sophisticated and integrated modern perspectives which allow for a variety of outcomes and acknowledge the role of the individual's interaction with their illness in determining outcome (Hogarty et al., 1995). Different generations of treatment approaches, reflective of the changing perspectives on serious mental illness, can be identified. Initial attempts at psychological intervention in mental illness were based on psychoanalytic theory (May, 1968) and were strikingly unsuccessful (Mueser & Berenbaum, 1990). Following this, behavioural treatments such as social skills training (Bellack & Hersen, 1979), family interventions (Falloon, 1985), and independent living skill programmes (Liberman et al., 1994), which targeted negative symptoms and disabilities, demonstrated more efficacy but failed to acknowledge the central role of personal characteristics, self-esteem, and individual attributions, in determining the impact of psychological treatment approaches. More recent treatment approaches, emanating almost exclusively from the United Kingdom, focus on the positive and negative symptoms of psychosis and emphasize the experience of the individual (Bentall, Haddock & Slade, 1994; Chadwick & Birchwood, 1994; Fowler, Garety & Kuipers, 1995). Such therapies have begun to demonstrate the effectiveness of psychological techniques in modifying psychotic symptoms, contrary to previously held beliefs that such symptoms were not amenable to psychological intervention. Finally, more comprehensive and integrated therapies, such as Hogarty et al.'s (1995) personal therapy, the constructivist approach of Perris (1989), or cognitively oriented psychotherapy for early psychosis (COPE) (Jackson et al., 1996), incorporate many of the successful components of earlier therapies and attribute a much more central role to the self and the bolstering of self-efficacy. This acknowledges that it is the interaction between the person, his or her illness, and society which determines outcome, and that there is a wide variety of courses for mental illnesses. It is no longer assumed that there is a simple relationship between symptoms, deficits and outcome, because impairments, strengths and opportunities interact in complex ways which are unique to each individual (Strauss et al., 1987).

The important difference for first-episode patients, as opposed to patients with established longer-term illnesses, is that disability and subsequent handicap may not have become entrenched, and there are greater opportunities for preventive work and developmental progression as opposed to remediation. This suggests that the focus should be on recovery work as opposed to rehabilitation. The former ascribes much more potential for change to the person or consumer and attempts to change positively their sense of self-efficacy. This is in accordance with the general trend in psychological treatments and psychosocial rehabilitation discussed above. Providing separate programmes for young first-episode patients in order to protect them from the potentially damaging stereotype of chronic mental illness, or 'negative and feared possible self' (Markus & Nurius, 1986), fits with this recovery focus of enhancing self-efficacy. In addition, the idea that there is a critical period of two to five years following the onset of psychotic illness and entry to treatment, during which there is the maximum possibility of deterioration and therefore the greatest role for preventive intervention (see Chapter 9) (Birchwood & Macmillan, 1993), suggests that an important function for treatment services is to provide an environment for the *maintenance* of skills, confidence and relationships during this period. Group-based programmes would seem to be ideally suited to the task of preventing deterioration in social skills, confidence and social networks during this critical period when the effects of the illness are likely to be the most severe.

Facilitating recovery: a new perspective

Recovery from mental illness is an emerging concept, described by Anthony (1993), as the new vision for the mental health service system of the 1990s. Citing consumers as major discussants of the concept, Anthony reported that: 'Recovery is described as a deeply personal, unique process of changing one's attitudes, values, feelings, goals, skills, and/or roles. It is a way of living a satisfying, hopeful, and contributing life even with the limitations caused by illness. Recovery involves the development of new meaning and purpose in one's life as one grows beyond the catastrophic effects of mental illness' (p. 15). Clearly, the aim of promoting recovery from a serious illness is to help the individual to regain independence and self-determination in achieving effectiveness and fulfilment in their various life domains, e.g. social, occupational, and leisure. For the person who has experienced the onset of a serious mental illness, it is particularly important to protect or reconstruct an enduring sense of self with which to interact with the world, and to influence positively his or her recovery (Strauss et al., 1987). This is because the experience of mental illness and especially psychosis, is likely to have changed the individual's view of the world and their safety within it, and diminished the individual's sense of personal control or self-efficacy (Bandura, 1977, 1986). Davidson and Strauss (1992) reported the results of a series of interviews conducted with people struggling to recover from serious mental illness. These research subjects frequently reported that the rediscovery of a sense of self was integral to their improvement: 'They note that an enhanced sense of self provides them with both a refuge from their illness and a foundation upon which they may then take up the work of recovery in a more active and determined fashion' (p. 131). For the first-episode patient it may be more a matter of preservation of the sense of self in the wake of the experience of psychosis.

Davidson and Strauss (1992) described four aspects of the recovery process which involve reactivating a functional sense of self. These are: discovering the potential to be active; assessing personal strengths and weaknesses and possibilities for change; performing actions to establish capabilities; and using the sense of self to enhance coping with symptoms and stigma. This list, derived from follow-up interviews with 66 recovering patients, thus provides a framework for the development of interventions to enhance these processes of recovery. However, since little information is given in the report about the chronicity of the sample, the relevance of these findings to the first-episode group is unknown.

McGorry (1992) reviewed a number of theoretical models relevant to the concept of recovery and derived a series of principles to guide the provision of clinical care. Originally applied only to the development of an inpatient programme for people recovering from early psychosis, these principles have formed the basis for the EPPIC approach (Edwards et al., 1994), and those which have particular relevance to the day programme are highlighted here. Following Strauss et al. (1987), McGorry (1992) suggested that the role of the patient in the recovery programme should be as *active* as possible. As emphasized by Leete (1989), the *active role* which patients play is generally poorly recognized, and is frequently hampered by the structures of services and the attitudes of treating professionals and the community at large. Thus a *collaborative* and *active* role is encouraged for all participants.

Secondly, the *type and quality of the milieu* in which the person is cared for constitutes the interface between the person and the social environment, and directly influences whether it will prove to be a recovery environment. Establishing an appropriately respectful and welcoming service model was listed by McGorry (1992) as essential for a recovery-

15 THE ROLE OF DAY PROGRAMMES IN RECOVERY

focused clinical programme. Thus, creating the type of environment that young people find comfortable is an important consideration in establishing recovery programmes. Finally, it is important to focus on *the strengths and attributes* that people possess which can often be called upon to assist in their recoveries. This accords with the ideas of Davidson and Strauss (1992) discussed above.

Other factors that have been cited as important in facilitating recovery from an episode of serious mental illness are: social relationships, goal setting and establishing routine and structure in the use of time. Breier and Strauss (1984), again drawing on material elicited in interviews with people recovering from psychotic illnesses, identified 12 functions of social relationships that have been found helpful in the recovery process. It was noted that these social needs changed through the course of ongoing recovery, and could be described by two overlapping phases: convalescence and rebuilding. The initial period following an episode of psychosis, or convalescence, is characterized by the need to reintegrate the self in the wake of the disruption caused by the illness. During this phase, patients listed ventilation, reality testing, social approval and acceptance, material support, problem solving, and constancy, or the re-establishment of relationships from before the episode, as the most helpful functions of social relationships in facilitating their recovery. Relationships during this phase were seen as more dependent and one-sided as the patients were struggling to regain their equilibrium. Patients reported being more comfortable maintaining relationships formed during the episode with co-patients and staff rather than entering new situations away from the treatment setting. Clearly, many of these functions are fulfilled by group-based interventions designed to facilitate the building of social relationships and self-esteem.

The second phase of recovery described by Breier and Strauss (1984), rebuilding, occurs once the individual has recovered a certain amount and feels somewhat stronger. This phase sees the patient moving away from a reliance on family, treating staff and fellow patients, to begin to develop new relationships. The functions of social relationships identified as important to continued recovery during this phase, were motivation, reciprocal relating and symptom monitoring. This paralleled the subjects beginning to take more responsibility for managing their illness and enlisting the help of others in this. Providing recovering patients with the opportunity to form or maintain social relationships and reinforcing the skills entailed in maintaining social networks, stands out as an important component of any programme aimed at facilitating recovery from psychosis. This task may be different for patients with chronic illness who may require help to build new or prosthetic relationships, whereas first-episode patients are more likely to have existing social networks that can be restored or maintained. However, social networks have been found to be impoverished even early in the course of psychotic illnesses (Jackson & Edwards, 1992), and to be at risk of further deterioration as illness continues. Restricted social networks and support have been shown to be related to poor prognosis in psychotic disorders. Group-based interventions that emphasize social interaction between young people are likely to be an important resource for protecting social networks through maintaining social skills and confidence and allowing first-hand experience of the benefits of social support during recovery from psychosis.

The importance of goal setting and developing structure and routine in coping with serious mental illness has been eloquently described in a first person account by Esso Leete (1989). Although describing her experience of coping with schizophrenia over a 25-year period, her observations give us important insights into strategies and skills helpful in overcoming a psychotic illness that are relevant to sufferers of early psychosis. Leete emphasized that structured activity, an organized daily routine, and goal setting were important in maintaining her 'wellness'. These factors constitute an important strategy for re-establishing the self as an instrumental and effective person, which in turn is crucial for recovery. Other factors regarded by Leete as important in her recovery and maintenance of 'wellness' were stress management, education about the illness, and an ongoing and reliable social support system. To this end, she established a peer-run support group that she believes has been important in her learning to cope with her illness. Thus, again the importance of social support is emphasized for those recovering from serious mental illness. That such support is an important part of the therapeutic value of group-based day treatment programmes for recent-onset psychosis was eloquently described by a young woman attending the EPPIC day programme.

> A 22-year-old single mother had experienced six months of social isolation and withdrawal prior to commencing treatment at EPPIC. Referred to the day programme by her case manager, she drew great comfort from being able to speak openly about her frightening psychotic symptoms with others who had experienced similar symptoms, and gradually built friendships with others attending the programme. She reported that group sessions that involved practical activities like cooking and recreational outings helped her to regain her confidence in being with other people, and she slowly increased

her social activities outside the programme. This began with outings with others from the programme, and then progressed to old friends and new acquaintances as her recovery advanced. She believes that the opportunity to participate in group programmes was the most important component of her treatment in facilitating her recovery.

From principles to practice: a day programme for recovery: the EPPIC day programme

In designing the EPPIC day programme as a part of the comprehensive multi-component service of EPPIC, a basic philosophy based on the perceived needs of the recovering young person was adopted. This was in keeping with the fundamental aim of the EPPIC service: to implement early intervention and preventive strategies, here within a group context, for young people in the post-acute and recovery phases of their first episode of a psychotic illness. The programme was to emphasize the important role of the recovering patient in guiding their improvement, and this was to be facilitated by focusing on strengths and collaboratively defining goals. Previous competencies were not considered 'lost' but 'temporarily out of order', and the view that these would return with support, encouragement, appropriate interventions, and realistic expectations, was espoused. Given the age of the participants, a consideration of each individual's specific developmental needs and the provision of opportunities to complete developmental tasks, were to be given high priority. Thus, the collaborative development of individualized programme plans, derived directly from each participant's stated needs and goals, was to ensure a meaningful and empowering experience.

This basic philosophy of practice was then translated into specific goals for the EPPIC day programme. These goals are listed in Table 15.1, and, together with the factors thought to be important in facilitating recovery from psychosis, guided the development of the content and operating procedures of the EPPIC day programme.

EPPIC day programme: structure and content

The day programme provides a range of group and individual experiences that are selected to meet each individual's specified goals. It places emphasis on self-direction and responsibility and, as such,

Table 15.1. *Goals of an early psychosis day programme*

Promote recovery from a psychotic episode
Facilitate recovery of previous competencies and the development of new skills
Prevent the development of secondary morbidity
Prevent, delay or reduce the severity of relapse
Facilitate maintenance of community connections and foster reintegration into the community
Minimize disruption and conflict within the individual's social network
Assist adjustment to, and working through, developmental stages
Enhance independent functioning
Maximize life satisfaction
Minimize effects of stigma

supports the recovery process. Day programme staff adopt a non-directive and supportive role in encouraging people to explore issues, identify goals, and reinforce the individual's primary responsibility in the decision-making process (see Figure 15.1).

Referral and assessment

Individuals are referred to the day programme by their EPPIC case manager. Attendance at the day programme occurs in addition to ongoing case management and usually begins towards the end of the acute phase of illness. Potential participants and interested family members and friends are invited to an introduction to the day programme session, at which all the groups offered and procedures of the programme are explained. Following this session, participants are asked to complete a comprehensive self-referral form, which covers the domains of social, domestic, leisure, educational, and occupational functioning. In completing this self-referral form, individuals need to consider their goals for attending the day programme in relation to the many domains of functioning that can be addressed. Individuals then have an assessment interview with a day programme staff member who has been assigned as their 'key worker' to decide which parts of the group programme they will attend, and any individual work that is deemed appropriate, in accordance with the goals that they have identified during the intake process. All of this collaborative work serves to ensure that each participant has chosen to become involved in the day programme in the way that is most relevant and useful to them, and that promotes the themes of self-determination and responsibility. These procedures are used flexibly in order to encourage as many recovering young people to attend the programme as possible. The

15 THE ROLE OF DAY PROGRAMMES IN RECOVERY

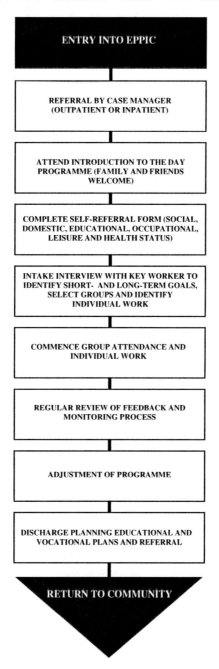

Figure 15.1. Client pathway through the day programme and role of the key worker.

client pathway through the day programme is summarized in Figure 15.1. However, it is likely that those with severe social anxiety or marked negative symptoms may be reluctant to complete the referral process until their symptoms have reduced. In these circumstances, case managers can assist in gradually introducing participants to the day programme, as illustrated in the case of 'Wayne' later in the chapter. In practice, younger participants who share common interests seem to utilize the programme the most. Older and female clients tend to be less represented, which suggests that the needs and interests of these clients are different. Specific therapeutic needs, or special client groups, are addressed through the provision of special groups called 'focus groups', which represent an expansion of the core day programme service to be described in detail below.

Structure

The core programme operates on Mondays to Fridays for about three to five hours per day. Individual assessment determines which parts of the programme each participant attends, and this varies from one group per week to attendance at nearly all of the groups offered each week. All groups are 'open' and welcome new members at any stage. However, the programme operates with four terms each year, and thus an approximately ten-week cycle occurs. This enables participants who commence during a term to attend the sessions that they missed in the following term. It is also felt that this structure contributes to the normalization of the day programme, in that it parallels the term structure of schools and tertiary institutions, with which young people are familiar.

Content

Group programmes offered in the day programme are divided into five categories or streams which relate to the perceived needs of recovering young people, the factors thought to facilitate recovery, and the particular challenges faced by the adolescent or young adult with early psychosis. The stream structure also ensures that, at any particular point in time, there is always a broad range of activities on offer to cater for the diverse needs and interests of participants. Each of these streams will be described in turn.

The social recreational stream
Social isolation and inactivity are common and persistent problems for people with serious mental illnesses and have been frequently ob-

15 THE ROLE OF DAY PROGRAMMES IN RECOVERY

served to be the most pressing initial problems experienced by the recovering first-episode patients treated at EPPIC. There are two groups that have been specifically designed to facilitate social interaction and increase general activity level, as well as foster a sense of hope for an enjoyable future. They are the 'out and about' group and the drop-in session. However, all day programme activities involve social interaction and some level of activity, and thus can also be seen as targetting these goals. The social recreational stream focuses on providing enjoyable social activities to maintain and develop social skills and networks, and to encourage access to community activities and resources.

(1) 'Out and about'. This is an outing group in which participants choose a place or exhibition to visit, or an activity to try out. The focus is on finding accessible and affordable activities in the local community, developing new leisure interests, and socializing in a group. It is run weekly for approximately three hours and utilizes public transport and local facilities. Obviously, this group provides the opportunity for the development of friendships and greater use of local recreational resources.

(2) Drop-in session. This is an unstructured session during which day programme participants can use the house facilities and spend time getting to know each other, play games, or get involved in creative activities. Staff are available to provide support and to suggest activities as needed. The unstructured nature of this session allows participants the opportunity to choose a comfortable level of intensity for their interactions with others, and often serves as a useful introduction to the environment, staff and other participants, for newcomers. The following case vignette illustrates the value of the drop-in session as an easy introduction to the day programme.

Wayne experienced his first episode of psychosis with affective features in his first year after leaving school. He gradually lost contact with most of his friends and spent several months confined to his bedroom because he was too frightened to leave it. After commencing treatment at EPPIC his psychotic symptoms resolved, but he was left feeling shattered and unable to resume his friendships because he was afraid of how his friends would react to him. His case manager recommended that Wayne attend the day programme in order to regain his social confidence. However, Wayne felt too frightened to join the programme at first. His case manager then arranged for Wayne to have his regular review appointments immediately before the drop-in session, and suggested to Wayne that they visit the programme together after their session. After a couple of visits, during which Wayne met and played cards with other participants and his case manager, Wayne felt confident to go along on his own, and gradually began to attend other parts of the programme, starting with 'out and about'. After a couple of months in the day programme Wayne began to re-contact his old friends and has been considering applying to go to a TAFE College next semester.

Vocational stream

After a period of illness and inactivity that may have included a significant period of deterioration prior to the psychotic illness being recognized and treated, many young people have lost their vocational path and need help to develop confidence in their ability to be active and productive (Jones et al., 1993; Kessler et al., 1995). The vocational stream focuses on minimizing the loss of work and study skills, encouraging the development of prevocational skills, and establishing realistic vocational plans based on knowledge of the available options and recognition of personal interests, skills and values. Successful vocational placement has long been a stated goal of psychiatric rehabilitation programmes and is often used as the ultimate indicator of the success of a programme (Bond, 1994). Groups in this category provide the opportunity to become more active and develop new interests in preparation for a return to training or study, or (re)entry to the workforce. They are: the vocational group, community lunch and catering project, and gardening.

(1) Vocational group. This group is for people getting ready to enter the employment market. It covers job selection, training options, community resources and services for the job seeker, resumé and application writing, and interview behaviour. In particular, strong links have been established with the Commonwealth Rehabilitation Service.

(2) Community lunch and catering project. This group involves participants in all of the steps entailed in preparing and serving lunch which is then offered to staff and clients of the service for a small charge. Participants learn basic cooking skills, as well as budgeting, food preparation, marketing, and basic kitchen management. It can be used as a stepping stone for those thinking about a career in catering, or just to gain confidence in basic cooking and working

as part of a team. Obviously, as with most day programme sessions, socialization is encouraged through such activity, and self-confidence is gained through mastery of tasks.
(3) Gardening. Through maintaining and enhancing the gardens around the day programme house, participants learn gardening skills that can form the basis of later vocational or leisure pursuits. Participants are also contributing to the upkeep of the programme which fosters a sense of ownership. Income generated through the sale of plants and produce has been used to fund extra activities such as summertime camps at beach resorts. 'Completers' now have the option of receiving a diploma in horticulture from a local tertiary college.

An 18-year-old man from a very disadvantaged background, including several periods of institutional care during his childhood, came to the EPPIC service when psychotic illness developed. He responded well to medical treatment but experienced many social difficulties, including homelessness and minor legal charges, and had no idea of a vocational direction for his life that might help to break his cycle of difficulties. Over time, he was engaged in the day programme, formed supportive relationships with staff and other participants, and discovered a strong interest and flair for gardening. This interest was encouraged and he was accepted into a vocational training programme for local government outdoor workers. This provided the opportunity for future employment and thus the opportunity to 'break the cycle'.

Creative expression stream

The creative expression stream utilizes a range of media through which participants can express their creativity and enhance their self-esteem. Participants usually enjoy these activities and subsequently have increased motivation to be active. The groups offered in this stream are: the 'rhythm of life' group, the creative writing group and the creative activities or 'studio 21' group.
(1) 'Rhythm of life'. This group aims to build self-confidence using movement, music and drama to encourage self-expression and awareness. There is also a focus on working with other people and having fun.
(2) Creative writing. This group either writes and produces a regular day programme newsletter or encourages group members to

pursue their own creative writing interests. Skills developed include: writing, word processing, layout, photocopying, drawing, and all the social skills involved in working in a team. These skills may contribute to the development of vocational interests and general self-confidence.

(3) Creative activities or 'Studio 21'. This group provides the opportunity for attendees to experiment with a variety of artistic techniques and media. Painting, papier mâché, clay sculpture, fabric printing, and any other creative activity suggested by participants is explored, and the sense of satisfaction in producing something contributes to enhanced self-esteem. The group also explores community art and craft groups that participants may wish to join if they find they develop a special interest in particular techniques.

Health promotion stream

The health promotion stream focuses on broad issues of physical and mental health with particular emphasis on those issues pertinent to the age of the population such as sexuality, physical fitness and nutrition. This stream includes the following groups: stress management, 'body and soul' group and 'fun and fitness' group.

(1) Stress management. As the title suggests, this programme presents an array of strategies for coping with stress and participants are encouraged to sample these during the sessions. These skills are considered vital to the achievement of recovery and the maintenance of 'wellness' within the stress-vulnerability model of psychosis (Nuechterlein & Dawson, 1984).

(2) 'Body and soul'. This group examines a wide array of issues and habits involved in maintaining a healthy lifestyle including diet, exercise, sleep patterns, substance use and goal setting. Poor physical health or co-existing physical disease has been reported frequently in people with mental illness (Kulkarni, Copolov & Keks, 1991) and this group aims to prevent unhealthy lifestyles and consequent poor physical health. It is particularly relevant to many young people who are at the stage of moving out of the parental home for the first time.

(3) 'Fun and fitness'. Through a weekly visit to a local gym and swim centre, participants are encouraged to experience the psychological benefits of regular exercise and establish or re-establish exercise routines. This is a general health promotion activity. In addition, the opportunity for casual conversation around a non-threatening activity is intended to help socially anxious young people to gain confidence in their ability to develop friendships. In

15 THE ROLE OF DAY PROGRAMMES IN RECOVERY

addition, those young people who possess particularly well developed physical skills or natural abilities, are able to use these to protect self-esteem in the wake of their psychotic illness. As illustrated in the following account provided by a day programme staff member, demonstrating mastery in one area of activity bolsters self-esteem and protects against self-stigmatization. Physical activities, offered in a number of day programme groups and associated camps, are important and salient areas of preserved skill for young people recovering from psychosis.

At 7.30 a.m. the door burst open and banged against the end of my bunk. A loud voice boomed out, 'When are we going fishing?'. I opened one eye to see David's outline in the doorway; it was the first morning of a three-day camp at a seaside town with ten young men from the day programme. I groaned and rolled over.

Fishing wasn't planned until that evening and we managed to engage David in the day's activities of swimming, body surfing and cricket, but he was just itching to catch some fish, and reminded us constantly.

I didn't go on the big fishing excursion; I stayed back with some of the others and played Scrabble. At 11 p.m., when they still weren't back, I was getting a little worried, but then I heard the minibus pull up outside. Everyone tumbled out of the bus in a state of high excitement and David presented himself with a huge smile, and a string of fish. Eyes were gleaming as people told the story of what had happened at the river. David had pulled out fish after fish; he truly was a master of his sport.

I had a glimpse of his genius the next day when we went yabbying. Armed with smelly meat, string and collanders we jammed our sticks into the sticky, muddy edges of the dam and, with mud oozing between our toes, we squatted down to wait for the small freshwater crustaceans to show themselves. It wasn't long before we were scooping them in; they were small and pale, thrashing around wildly before we threw them back.

David was still and silent and then, with a sudden graceful movement, he would scoop out big, black shiny monsters. We looked on in awe, and slowly moved our sticks closer and closer, trying to encroach on his territory. This didn't help – it was the skill that we were lacking.

David is a man who suffers from a psychosis, and who has watched

> his dreams crumble as he struggles to come to terms with his illness. On the water he is an expert and a master. He gained our respect and admiration for being a great fisherman, and I valued the opportunity to see him in that role.

Personal skills development stream
The personal skills development stream focuses on the development of a range of skills and strategies which enhances the person's ability to integrate the experience of psychosis, to cope with everyday life and to achieve optimum potential. The importance of psychoeducation and coping skills for the self-management of psychotic disorders has been increasingly emphasized in recent literature (Birchwood & Tarrier, 1992; McGorry, 1995). Clearly, understanding the nature, symptoms and treatments of one's illness, and having skills to cope with stress and meet life challenges, are important for maintaining 'wellness' and self-esteem. Within this stream lie most of the groups that most directly target interpersonal relationship skills, beyond those of basic interaction promoted by the social recreational stream. This set of groups addresses the important realm of interpersonal relationships. Perhaps the most commonly reported area of difficulty for people with psychotic disorders, especially schizophrenia (Halford & Hayes, 1991), it is seen as contributing to the inadequate role functioning of those seriously disabled by mental illness. Thus, social relationship and role-functioning skills are important areas to target in a programme of interventions aimed at the prevention of disability and the promotion of adaptive and independent lifestyles. Groups include: 'power to the people', discussion group and the 'secret of success'.

(1) 'Power to the people'. This is a psychoeducation programme conducted over ten sessions. Power to the people covers topics including the nature and treatment of psychosis, effects of drugs and alcohol abuse, social supports, stigma, early signs of relapse, and anxiety and depression. This knowledge is likely to be important in the overall psychotherapeutic process of psychoeducation (McGorry, 1995) that is aimed at promoting recovery and preventing relapse and secondary morbidity.
(2) Discussion group. Adapted from Yalom's (1983) model for inpatient group psychotherapy, this group is run weekly and uses a discussion format to foster the development of trust within the group, so that individuals can feel supported in facing up to, and dealing with, their problems. It is hoped that the opportunity to vent feelings and receive feedback from peers will help individ-

uals to enhance and protect their social networks. Increased understanding of the effects of their behaviours on others, and practice in dealing with conflicts, provide important learning experiences for participants.

(3) 'Secret of success'. This is a social skills training group in which skills are discussed, role-played and practised during sessions, often using games. Practice in the natural environment is encouraged through the use of homework assignments, fun rewards, and a participant-chosen 'end of term' activity. Social skills deficits are frequently reported in people with long-standing mental illnesses (Halford & Hayes, 1991). This group aims to encourage the utilization and development of social skills and to guard against social withdrawal and loss of confidence.

Focus groups

As mentioned above, a range of 'focus groups' have been developed in addition to the core day programme service to address particular needs identified for subgroups of EPPIC clients. These clients may or may not attend other parts of the day programme, and specific referrals are made to these groups as opposed to a generalized day programme referral. This option is appropriate for clients who are reluctant to join the overall programme, or who have particular circumscribed difficulties that are suited to group intervention. The following case vignette illustrates the latter situation.

Craig, a 27-year-old engineer, experienced his first episode of a manic illness with rapid onset and quick recovery. He recovered very well, kept in contact with his group of supportive friends, and returned to work after three weeks. However, he found that his illness experience had exacerbated the social anxiety that he had struggled with since he was a teenager. He was finding it increasingly difficult to address meetings at work, and had begun to avoid duties that were likely to place him in group situations. He worried that this problem was going to severely hamper his career. After discussions with his case manager, Craig completed a referral to the overcoming social anxiety focus group and attended the ten-week course which is based on cognitive–behavioural principles. He found that increased understanding of the basis of his social anxiety helped him to stop avoiding situations and that his anxiety began to improve.

The case of 'Craig' illustrates how a particular difficulty can be addressed through a focus group when wider involvement in the day programme was not indicated. Other areas in which focus groups are offered are: psychotherapy, for those wishing to more intensively explore interpersonal relationships; coping skills, for individuals interested in improving their resilience, problem-solving skills and positive thinking; and coping with psychotic symptoms, for the minority of clients who experience persistent psychotic symptoms. The focus groups have more limited selection criteria and clearly defined outcomes. The majority of the focus group programmes provide components of the personal skills development stream, although specific others, such as the vocational group, may also be focus group programmes in order to be accessible to a wider range of clients.

Monitoring progress

Regular reviews of goals and participation, with open access to feedback given by group leaders, occurs at review meetings between participants and their key worker. This ensures that progress is monitored, and goals and groups attended are adjusted accordingly. Day programme staff regularly review client progress at clinical review meetings and in individual supervision sessions. Mini case conferences are frequently held that include all clinical staff involved with a particular client. These may include the case manager, the key worker, the treating doctor and other clinicians involved.

Evaluation of the impact of the day programme

Regular feedback is received from day programme participants at review days held at the end of each term. This feedback from participants, together with consistent attendance and positive reports from case managers and others involved with EPPIC clients, suggests that the day programme seems to be a particularly helpful intervention for young people recovering from a psychotic illness. Preliminary outcome data from a study designed to evaluate the impact of the overall EPPIC programme would seem to support this contention.

The EPPIC follow-up study

Clients entering the EPPIC service, who meet the study inclusion criteria (i.e. reside in the catchment area of the service, are aged 16–30 years, are experiencing their first treated episode of psychosis, and are able to communicate in English) and do not meet the exclusion criteria (i.e. have an intellectual disability, or psychosis of organic origin), receive a comprehensive assessment package of psychopathological measures and an assessment of premorbid functioning. This assessment package is repeated at 6, 12 and 24 months after the original assessment, and also includes the Quality of Life Scale (QLS) (Heinrichs, Hanlon & Carpenter, 1984) conducted after the original assessment.

While not specifically designed to evaluate the day programme, it was possible to identify a group of day programme participants who had received the six-month follow-up package, and to compare them with a group of EPPIC clients who had not attended the day programme. Thus, the study was not a randomized clinical trial, but rather a naturalistic study of the effectiveness of the day programme. Thirty-four day programme participants (DP) were compared to 61 other EPPIC clients (NDP).

Table 15.2 reveals that there were no significant differences between the groups on the following baseline variables: age, sex, age of onset of psychotic disorder, distribution of diagnoses, duration of psychosis prior to treatment, level of education, marital status, or level of symptomatology at entry to EPPIC. However, the day programme group showed a trend towards having a higher level of negative symptoms (two-tailed t-test: t value $= -1.74$, $df = 93$, $p = 0.09$).

Interestingly, a significant difference was found between the DP and NDP groups in premorbid adjustment as assessed by the Premorbid Adjustment Scale (PAS; Cannon-Spoor, Potkin & Wyatt, 1982; two-tailed t-test: t value $= -2.40$, $df = 81$, $p = 0.02$). The day programme participants had significantly poorer premorbid adjustment than the comparison group (see Figure 15.2). (Note that higher PAS scores equal poorer performance.) This suggests that the day programme is providing psychosocial intervention to a particular subgroup of young people recovering from their first episode of psychosis. This group appears to exhibit poorer functioning prior to the development of their illness, in that they have a lower level of achievement of developmental goals.

In contrast, at the six-month follow-up point, no significant differences were detected between the two groups on any symptom measure, including the SANS or on the QLS, which assesses roughly similar domains to the PAS (QLS at six-month follow-up, ANOVA $F(1,93) = 0.94$, ns). Figure 15.2 displays group mean scores for PAS and SANS at study entry and QLS and SANS at the six-month reassessment. It should be noted that the QLS has been reverse scored for the purposes of comparison in Figure 15.2, and mean scores for all instruments have been z-scored to allow visual comparison. Thus, while the day

Table 15.2. *Baseline demographics and level of symptoms for the day programme and non-day programme groups at study entry*

Variables		Day programme	Non-day programme
Number		34	61
Mean age (years)		22.1	21.6
Mean age of onset (years)		21.4	21.3
Mean duration of untreated psychosis (days)		233.21	117.82
Percentage male		62	70
Percentage never married		94	88
Percentage with each education level	Completed secondary or less	76	85
	Trade qualification	6	7
	Completed tertiary	18	8
Percentage with each diagnosis	Schizophrenia	47	36
	Schizophreniform	18	18
	Schizoaffective	9	8
	Delusional	0	5
	Bipolar	12	20
	Depression	15	3
	Psychosis NOS	0	10
Mean scores on symptom scales:	Mean BPRS*	12.97	11.54
	Mean SANS*	29.8	22.6
	Mean BDI*	7.2	6.4

* BPRS = Brief Psychiatric Rating Scale; SANS = Schedule for Assessment of Negative Symptoms; BDI = Beck Depression Inventory

programme participants entered the programme with a lower level of psychosocial adjustment, it is possible that their participation has allowed them to achieve further development, which is a specifically identified goal of the day programme.

The data suggest that the day programme may be providing a service to an especially vulnerable group of clients in the 'critical period' following first-onset psychosis as described by Birchwood and Macmillan (1993) and McGorry (1995). These vulnerable young people may be at risk of deterioration in functioning, exacerbation of symptoms and development of disability, due to their poor level of premorbid adjustment.

The importance of early intervention in psychotic disorders through secondary prevention strategies to limit emergence of disability, and actively promote recovery, is emphasized at EPPIC. It is addressed through the provision of a comprehensive range of services, of which the day programme is an important component. The role of a group-based psychosocial programme in helping clients to contain and limit the negative effects of a psychotic episode or to develop a 'holding pattern' in which deterioration is prevented, may be significant. In addition to the preventive focus, a complementary role of the day programme is to promote recovery actively through a number of recovery goals and strategies as described above. Such interventions may have an impact not only in the short term but also in the longer term. As Birchwood and Macmillan (1993) stated: 'The implication is that efforts to contain and stabilise developing disabilities in functioning in these early years could have a disproportionate long term impact compared with interventions later in the course of illness' (p. 377).

It is also important to note that there were no significant changes in SANS and BPRS scores across the study period. Thus, there was no exacerbation of psychopathology in general, or worsening of negative symptoms, in the day programme subject group. It seems reasonable to predict that a group of patients with poorer premorbid functioning, as assessed by the PAS, would be highly vulnerable to the development of severe negative symptoms following the emergence of a psychotic illness. Results reported here suggest that the day programme may have contributed to the prevention of deterioration. The fact that the level of negative symptoms did not increase during the study period supports this notion.

Unfortunately, the QLS was not administered at the first assessment, thus requiring comparison with the PAS for an estimation of change over time. While this is a limitation of the present study, the two instruments do appear to be comparable in that there is considerable overlap in the areas they assess: social relationships, role functioning, independence, and involvement in the community (Heinrichs et al., 1984; Morice, Urbanc & McNicol, 1985). The finding that there was no significant difference between the day programme subjects and the non-day programme subjects on the QLS at the end of the study period, implies at the very least a stable rather than a deteriorating course. Again this is a surprising and encouraging result given the poor level of premorbid functioning indicated by the PAS.

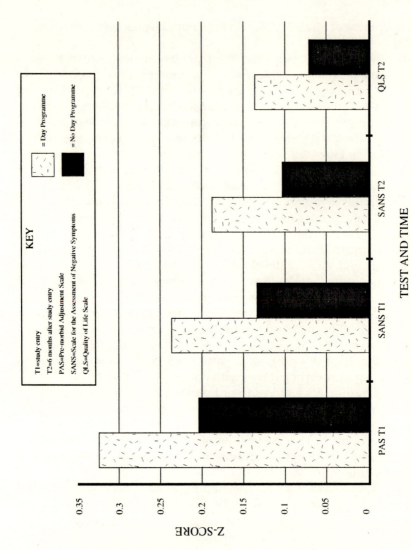

Figure 15.2. Mean PAS, SANS and QLS scores for the day programme group and the non-day programme group at study entry and after six-months.

Future directions

Further development of the EPPIC day programme can be considered from both a service delivery and a research perspective. First, in terms of service delivery, increased emphasis on the vocational aspects of the programme, with expansion of the staff to include trained teachers, further strengthening of links with community employment agencies, and the development of specific transitional employment programmes, is recognized as an important future direction. For many of the young people attending the programme, their stated aim (and a key index of recovery) is to find employment. The occurrence of an episode of psychosis during the important period of transition into adulthood has, for many, disrupted educational and vocational plans (Kessler et al., 1995), and re-establishing these is crucial for the maintenance of self-esteem. Providing work experience opportunities, through the development of local enterprises, is likely to be an important stepping stone into open employment for some young people.

An exciting new initiative being examined in the EPPIC day programme is the use of computer-assisted interactive learning to facilitate the psychoeducational process and programme evaluation. The fact that young people are generally familiar with, and attracted to, computers suggests that this learning method may facilitate engagement, sustain attention, and reduce the effects of social anxiety, thereby enabling young people recovering from psychosis to achieve maximum benefit from programme involvement. It will be important to monitor the influence of information-processing deficits that may be associated with psychosis in determining the success of this new technology, and computers can be useful in the assessment of this domain. The results of initial programmes utilizing computer-assisted learning are eagerly awaited.

From a research perspective, there are many important questions to be explored. The specific aspects of the day programme that have the most beneficial influence on outcome need to be explored in a component analysis, in order for the 'active' ingredients to be maximized. The psychological processes underlying positive change should be examined: are self-esteem and self-efficacy improved by attendance at the day programme? At a more basic level, we are not yet in a position to make recommendations about the optimal length and intensity of recovery-focused group interventions in first-episode psychosis. Clearly, there are more questions than answers at present, and further and more sophisticated research is required.

Conclusion

The rationale for, and the potential utility of, recovery-focused, group-based psychosocial intervention for young people following their first episode of a psychotic illness, has been presented, and the paucity of relevant research findings in this area has been highlighted. Emerging approaches in psychological therapies and psychosocial rehabilitation for those with serious mental illnesses that acknowledge the important role of the self and the social environment in recovery provide support for the further development of interventions using this format, which seems to be particularly appropriate for young first-episode patients. Preliminary outcome data has been presented that is encouraging and suggests that this day programme treatment modality may be an important component in an overall comprehensive service aimed at facilitating recovery from first-episode psychosis.

Acknowledgments

The author wishes to thank Mary Shannon, Deborah McDonald and Dianne Albiston, who have each had an important role in the development of the EPPIC day programme, for their assistance in the preparation of this chapter. Thanks also to Shelley McDonald for contributing the story 'David, the fisherman'.

References

Anthony, W. A. (1993). Recovery from mental illness: the guiding vision of the mental health service system in the 1990s. *Psychosocial Rehabilitation Journal*, **16**, 11–23.

Bandura, A. (1977). Self-efficacy: toward a unifying theory of behavioral change. *Psychological Review*, **84**, 191–215.

Bandura, A. (1986). *Social Foundations of Thought and Action: A Social Cognitive Theory*. Englewood Cliffs, New Jersey: Prentice-Hall.

Bellack, A. S. & Hersen, M. (eds.) (1979). *Research and Practice in Social Skills Training*. New York: Plenum Press.

Bentall, R. P., Haddock, G. & Slade, P. D. (1994). Cognitive behavior therapy for persistent auditory hallucinations: from theory to therapy. *Behavior Therapy*, **25**, 51–66.

Birchwood, M. & Macmillan, F. (1993). Early intervention in schizophrenia. *Australian and New Zealand Journal of Psychiatry*, **27**, 374–8.

Birchwood, M. & Tarrier, N. (eds.) (1992). *Innovations in the Psychological Management of Schizophrenia: Assessment, Treatment and Services*. Chichester, UK: Wiley.

Bond, G. R. (1994). Applying psychiatric rehabilitation principles to employment: recent findings. In *Schizophrenia: Exploring the Spectrum of Psychosis*, ed. R. Ancill, pp. 49–65. Chichester, UK: Wiley.

Breier, A. & Strauss, J. S. (1984). The role of social relationships in the recovery from psychotic disorders. *American Journal of Psychiatry*, **141**, 949–55.

Carpenter, W. & Strauss, J. S. (1991). The prediction of outcome in schizophrenia. V: Eleven year follow-up of the IPSS cohort. *Journal of Nervous and Mental Disease*, **179**, 517–25.

Cannon-Spoor, H. E., Potkin, S. G. & Wyatt, R. J. (1982). Measurement of premorbid adjustment in chronic schizpohrenia. *Schizophrenia Bulletin*, **8**, 470–84.

Chadwick, P. & Birchwood, M. (1994). The omnipotence of voices. A cognitive approach to auditory hallucinations. *British Journal of Psychiatry*, **164**, 190–201.

Davidson, L. & Strauss, J. S. (1992). Sense of self in recovery from severe mental illness. *British Journal of Medical Psychology*, **65**, 131–45.

Edwards, J., Francey, S. M., McGorry, P. D. & Jackson, H. J. (1994). Early psychosis prevention and intervention: evolution of a comprehensive community-based specialised service. *Behaviour Change*, **11**, 223–33.

Falloon, I. R. H. (1985). *Family Management of Schizophrenia*. Baltimore, Maryland: Johns Hopkins University Press.

Fineberg, B. L., Kettlewell, P. W. & Sowards, S. K. (1982). An evaluation of adolescent and inpatient services. *American Journal of Orthopsychiatry*, **49**, 337–45.

Fowler, D., Garety, P. & Kuipers, E. (1995). *Cognitive Behaviour Therapy for Psychosis: Theory and Practice*. Chichester, UK: Wiley.

Gabel, S. & Finn, M. (1986). Outcome in children's day-treatment programs: review of the literature and recommendations for future research. *International Journal of Partial Hospitalization*, **3**, 261–71.

Halford, W. K. & Hayes, R. (1991). Psychological rehabilitation of chronic schizophrenic patients: recent findings on social skills training and family psychoeducation. *Clinical Psychology Review*, **11**, 23–44.

Heinrichs, D., Hanlon, T. & Carpenter, W. Jnr. (1984). The Quality of Life Scale: an instrument for rating the schizophrenic deficit syndrome. *Schizophrenia Bulletin*, **10**, 388–96.

Hogarty, G. E., Kornblith, S. J., Greenwald, D., DiBarry, A. L., Cooley, S., Flesher, S., Reiss, D., Carter, M. & Ulrich, R. (1995). Personal therapy: a disorder-relevant psychotherapy for schizophrenia. *Schizophrenia Bulletin*, **21**, 379–93.

Hoge, M. A., Farrell, S. P., Munchel, M. E. & Strauss, J. S. (1988). Therapeutic factors in partial hospitalization. *Psychiatry*, **51**, 199–210.

Hoge, M. A., Farrell, S. P., Strauss, J. S. & Posner, M. M. (1987). Functions of short-term partial hospitalization in a comprehensive system of care. *International Journal of Partial Hospitalization*, **4**, 177–88.

Isenberg, D. P. (1983). A systemic–developmental model of day treatment for young adult chronic patients. *International Journal of Partial Hospitalization*, **2**, 113–24.

Jackson, H. J. & Edwards, J. (1992). Social networks and social support in schizophrenia: correlates and assessment. In *Schizophrenia: An Overview and Practical Handbook*, ed. D. Kavanagh, pp. 275–92. London: Chapman & Hall.

Jackson, H. J., McGorry, P. D., Edwards, J. & Hulbert, C. (1996). Cognitively-oriented psychotherapy for early psychosis (COPE). In *Early Intervention and Prevention in Mental Health*, ed. P. Cotton and H. J. Jackson, pp. 131–54. Melbourne: Academic Press.

Jones, P. B., Bebbington, P., Foerster, A., Lewis, S. W., Murray, R. M., Russell, A., Sham, P. C., Toone, B. K. & Wilkins, S. (1993). Premorbid social under-achievement in schizophrenia. Results from the Camberwell Collaborative Psychosis Study. *British Journal of Psychiatry*, **162**, 65–71.

Kessler, R. C., Foster, C. L., Saunders, W. B. & Stang, P. E. (1995). Social consequences of psychiatric disorders, I: Educational attainment. *American Journal of Psychiatry*, **152**, 1026–32.

Kettlewell, P. W., Jones, J. K. & Jones, R. H. (1985). Adolescent partial hospitalization: some preliminary outcome data. *Journal of Clinical Child Psychology*, **14**, 139–44.

Kiresuk, T. & Sherman, R. (1968). Goal attainment scaling: general method for evaluating comprehensive community mental health programs. *Community Mental Health Journal*, **4**, 443–53.

Kiser, L. J. (1991). Treatment-effectiveness research in child and adolescent partial hospitalization. *The Psychiatric Hospital*, **22**, 51–8.

Kiser, L. J., Pruitt, D. B., McColgan, E. B. & Ackerman, B. J. (1986). A survey of child and adolescent day-treatment programs: establishing definitions and standards. *International Journal of Partial Hospitalization*, **3**, 247–59.

Kulkarni, J., Copolov, D. & Keks, N. (1991). Biological investigations. In *Mental Health and Illness: A Textbook for Students of Health Sciences*, ed. R. Kosky, H. S. Eshkevari & V. Carr, pp. 136–42. Sydney: Butterworth-Heinemann.

Leete, E. (1989). How I perceive and manage my illness. *Schizophrenia Bulletin*, **15**, 197–200.

Lefkovitz, P. M., Morrison, P. P. & Davies, H. J. (1982). The assessment of current functioning scale. *Journal of Psychiatric Treatment and Evaluation*, **4**, 297–305.

Liberman, R. P., Wallace, C. J., Blackwell, G., Eckman, T. A. & Kuehnel, T. G. (1994). Skills training for the seriously mentally ill: modules in the UCLA social and independent living skills program. In *Schizophrenia: Exploring the Spectrum of Psychosis*, ed. R. Ancill, pp. 35–47. Chichester, UK: Wiley.

Malamud, T. J. & McCrory, D. J. (1988). Transitional employment and psycho-social rehabilitation. In *Vocational Rehabilitation of Persons with Prolonged Psychiatric Disorders*, ed. J. A. Ciardello & M. D. Bell, pp. 150–165. Baltimore: Johns Hopkins University Press.

Markus, H. & Nurius, P. (1986). Possible selves. *American Psychologist*, **41**, 954–69.

May, P. R. A. (1968). *Treatment of Schizophrenia: A Comparative Study of Five Treatment Methods*. New York: Science House.

McGlashan, T. (1984). The Chestnut Lodge follow-up study: II. Long-term outcome of schizophrenia and the affective disorders. *Archives of General Psychiatry*, **41**, 586–601.

McGorry, P. D. (1992). The concept of recovery and secondary prevention in psychotic disorders. *Australian and New Zealand Journal of Psychiatry*, **26**, 3–17.

McGorry, P. D. (1995). Psychoeducation in first-episode psychosis: a therapeutic process. *Psychiatry*, **58**, 313–28.

McGorry, P. D., Chanen, A., McCarthy, E., Van Riel, R., McKenzie, D. & Singh, B. S. (1991). Posttraumatic stress disorder following recent-onset psychosis: an unrecognised postpsychotic syndrome. *Journal of Nervous and Mental Disease*, **179**, 253–8.

Morice, R., Urbanc, S. & McNicol, D. (1985). The Premorbid Adjustment Scale (PAS): its use in an Australian study. *Australian and New Zealand Journal of Psychiatry*, **19**, 390–5.

Mueser, K. T. & Berenbaum, H. (1990). Psychodynamic treatment of schizophrenia. Is there a future? (Editorial). *Psychological Medicine*, **20**, 253–62.

Nuechterlein, K. H. & Dawson, M. E. (1984). Vulnerability and stress factors in the developmental course of schizophrenic disorders. *Schizophrenia Bulletin*, **10**, 158–200.

Perris, C. (1989). *Cognitive Therapy with Schizophrenic Patients*. New York: Guilford Press.

Rice, K. G., Herman, M. A. & Petersen, A. C. (1993). Coping with challenge in adolescence: a conceptual model and psycho-educational intervention. *Journal of Adolescence*, **16**, 235–51.

Rosie, J. S. (1987). Partial hospitalization: a review of recent literature. *Hospital and Community Psychiatry*, **38**, 1291–9.

Strauss, J. S., Harding, C. M., Hafez, H. & Lieberman, P. (1987). The role of the patient in recovery from psychosis. In *Psychosocial Treatment of Schizophrenia: Multidimensional Concepts, Psychological, Family and Self-Help Perspectives*, ed. J. S. Strauss, W. Boker & H. D. Brenner, pp. 160–166. Toronto: Hans Huber.

Yalom, I. D. (1983). *Inpatient Group Psychotherapy*. New York: Basic Books.

Part IV
Conclusion

16

Sharpening the focus: early intervention in the real world

PATRICK D. MCGORRY, JANE EDWARDS AND KERRYN PENNELL

Introduction

> Very early schizophrenia still constitutes a relatively unexplored territory. Entry into this territory calls for new ideas on the social problems involved in bringing the early schizophrenic under treatment, or where the treatment should be carried out and in what it should consist.
> (Cameron, 1938, p. 577)

Until recently, the attractive notion of early intervention in schizophrenia and related psychoses had not progressed any further than in Cameron's day. The previous chapters in this volume have begun to fill in some of the gaps on a previously blank canvas, yet there is much that remains to be done. The hypothesis that early detection and optimal treatment in psychosis has a prominent effect upon the medium- to long-term course and outcome of these disorders has not been conclusively confirmed, yet the evidence that does exist has created sufficient momentum for a genuine reappraisal of theory and practice. A preventive model is consistent with conceptions of the other complex medical disorders and has impeccable logic, yet it continues to face significant obstacles; and its status will ultimately be determined by the evidence which will gradually emerge.

The potential for reducing the suffering and lost opportunities for young people which flow from untreated or partially treated psychosis is great, at the very least in the short term, since these illnesses are highly treatment-responsive in most people (notwithstanding the fact that some individuals develop a variable degree of treatment resistance and that relapses are common). In the short term, then, for most patients early detection will limit psychosocial damage if treatment is offered, accepted, and the treatment provided is effective. The notion that early intervention may minimize or defer biological change is more speculative, as are the explanatory mechanisms advanced to explain such biological protection. Moreover, such biological processes, while they would add great force if proven, are not essential to sustain the argument for early detection and treatment, since this is robust on psychosocial grounds alone (see Chapter 3).

In economic terms, the potential benefits to society are correspondingly far-reaching and, within the current zeitgeist of economic rationalism, could become the main source of the momentum which will be required to restructure services systematically around an early intervention focus. Moscarelli, Capri & Neri (1991) identified an association between longer duration of untreated illness and higher subsequent health costs over the following three years. McGorry, Mihalopoulos & Carter (in press) found that an early intervention programme was highly cost-effective, even within its first year of operation. In this study, outcomes were substantially improved with a halving of inpatient costs, although outpatient costs needed to be markedly boosted to obtain both the savings and the better outcomes. The improved outcomes for individuals experiencing early psychosis were almost certainly due to greater intensity of community aftercare rather than a reduction of the duration of untreated psychosis, which was modest. Young people in this phase of illness appear to cost substantially more than middle-aged patients with established or chronic phases (Cuffel et al., 1996), even though they may experience serious problems in accessing services (Mental Health Branch, 1997). The increased costs are probably because the illness is more severe at this phase, adaptation and illness self-management remains problematic, and relapses and disability are more prominent. These aspects tend to improve with time, as does the severity of illness for the group as a whole, although costs again rise in the elderly. A rational approach would be to structure funding by phase of illness and developmental stage in a proactive way, since this is likely to be more cost-effective than the current pattern which has a reactive or 'catch-up' nature.

Andrews (1997) has recently proposed that, as a society, we should be shifting health care resources to types and phases of disorder where cost effectiveness has been demonstrated. He proposed a blend of burden (i.e. 'seriousness') and cost-effectiveness as the key parameters determining resource allocation within a capped budget. The only problem with this argument is that data underpinning indices of burden and cost-effectiveness are sparse and inadequate. Specifically, appropriate long-term cost-effectiveness studies in psychotic disorders have not yet been conducted. Short- and medium-term efficacy studies have shown that treatment in schizophrenia and other psychoses can be very effective, at least under favourable conditions. It is the real-world effectiveness that is more difficult to achieve, as it is for most disorders, and this has probably contributed, among other factors, to the rather gloomy (and probably exaggerated) conclusion that the course and outcome for schizophrenia has not changed since the time of Kraepelin, despite our claims of advances in treatment (Hegarty et al., 1994). In any event, in the presence of adequate systems of health care delivery and adequate specialist skill levels, we should be able to improve the quality and efficiency of care significantly. Within such systems, the logic of focusing treatment and resources on phases of disorder where there is likely to be maximum cost-effectiveness is sound. Such an approach makes sense in a range of medical and psychiatric disorders, for example hypertension, arthritis, breast cancer, eating disorders, and obsessive–compulsive disorder. It is a striking legacy of Kraepelin and the alienist tradition that the realm of psychotic illness has been so impervious to models of preventive medicine. A possible outcome of prioritizing the early phase could be a shrinkage in the size of the treatment-resistant group, a reduction in relapse frequency and severity, and a dimensional reduction in levels of impairment and disability across the board. The resulting savings could be utilized to further enhance the quality, depth and breadth of mental health services for all cases.

There are many obstacles to be overcome before the above scenario will become achievable. These will be discussed below; however, the major ones relate to mindset and funding. Even though there is some momentum behind the notion of early intervention, it is striking how difficult it can be to implement in real world settings. Nihilism, powerlessness, underfunding, the burden of existing cases, practical difficulties, low skill levels, a lack of support for specialization within a generic system, and inappropriate service boundaries, commonly conspire to inhibit reform. The following is an extract from a letter written soon after relocating to another region by one of our nursing colleagues who had worked for some years in our inpatient and home treatment services:

> Work is quite a challenge... The value of (my experience) was poignantly illustrated in some recent experiences with patients in the hospital where I now work. One was with a young man, psychotic and admitted for the first time. As I was escorting him to his room, assigned at the end of the high dependency (closed) section, he was glancing side to side along the corridor, flanked by heavy double locked doors of bedrooms which double as seclusion rooms. In one room he saw a patient sitting with her

arms folded. He looked at me, alarmed, and I knew straight away he had briefly thought he had seen someone in a strait-jacket. Paranoid, they called him; what about just plain old frightened? I'm a bit of a lone voice, but I'm on a mission in there. A rescue mission. I just have to be careful to balance these special needs against my own credibility in an atmosphere of entrenched attitudes.
(Colin Nicholson, personal communication, 1997)

Nevertheless, in our experience, such attitudes can be changed, and dramatically so over time. Sufficient expertise to improve outcomes does exist and is growing rapidly. A series of systematic studies should yield data which can be utilized within an evidence-based medicine (EBM) paradigm to improve the quality of clinical care in early psychosis. A second and more complex challenge will be to deploy this growing expertise in detection and treatment in the routine clinical practice. The failure of this latter step in many settings has allowed the claim to be made that treatment is not cost-effective. A similar delivery failure is responsible for the reduced impact of highly effective treatments such as lithium on the course of bipolar disorder, rather than a lack of efficacy of the treatment itself (Moncrieff, 1997), and of family interventions in psychotic illness (Kavanagh, 1992).

The key messages of this chapter are as follows. First, an early psychosis service or focus can be developed in many different ways. Diversity and creativity are to be encouraged and models can be developed in ways which are congruent and synergistic with the local setting. Indeed, a range of approaches already exist. What is common to these is a set of goals (see below). Secondly, planning is essential in terms of objectives (what you want to do and why), and strategy and tactics (how you will implement the planned changes). It is worth striving for a careful balance between process and content without neglecting or favouring either. Thirdly, evaluation of outcome and quality of care are central to the success of new initiatives. Evaluation allows clinicians to judge the value of their interventions; outcome data can have a powerful influence on policy makers and, importantly, on the practice of other clinicians. It is important to ensure that such evaluation and quality assurance activities are genuine. If the process is superficial or remote from true indicators of good clinical care, or if the data are invalid or unreliable, the process can cause harm: cynicism will emerge and inappropriate conclusions are drawn, resulting in poor planning decisions. Good evaluation and feedback are the lifeblood of an evolving service, and worthy of investment and nurturing: they are a means of protecting genuine efforts at improving the quality of the service from the ubiquitous superficial and dubious variants which are ultimately unhealthy for the organization.

The process of getting started in this area of work will be outlined in this chapter, and how to draw on positives in the local environment and to confront common obstacles will be discussed. Some examples of emerging and existing early psychosis programmes will be briefly described and future directions foreshadowed.

First steps: establishing an early psychosis focus

The first question to be answered is 'do we really want to do this?' If the answer is 'yes', then ask 'how much do we want to do it?' In other words, what is the level of motivation for the task. The question of 'why' is also important. In addition to the arguments already presented in favour of a preventive approach, it is worth remembering that any service focusing on 'serious mental illness' is likely to become responsible, at some point, for all the new cases of psychosis (except the most transient and self-limiting) presenting in the relevant region or sector, provided the service operates on a catchment area basis. Ultimately, over a period of several years, this cohort will give rise to the subgroup of regular or prolonged users of the service, i.e. the majority of the patients. Hence, it makes sense for a service of this kind to devote specific attention to the needs of new consumers. Nevertheless, logic is one thing and motivation another. It is worth asking yourself the above questions before embarking on a significant change in service delivery which will require energy, patience, and long-term commitment. It needs to be kept in mind that service reform operates on a continuum and the level of motivation needs to be matched with the scope of the endeavour.

A three-step model for getting started

If the initial motivational barrier is passed, then following the three steps outlined below should help to get things underway.

Step 1: Scoping
This involves a careful assessment of the incidence of psychotic disorders within the catchment area or sector. Examination of data from the World Health Organization (Jablensky et al., 1992) would be a useful starting point. The WHO figures provide only a guide, since there is a range of incidence rates, particularly for broadly-defined schizophrenia; nevertheless, it is useful to obtain estimates of the maximum and minimum levels. It will be necessary to define an age band

upon which to focus, either adolescent–young adult (e.g. 12–25, or 16–30 years) based on the period of maximum risk, or 16–45 or 16–65 years even; the latter might be linked to adult mental health service criteria. It should be recognized, however, that much of the power and clinical face validity of the early psychosis paradigm derives from the synergy of the preventive and developmental perspectives, hence focussing upon adolescent and young adults may work best. General population figures for that age group and area will need to be obtained (i.e. using census data), and then the expected incidence of psychosis calculated. Any marked discrepancy in existing inception rate into the service from the expected incidence levels should be noted and considered as a potential indicator for future evaluation of quality of access. For example, EPPIC's catchment area is approximately 820 000, covering the Western Metropolitan Region of Melbourne; census data indicated that in 1991 the number of people within EPPIC's catchment area and age range was 208 104 (Australian Bureau of Statistics, 1991). We estimated that a mid-range figure for incidence would be about 200 new cases of psychosis per annum; in fact, the actual rate has been stable for five years at approximately 230–250.

Once an estimate of numbers is obtained, the specific needs of this group in the local setting need to be clarified by an exploratory approach using a combination of quantitative and qualitative approaches. How many early psychosis cases do the mental health services currently see or not see? Are the individuals who are not seen by mental health services being well serviced by the private sector or primary care? If so, does this present opportunities for collaboration or suggest the need for specific specialization. Consideration needs to be given to the duration of service provision that is feasible before internal or external transfer of agency care. This will not necessarily be an issue depending on the level of specialization and segregation of the service in relation to mainstream mental health services. However, to maintain the early psychosis focus, some estimation of duration of service provision allied to the notion of the 'critical period' (see Chapter 9), and taking into account referral rates and available or anticipated human resources, will need to be made. For example, within EPPIC, treatment is currently provided for an 18-month period only, with a standard service case load of 320 patients; case managers manage approximately 35–40 individuals, in fact an excessive number. This relatively short time frame is not ideal; however, it allows us to seek, accept and manage all new cases within our catchment area – a 'front end' approach. If there were changes in the size of the catchment area, the age criteria the service has contracted to service, or the numbers of staff employed (i.e. funding), then re-assessment of the time frame which has been adopted would be required.

Table 16.1. *Core goals of a preventive intervention strategy*

1. Reduction of the duration of untreated psychosis	*Specific focus on that subgroup at high risk of delayed treatment*
2. Comprehensive expert treatment of the first episode of psychosis	*'Starting off on the right foot' e.g. slow introduction of low-dose medication (see Chapter 15 for strategies)*
3. Reduction of the duration of active psychosis in the first episode and beyond	*Maximize remission rates (identify slow responders and early treatment resistance)*
	Focus on relapse prevention in the critical period (2–5 years)
4. Maximize recovery, reintegration and quality of life	*Focus on the important concepts of recovery (early and prolonged) and recognize the validity of holding patterns for slower and less complete recoveries*

Step 2: Defining a focus

The second step involves defining the extent and complexion of the special focus. A recap on the core goals of a preventive intervention strategy in early psychosis is outlined in Table 16.1.

Some or all of these goals can be tackled, depending on the proposed scope of the strategy. It is possible to create an early psychosis focus or service even if resources are limited in scale or time. Possible spheres or levels of development are depicted in Figure 16.1. Within the enhanced service sphere, proposal could include, for example, a detection and assessment service, a strategy targeting young people with slow or prolonged recovery, a staff development and training programme, a high-risk clinic, or a recent-onset family intervention.

In some settings it will be possible to attempt ambitious and far-reaching reform of the service system, where historical and/or local political factors are favourable. Elsewhere, common features found in most service systems (e.g. an adolescent or youth mental health programme), can be built upon in creating an early intervention strategy. The coincidence of the epidemiological emergence of psychotic disorder and the developmental phase of adolescence provides natural momentum for such a strategy, although the close linkage in many countries of adolescent psychiatry with child psychiatry may be constraining (McGorry, 1996; Parry-Jones, 1995; Patton, 1996). In determining the scope of the change a number of specific factors need to be considered.

First, the level of support and capacity of health planners/administra-

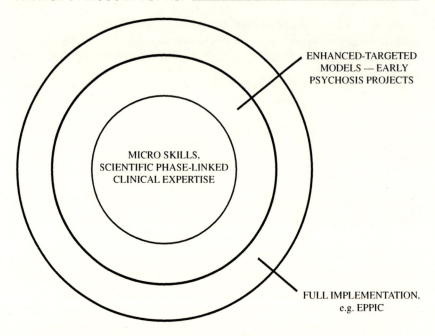

Figure 16.1. Spheres of action for preventive intervention in early psychosis.

tors and politicians to respond to the challenge is a key variable since it determines the level of resources which will be devoted to the focus, either through new funding or reallocation of resources. Consultation with health planners, policy makers, and management/executive groups helps to sell the concept, and this is probably the rate-limiting step for substantial and lasting service change. This phase might also involve discussion with affiliated academic departments, assessing the potential for interest and/or collaboration in potential research endeavours. Secondly, the attitude and morale of local clinicians and their potential to respond positively is critical. It is likely that this can be readily mobilized if some new resources can be obtained to initiate reform, and it may prove to be a powerful force for change. The level of interest of local clinicians can be assessed through the response to awareness-raising lectures and/or workshops. The early intervention strategy involves rekindling and harnessing the altruism and energies of mental health workers, which have often become blunted or extinguished in many service systems. We have generally been surprised by the widespread endorsement of the early psychosis paradigm. It seems that many clinicians have been waiting for an approach which offers a pragmatically preventive antidote to decades of withering pessimism. This pessimism has prevailed whether or not the patients have been treated in asylums or in the community. It has also been previously reinforced by outbreaks of false optimism. The latter include the antipsychiatry paradigm and other well intentioned reactions to the traumatic and dehumanizing aspects of front-line public psychiatry. All of these reactions contained very positive elements, but ultimately foundered on the rocks of reductionism or remained too marginalized to impact on the wider service system. While we believe the early psychosis paradigm is more soundly based, the current remoralization can be subject to potential threats, especially perceived additional burdens or externally imposed change.

Thirdly, key clinicians capable of driving or facilitating the venture need to be identified. Frequently, these individuals declare themselves during staff training activities. Fourthly, the capacity to attract additional project or research funding to catalyse a restructure of the service system and enhance clinical expertise is a further element which can influence the process. It is often difficult to pursue a new initiative without some allocation of dedicated resources. Even the securing of sessional clinical input for a time-limited period can be extremely helpful in getting started, a relatively inexpensive catalytic manoeuvre. Fifthly, consideration of the level of resources needed to support the process as the project develops, especially in terms of clinical supervision and training, is important. Are there sufficient resources within the service? Do any individuals have relevant expertise? The potential for collaborative ventures in training and supervision across neighbouring services could be examined. Finally, an estimate of the organization's overall level of health, energy, appetite for change, and capacity to manage effectively a change process of the scope envisaged needs to be made.

Use the population data from the needs assessment of the catchment area to help decide what the focus of your service should be. For example, are the numbers for first-episode psychosis sufficiently high to warrant development of a dedicated service? Alternatively, joint ventures with neighbouring services may be a fruitful option. Is there a relatively high number of young people with already established or chronic psychotic illness – does this therefore suggest that a preventive or early intervention service is needed?

In rural or remote areas it may be necessary to target *young people* with psychotic disorders within a certain age group, including individuals who have experienced multiple episodes in order to achieve a critical mass of recent onset cases, rather than focusing solely from the first episode onwards. In the situation of particularly low prevalence, detection of first-episode cases is likely to be assisted by adopting a 'broader net', given the low number of first-episode cases likely to be seen by any one service at any one point in time. Alternatively, linking with other services on a national or international basis may achieve the same goal under these circumstances. Some of the ideas and models adopted by the Scandinavian countries (Alanen et al., 1994), and the network of initiatives spawned by the Australian National Early Psychosis Project (Pennell et al., 1997) could be useful here. Where financial resources are time-limited, there is an argument to avoid using them to set up structures which the general mental health service will not be able to continue to fund once the specific project funding is withdrawn. This usually means focusing on training in the short term, unless a strategy can be developed to attract or assign 'hard' funding for continuation of the new service or the service can be reconfigured to shift resources from other patient groups. Another possibility is to focus on policy and procedure issues, developing treatment protocols which can be incorporated in mainstream systems, thus leaving tangible legacies. These must be living legacies rather than elegiac pronouncements, and further growth and evolution is essential.

Step 3: Pilot phase

Plan for a pilot phase of operation with evaluation of outcome as a component of the pilot. In preparation for this pilot phase, gather appropriate resource materials to form an 'early psychosis resource centre' and disseminate these to relevant clinicians, researchers, managers, etc. In addition, tap into local networks (e.g. internet discussion groups) and link with national or international associations (see below). This is a crucial step since written and visual resource materials, whether they are academic papers, practical manuals, or patient information tools such as videos and web-site addresses, have been found by others attempting to create an early psychosis focus to be highly influential. Considerable effort needs to go into a strategy for making these resources readily available for clinicians to use with early psychosis patients and their families. A separate issue concerns whether or not clinicians actually use the materials, once they have been made available; this can become a focus for clinical audits (Edwards & McGorry, 1998).

Obstacles to successful implementation of prevention strategies

General

Mind set

Pessimism is common among clinicians about the efficacy of treatment for psychotic disorders, especially schizophrenia, and not all clinicians recognize or acknowledge the importance of phase and duration of illness in terms of influencing outcome. Successful implementation of a preventive approach will require provision of antidotes to this pessimism. Resistance to change or, conversely, 'change fatigue' can also be barriers to achievement of objectives.

Money

Resources in mental health services are finite and generally scarce. Even when resources are seemingly abundant it seems to be a universal priority to provide for patients with established disorder and to continue to configure services to cater for such patients. This has also been a problem in the mainstream health system, where expensive high-tech interventions are delivered to patients with end-stage chronic disease, while preventive interventions in the earlier stages fail to receive adequate support. Older psychotic patients with significant disability tend, not unreasonably, to be seen as 'more severe', and their characteristics contribute almost exclusively to the definition of 'serious mental illness'. A more dynamic model of disorder enables the preventive possibilities to be grasped. The current prioritizing of the (sizeable) minority of established cases ignores the future chance to shrink the size of this group and reduce the need in due course for belated 'rescue' or palliative therapies. For example, the yield in trying to provide family intervention several years after the onset of illness against a background of neglect, detachment or high expressed emotion is almost certainly much lower in terms of cost-effectiveness, particularly if the patient no longer lives with the family. Families need phase-appropriate help during the early course of the disorder. Unfortunately, there will inevitably be a lead time before such improvements in outcome and service savings occur. Thus, a certain amount of vision in service planning, and longer-term budget cycles are required.

Morale

The degree to which people working in front-line clinical services can be inspired to embrace a more optimistic approach is a crucial factor in the success or otherwise of implementing change. Although there is a high level of burnout in many services which breeds cynicism, it is generally surprising how readily staff tend to be attracted to these preventive strategies. It is important not to over-sell what can be done and not to raise expectations too high. Many staff are aware of the danger of 'rescue fantasies', but the pessimism in the management of schizophrenia, in particular, has been extreme and a substantial degree of realistic optimism can be justified. An optimistic approach in early psychosis is not only justifiable but essential. It is not only dependent upon, but also breeds and sustains, morale in a service. The optimism translates to the patients and this attitude not only actively promotes recovery (Kuipers et al., 1997) but also, it could be argued, leads to improved outcomes.

Specific

Lack of specific skills

Overcoming this obstacle requires resources, staff development mechanisms, adequate supervision, and quality assurance mechanisms. Practical details of how EPPIC approaches many of these issues are provided in the *EPPIC Information Package*, a staff information document which is updated and distributed to all staff at six-month intervals (Edwards & McGorry, 1998).

Lack of focus

There is a need for a capacity to create specialist foci within a generalist service, even one which is already targeting psychosis or 'serious mental illness'. This may be limited by ideology or, more commonly, by cost or the size of the service, i.e. the critical mass for specialist endeavours may be difficult to create and maintain in the face of competing demands. Essentially, it involves valuing and implementing a division of labour model, and works against a lowest common denominator effect. The costs of increased specialization of this kind need to be identified, since it may prove more expensive, at least in the community setting. In such an exercise, the overall degree of cost-effectiveness in the medium- to long-term is the key issue.

Lack of appropriate operational/organizational structure

Any 'special focus' service benefits from being set up with a specific programme structure rather than being discipline-based. The existence of a service co-ordinator (ideally, an experienced senior clinician), with a clear statement of goals and remit for action, can help focus resources on particular tasks; specialist expertise from given disciplines can then be fed into the programme and deployed within the context of a multidisciplinary team.

It is important that individuals are mandated to undertake leadership roles. Working parties and committees need to identify convenors clearly, operate with terms of reference, and appoint chairpersons. There needs to be formal recognition of the time required to undertake co-ordination roles. Managers and/or funding providers need to acknowledge that resources must be allocated for such tasks to enable effective clinical leadership to occur. This usually requires a combination of logic, persuasion and lobbying skills.

Age barriers

Services are frequently established for children (0–18 years), adults (16–65 years), and aged persons (> 65 years). Approximately 20% of new early psychosis cases will fall in the < 19 years age group. This 'age barrier' does not fit with the early intervention model (Rutter, 1995). Considerable inefficiencies are evident in the transfer of young people from one service to another when a certain birthday is reached, co-ordinated approaches to early identification are missed, and opportunities for staff training which span the age barriers (i.e. developmental issues) are lost. Furthermore, the cultures of care and skill mixes across child and adult services are frequently radically different. A serious approach to early intervention in psychosis needs to confront the issues around the organization of systems of care. A strategy which has face validity and which we have been pursuing is the forging of a youth mental health service (for those aged 12–25 years), focussing on prevention across a broad range of disorders and blending elements of child and adult psychiatry (McGorry, 1996).

Pathways to care: the structure and quality of the primary care system

A service that has prevention and early intervention as its focus will not succeed unless good links exist or are established with the primary care services in the sector or region within which the service intends to operate. If existing links are not optimal, then one of the first tasks is to develop these. Primary care practitioners are the gatekeepers to health care in most systems and the first helping contact for most people. Their role is essential in early recognition and initial treatment of psychosis (see Chapter 3).

Training, consultation and education

Training, consultation and education are all necessary to bring about change within a service and to develop a new approach successfully. Investment in staff in terms of training and education is probably one of the single most important factors to consider when setting up an early psychosis service. Interventions can range from simple distribution of relevant academic papers to more comprehensive programmes.

Staff training

One of the most important elements in the provision of training and professional education is the matching of the content to the needs of the participants. Significant consideration should be given to the format and content to be used by the trainers. Much of what can be taught about early psychosis is reflected in this book but it is essential to match the topic and complexity of the information to the participants' needs. For example, with a large group with very little background in early psychosis, it will be important to discuss the philosophical underpinnings of the preventive approach and the rationale for early intervention before moving on to cover more specific issues such as at-risk mental states and assessment. With a group with some background in the area, or with particular professional skills (e.g. psychotherapy), it will be possible to address even more specific areas within the field, such as cognitive behavioural therapy or family work. We have developed a 'train-the-trainer' package for early psychosis (McGorry & Edwards, 1997) which is aimed at assisting with this training process.

It is useful to build in opportunities for the training group to reconvene at regular intervals to discuss how they have been able to implement the new skills and knowledge developed during the training sessions and to use the process of group discussions to work through the challenges and dilemmas that they may have faced. One approach is to form a peer support/supervision group or a mentor/buddy system whereby two or three participants support one another in the early stages after a formal training programme as they begin to use their new skills. Distance learning via video conferencing, internet-based packages, or using video and audio tape training materials, can also be used effectively. More extended postgraduate education is an additional component, and this can be provided through creating a module within broader courses and programmes. Examples of this include the graduate diploma in young people's mental health offered via distance education within the Department of Psychiatry at the University of Melbourne in collaboration with EPPIC, and the Community Mental Health Diplomas offered by the Universities of Wollongong and Melbourne, and Monash University in Australia. Written materials in the form of key references, handouts, clinical guides, work books, and practical manuals can all be used to enhance people's knowledge independently of workshops or lectures.

Site visits and the use of expert speakers

Site visits whereby clinicians can exchange expertise, experience and challenges are helpful. Many of the services described below, including EPPIC, encourage site visits. Furthermore, some of these services have organized national conferences on early psychosis issues (e.g. Australia, the Netherlands, Scandinavia, and the UK); these can be an important tool in influencing policy makers and other clinicians, and offer the host service an opportunity to access external expertise (e.g. from expert speakers) for the benefit of their own staff in a cost-effective manner.

Consultation

Consultation is a powerful educational strategy which promotes a collaborative partnership through which solutions are identified. Mental health consultation involves client-centred case consultation (which relates to the management of a particular case or group of cases), consultee-centred consultation (which aims to help the consultee to improve knowledge and skills), and programme-centred consultation (which involves improving planning, administration and programme development).

It is necessary for the individuals providing the consultation to be closely allied with a clinical setting from which they can act as a conduit, specifically drawing on the clinical experience of the clinicians at that service. The drawback of this model is that it needs a home base from which trainers and experts can be drawn, and such a base must be able to fund and resource extramural activities. There are several strategies which can be used; however, a mandate from the purchasers of services together with appropriate funding is an essential foundation. A broader range of activities can be funded on a fee-for-service basis.

Provision for consumer involvement

Any provision for consumer involvement in the development of an early psychosis service needs to recognize that carers and consumers in early psychosis have a different perspective on the issues surrounding psychiatric illness, from those experiencing chronic illness, and therefore their role needs to reflect these differences rather than following a standard model of consumer participation. Many individuals who experience early psychosis are relatively brief users of the service and may not find the adoption of a consumer-participation role relevant or meaningful. Others find themselves struggling to cope with the whole experience of the illness and its treatment, and consequently may find it difficult to contribute to consumer input into the service. Nevertheless, it is essential to ensure that there is a strong consumer influence on the service, since this maximizes respect for consumers and carers, and enhances the ambience and quality of care. It may be best to involve and consult with recent 'graduates' of the early stages of illness and treatment.

Evaluation and quality assurance

Evaluation and quality assurance in health services is becoming an increasingly important issue as those who fund services, those who provide services, and those who use services, want to know whether the services provided are effective and delivered in the best possible manner. Mental health services, previously neglected because of presumed difficulties in measuring outcome, are no exception to this emphasis on evaluation. Because preventive intervention in early psychosis is a relatively new area, evaluation of outcome and quality control in service provision are particularly important, not only for their intrinsic value, but also as a powerful tool to influence policy makers and other clinicians.

Naturalistic studies of a treatment intervention or programme of care in a mental health service, rather than studies of efficacy in controlled experimental conditions, are probably most useful in determining effectiveness, as any interventions adopted as a result of positive outcome data will be implemented in similar real-world clinical settings. Ideally, such naturalistic studies are comprehensive and measure effectiveness in several different ways, including measures of effect on the patient (psychopathology, social functioning and quality of life) and measures of effect on the wider service system, and ultimately the community (cost analyses, service utilization analyses, etc.). However, on a smaller scale, it is possible to use existing clinical audit and quality assurance to measure the effectiveness of specific interventions and to monitor the quality of care being provided.

Clinical practice guidelines

The development of clinical practice guidelines is an integral part of the evaluation process that can help direct resources and smooth out inappropriate variation in clinical practice (Grimshaw & Hutchinson, 1993). In the context of an early psychosis service, clinical guidelines have a particular role in providing parameters by which clinicians working in a new field can monitor and adjust their own practice.

Clinical guidelines need to be drawn up as a result of a consensual multidisciplinary process or their chances of implementation will be limited. Without suitable clinical guidelines and linked auditable parameters, any evaluation attempt will be doomed as the number of variables will be too great to allow proper assessment of the interventions proposed.

Guidelines need to be specific and related to the different phases of

Table 16.2. *Examples of clinical guidelines and measurement indicators used by EPPIC as part of the EPPIC: Standards of Quality in Clinical Practice (contained in the EPPIC Information Package, February 1997)*

Guideline	Indicator
EPACT will undertake urgent assessments within 1 hour	Mean number of minutes between receipt of urgent referral and action taken
Non-urgent assessment will occur at a mutually convenient time for the client and EPACT	Mean number of days between receipt of urgent referral and action taken
Referring agency will be informed (in writing) of outcome within 48 hours of the initial assessment	Percentage of referrers contacted within 48 hours
The location of acute treatment should be in the least restrictive environment	1. Admission/readmission rates per last quarter 2. No. of referrals to HBT for acute episodes 3. Average no. of bed days/patient/year 4. Mean LOS 5. No. of patients on CTOs/quarter 6. Average length of stay on CTOs 7. Episodes of seclusion/month.
All new HBT patients should have a neuroleptic-free period for 24 hours	1. Percentage of clients not medicated with neuroleptics in first 24 hours of any HBT plan
All new inpatients should have a neuroleptic-free period for 48 hours	2. Percentage of clients not medicated with neuroleptics in first 48 hours of any admission
Daily dosage of neuroleptic should not exceed 2 mg HPD equivalent within the first 3 weeks	1. Percentage of clients receiving 2 mg HPD equivalent in first 3 weeks 2. Mean daily dose of neuroleptic medication in first 3 weeks of treatment of all first episodes

CTO = community treatment order; EPACT = Early Psychosis Assessment and Care Team; HBT = home-based treatment; HPD = haloperidol; LOS = length of stay.

management (referral, assessment, acute treatment, recovery interventions, discharge) and it must be possible to develop related measurement indicators for the guidelines to be useful as part of an evaluation and quality assurance process. Table 16.2 gives examples of clinical guidelines and measurement indicators developed by EPPIC to evaluate service provision for clients in the acute phase of illness. The

Australian National Early Psychosis Project has also produced a set of clinical practice guidelines (NEPP, 1998).

Evaluation techniques

With respect to an early psychosis service, evaluation should focus, first, on how well the programme is being delivered, i.e. *process* evaluation and, secondly, whether the programme is achieving its specified outcomes or effects, i.e. *impact* and *outcome* evaluation.

Any evaluation model should be realistic and achievable within the constraints of a busy clinical setting. How this is undertaken depends on a number of issues including resources, programme design and the constraints of naturalistic settings (see Thornicroft & Tansella (1996) for suggestions of ways of measuring outcome in mental health).

Preliminary evaluation at EPPIC (McGorry et al., 1996) used a quasi-experimental research design whereby the initial 51 consenting patients from EPPIC and 51 matched control patients from our earlier more generic early psychosis model, were assessed and followed-up at four different time points using a battery of outcome instruments to determine whether a service oriented around intensive early intervention, with a strong community focus, does improve outcome compared with relatively (but not typical) generic psychiatric care. Measures used included the Royal Park Multidiagnostic Instrument for Psychosis (RPMIP) (McGorry, Copolov & Singh, 1990; McGorry et al., 1990), the Brief Psychiatric Rating Scale (Overall & Gorham, 1962), the Scale for the Assessment of Negative Symptoms (Andreasen, 1983), and the Quality of Life Scale (Heinrichs, Hanlon & Carpenter, 1984). Fuller economic evaluation (e.g. cost-effectiveness and service utilization) of the early detection and biopsychosocial interventions used at EPPIC has subsequently been carried out (McGorry, Mihalopoulos & Carter, in press).

Another example is the Melbourne-based Central East Early Psychosis Project (Haines et al., 1997), which is training clinicians within a mainstream service to provide specialist care for young people with early psychosis. Process and outcome evaluation in this project uses markers such as minimal use of police in hospital admissions and various indicators of the quality of follow-up of first-episode patients as benchmarks of best practice. Data collection for this evaluation process is carried out by a full-time research assistant for whom funding from the state health department has been provided. The project research assistant is also collecting concurrent clinical data related to patient outcomes from a neighbouring mainstream service, in which no specialist focus was developed, for purposes of comparison.

Other approaches to evaluation of early psychosis services are given in the examples of early psychosis services/projects outlined below.

Examples of early psychosis services/projects

During the 1970s and 1980s in Scandinavia, particularly in Finland, there has not only been a serious commitment to prevention in schizophrenia, but also a significant impact of these preventive ideas on the service system (Alanen et al., 1994). Unfortunately, this integrated approach with an emphasis on psychotherapeutic methods, while including biological therapies (although these were somewhat de-emphasized until recently), is not widely known or appreciated in other countries (Alanen, 1997). Building on this substantial first generation of effort in moving towards a preventively oriented system which values biological and psychosocial treatments equally, we will continue by describing some of the current generation of projects which, thanks to a range of recent enhancing factors, is at last achieving significant international momentum. This has reached the point that, at the first large-scale international conference on the subject held in Melbourne in 1996, 'Verging on reality: preventive strategies in early psychosis', the establishment of an International Early Psychosis Network was proposed, and a preliminary statement of principles regarding the detection and treatment of early psychosis was agreed upon (see Appendix 1 to this chapter). A global network to be known as the International Early Psychosis Association has now been formed which will disseminate information, publicize conferences and other professional meetings, and facilitate research in the field and the development of a collection of educational and scientific resources relevant to the field. To guide its early development, an international advisory group has been established. Readers who are interested in becoming a member should complete the form contained in Appendix 2. The early psychosis projects described below are all affiliated with the network and have provided information on their services as a means of encouraging and supporting other clinicians and researchers in new initiatives.

Australian National Early Psychosis Project
Contact: e-mail eppic@vicnet.net.au
WorldWideWeb http://ariel.unimelb.edu.au/~nepp.
The Australian National Early Psychosis Project (NEPP) has been a collaboration between the Commonwealth, State and Territory Governments of Australia to develop and promote a national model of best

practice in early intervention in psychosis (Pennell et al., 1997). It was established in early 1996 as a key initiative of the landmark National Mental Health Policy and Plan (AHMAC Working Group, 1992), which has strongly emphasized prevention and early intervention. NEPP operated as a national network with a project co-ordinator based in each state and territory whose role has been to progress the project in conjunction with government departments, mental health professionals, consumers and carers, and other key stakeholders. These co-ordinators worked with existing early psychosis projects such as those already described, as well as promoting the development of new initiatives. This has involved a synergistic equilibrium of 'top down' and 'bottom up' forces (NEPP, 1998) which have catalysed a major shift in thinking and a patchwork quilt of service reform. The ultimate measure of the success of the initiative will be the extent to which an enduring systemic restructure of mental health services occurs which can deliver better outcomes and quality of life to young people with early psychosis.

The project had three key foci:

(1) Service and policy development including the provision of tertiary consultation, ongoing support, advice, information, and access to expertise to aid mental health service providers and policy makers to incorporate a best practice approach.

(2) Professional education and training which involved provision and distribution of a range of professional development resources and activities facilitated by project coordinators.

(3) Provision of information and promotion of best practice policies via a variety of means including a newsletter, the project resource centre (located on the WorldWideWeb), and development of clinical practice guidelines.

The project was funded until January 1998 and several elements continue. During its lifetime, it established a network of interested individuals who have continued to work on the development and promotion of best practice in early psychosis.

EPPIC Statewide Services
Melbourne, Victoria, Australia
Contact: e-mail eppic@vicnet.net.au
WorldWideWeb http://www.vicnet.net.au/~eppic

A subprogramme of EPPIC, Statewide Services, has developed a model of professional training, development and consultation that aims to ensure all mental health agencies in the state of Victoria, Australia, can have access to clinical skills, expertise and knowledge in the field of early psychosis (Haines et al., 1997). The team focuses on providing assistance to other mental health teams through a range of specific services that include: secondary and tertiary consultation, professional education and training, resources development, community education, and the facilitation and development of early psychosis projects. Moving sequentially across the state, these latter projects make effective use of standard staffing levels by providing a concentrated and intensive exposure focusing upon early psychosis over a six-month training period within the mental health service the team provides for a discrete region. The team initially seeks the support of the local management and clinical leaders and, with the mandate of the state director of mental health, works in collaboration with local services to develop models of practice and protocols of care. They aim to develop models which are responsive to local needs and mesh well with the regional services organization, direction, and way of working.

Early Episode Psychosis Project: a system of care
Freemantle; Armadale/Kelmscott; Rockingham/Kwinana, Western Australia
Contact: South Metropolitan Health Authority, Locked Bag 3, Post Office, Applecross, Western Australia
This project was set up in recognition of the need for new thinking and a more optimistic outlook in the treatment of psychotic disorders. It uses a partnership model between different service providers. The project aims to create a mechanism for general practitioners and psychiatrists in the private sector to access public mental health services and publicly-funded services in the non-government sector; expand the role of the non-government sector to include clinical services in addition to their more traditional support services; involve general practitioners in providing services to the seriously mentally ill from initial assessment through all stages of treatment, rather than the traditional model where patients would return to their general practitioner after treatment in the public mental health sector; and offer patients greater choice about receiving services through the private, public or non-government mental health sectors. The model is community-based with an emphasis on a range of psychosocial interventions, a low-dose medication approach and reduced emphasis on inpatient treatment. When needed, inpatient treatment is given in specially-designated units supervised by psychiatrists with a special interest and expertise in psychosis. Training is provided to general practitioners and others working within the model to ensure that they are able to deliver the system of care.

This 'system of care' model was developed in early 1995 by a project officer and members of the project's steering committee (representing a wide range of organizations) in consultation with other West

Australian early psychosis groups. Implementation of the model has been on a district basis as this best suited the existing health care structure of the area and its future needs based on estimates of population growth.

Early Psychosis Prevention and Intervention Project
James Fletcher Group of Services (JFGS), Newcastle, New South Wales, Australia
Contact: FAX +61 49 246 724
This project operates within Newcastle and the Hunter Valley in New South Wales, Australia, which has a catchment area of 120 000 persons between 16 and 30 years of age within a total population of 500 000. The early psychosis project, supported by the service and academic leaders of the region, has been co-ordinated by a sole practitioner and has focussed on education and skills development. It has drawn heavily on a train-the-trainer model using several key mental health professionals from local teams and providing them with theoretical and skills training in early psychosis work so that they could assume the role of early psychosis liaison worker. The team of early psychosis liaison workers are responsible in turn for training their local teams and facilitating development of local referral, assessment and treatment protocols. A central part of this project was the generation of an early psychosis library which circulated journal articles on early psychosis and provided written material on relevant issues as requested. Evaluation is an integral part of the project. The project has now developed an early intervention assessment service to try to reduce the delay before treatment and gather knowledge about the early stages of psychotic disorders, particularly the pre-psychotic phase. Linkages with primary care have been a key feature of this latter initiative.

New Zealand National Early Intervention Interest Group
New Zealand operates a purchaser–provider model of funding and so the New Zealand National Early Intervention Interest Group has focused on the development of a draft consensus statement on early psychosis service structures and specifications. This group has harnessed local interest to develop a document that can guide service funders about the clinical and organizational steps needed to provide a specialist early psychosis clinical programme. Early psychosis programmes are now in existence in Wellington, Auckland and Christchurch.

The Early Treatment and Identification of Psychosis (TIPS) project
Stavanger, Norway
Contact: < tklarsen@online.no >
This project is embedded in a high quality global service system with

close involvement with the local community, anti-stigma initiatives, and strong leadership. The TIPS project is a prospective longitudinal five-year study designed to see whether early identification and optimal treatment of first-episode psychosis leads to better long-term prognosis. Three different sites will be compared: one test site (early detection) in Rogaland (Norway) and two control sites in Oslo (Norway) and Roskilde (Denmark). The project has expert research support and collaboration involving Yale University and the University of Oslo (Johannessen, 1996; Larsen, McGlashan & Moe, 1996; McGlashan, 1996). The test programme includes education, networking and clinical early detection teams. A well-funded, large-scale, total community education programme aims to increase awareness of early signs of psychosis among health care workers, teachers, and the general public. Training in early detection for all general practitioners and social nurses will be provided using lectures, videos, rating manuals, and information brochures. Networking will involve contacting, educating and recruiting primary care providers to the early detection programme. The early detection teams are multidisciplinary and are led by clinicians whose primary responsibility is the early detection of untreated first-episode functional psychosis. The standard treatment protocol at all three sites includes three core elements: supportive psychotherapy with active outreach, a standard low dose medication regimen, and family work. Evaluation will occur at baseline, three months, and one, two, and five years. Assessment will include diagnosis, premorbid functioning, duration of untreated psychosis, level of symptoms, social interaction, quality of life, and global functioning. Neuropsychological assessment will also be carried out at three months, and one, two, and five years.

'The Parachute Project': need-adapted treatment for first-episode psychosis – a Swedish multicentre project
Contact: Fax no. +46 8 616 52 18 @Stockholm Söder Hospital
In January 1996, 18 psychiatric clinics in Sweden (sectors) began a two-year project to collect data on their first-episode psychosis patients. The total catchment area covers a population of approximately, 1 200 000 persons, with an expected incidence of non-organic, non-drug-related psychosis of 350–400 cases per year in the 18–45 age group. Staff were trained on the research instruments in the year preceding the project start, following a pilot period of investigation (Cullberg, Levander & Claes-Göran, 1997). The participating clinics aim to fulfil the following six therapeutic and care principles:

(1) Early intervention: Specific treatment begins immediately a first-episode patient has been identified. Project staff see patients and their

families, preferably in their homes, and follow the patient through the course of treatment.

(2) Crisis and psychotherapeutic approach: Each patient is treated as being in an acute crisis situation (while acknowledging the biological aspects of psychosis), i.e. possible environmental stress factors and the stressful nature of psychosis itself are recognized and addressed.

(3) Family approach: The family is invited to take part in weekly 'family meetings' in the early stages of a family member's illness. These are less frequent as recovery proceeds. These family meetings aim to assess ongoing stressors, provide support and information and assist promotion of more constructive relationships where these are dysfunctional.

(4) Continuity and easy accessibility: Change of treatment team is avoided as far as possible so that knowledge of a patient's history, abilities, and specific problems is retained within the treating team, thereby allowing optimal chance for constructive help if the patient relapses. Continuity and easy accessibility are a high priority during the first five years after a psychotic episode because this is the high-risk period for relapse.

(5) Lowest effective neuroleptic medication: Immediate neuroleptic medication is avoided if the clinical situation allows. Benzodiazepines are used for anxiety symptoms and low-dose neuroleptics are used for psychotic symptoms that do not resolve in the short term (with slow-dose titration to the minimum effective dose). Those patients who do not respond to this strategy are treated with atypical neuroleptics or lithium combinations.

(6) Flexible, home-based treatment: Efforts are made to support patients remaining in their own homes during the episode of illness. If supervised accommodation is needed, a special more personal unit is available in several, but not all, clinics. A mobile unit is also available.

Clinics involved in the project are taking part in a five-year research programme which includes a naturalistic long-term follow-up study designed to differentiate better between clinical and personality subgroups with different background factors, treatment needs and prognosis. A large set of baseline diagnostic tools is used including symptom check lists, neuropsychological tests, projective tests, family climate scales, MRI or CT scan, EEG, and records from the patient's referring clinic. Follow-up investigations will be done at one, three, and five years. A comparison will be undertaken with 'ordinary care' using a group of patients from the same areas, collected using the same criteria, but who had their first episode of psychosis three years earlier. These retrospective cases will be compared with project cases in terms of diagnosis, consumption of care, and prescription of neuroleptic medication. Efforts are also being made to include a prospective control group from an adjacent geographical area.

Birmingham Early Psychosis Service
Birmingham, UK
Contact: e-mail BIRCHMJZ@novell1.bham.ac.uk
The Birmingham Early Psychosis Service focusses on young people in the early stages of psychosis and considered to be at high risk of early relapse and disability. Originally commencing at the Archer Centre, a psychosocial programme based within a large state psychiatric hospital, the programme focussed on younger people, initially including many with more established psychosis. The programme was the base for an important study highlighting the role of cognitive therapies in promoting recovery from acute episodes of psychosis in an inpatient setting (Drury et al., 1996). Since 1995, the project has developed into a dedicated service for young people experiencing psychosis for the first time providing vocational, cognitive and psychosocial interventions, embedded within a broader assertive outreach programme and system of care. The service operates in an inner-city area (population 300000) with a known high morbidity of psychosis (50 new cases per 100000 population per year on average), high social deprivation, and a wide ethnic mix. The service is part of the local UK National Health Service mental health provision which includes psychiatric emergency and home treatment teams, assertive outreach and continuing needs services. The Early Psychosis Service draws its clients from emergency psychiatric admissions and referrals from primary care liaison teams.

The service has two core components – the assertive outreach team and the residential/respite unit, but is expanding. The former has ten case managers, trained to implement core cognitive, psychosocial and pharmacological treatments, who have a maximum case load of 15. Treatment programmes include cognitive therapy, family intervention, vocational training, and dual diagnosis interventions which are led by staff with special responsibilities. The residential/respite unit is a small community-based unit targeted at clients needing intensive input because of prolonged recovery and who cannot be managed within the community; for example, those at high suicide risk or with major interpersonal problems that means they cannot remain at home. Clients are maintained within the service for up to three years and outcomes are monitored carefully. Research and evaluation are an integral part of the service. The effectiveness of the service is evaluated within an agreed protocol including intake, assessments and follow-up assessments (including vocational outcomes) at one, two and three years.

The Bern First Episode Programme
Universitäre Psychiatrische Dienste Bern (UPD)
Bolligenstrasse 111, CH – 3000 BERN 60
Contact: Dr. Marco C.G. Merlo
Phone: +41 31 930 91 11
Fax: +41 31 930 94 04

This inpatient programme was one of the earliest to be established, commencing in 1989. The programme is part of a larger university psychiatric hospital and features low dose neuroleptics, psychotherapeutic and family therapies, and early use of clozapine. The clinical service is well integrated with basic research and is part of a centre with an excellent reputation for research in schizophrenia and related disorders.

The Amsterdam Adolescent Psychiatry Unit
Academisch Ziekenhuis bij de Universiteit van Amsterdam
Academisch Medisch Centrum
Psychiatrisch Centrum
Tafelbergweg 25, 1105 BC Amsterdam
Contact: Dr. Don Linszen
Phone: +31 20 566 2311
Fax: +31 20 691 9139

This programme for young people (aged 14–26) focusses upon recent onset psychosis and is a referral centre for a large population base. The group have carried out a series of high-quality psychosocial research studies, focusing particularly on family interventions and the relationship of cannabis usage to relapse (see Chapters 13 and 14).

Other substantial projects and established centres also exist throughout Australia, New Zealand, Denmark, Canada, Germany, Finland and the USA. A more complete account appears in Edwards & McGorry (1998). The above selection by no means does justice to the range and quality of emerging and established programmes. It merely gives a flavour of the extensive efforts which are occurring with increasing momentum around the world.

Conclusion

> At first people refuse to believe that a strange new thing can be done, then they begin to hope it can be done, then they see it can be done – then it is done and all the world wonders why it was not done centuries before
> Frances Hodgson Burnett, 1849–1924, English born US writer

While several authors have pointed to the potential of a preventive approach, it has not seemed a realistic possibility until very recently. The logic and best available evidence supporting an early intervention approach have been exhaustively considered in this volume. The paradigm is not only likely to lead to enhanced and more cost-effective care in psychotic illness, but is capable of extension to a wider range of potentially serious mental disorders (McGorry, 1996). However, in bringing about macroscopic change in service delivery, logic and evidence are frequently not sufficient. There are numerous examples of cost-effective initiatives which have lost funding or were not widely implemented. Even clearly efficacious specific treatments are not efficiently deployed. Additional forces need to be mobilized, and these fall under the rubric of ideology (Saul, 1997). The elements required include an attractive idea, promotion and community development around the idea and its implementation, and the backing of political and clinical leadership. It also helps for there to be real-world examples of successful implementation, i.e. beyond demonstration projects. For these reasons, it is becoming increasingly apparent that, just like any other reform process, an 'early psychosis movement' must have a political element – since the systems of psychiatric care which have targeted 'serious mental illness' pose an intrinsic barrier to early detection and intervention, through their concentration upon established cases. Even when devolved to the community, they focus on a similar spectrum of patients as the old state hospitals. Barriers to early intervention are even more powerfully at work in developing countries where resources are scarce, but are increasing in many developed countries too, where the ideology and impact of economic rationalism is eroding the quality of health care. This is paralleled by a shrinking commitment by governments to shared community values and 'the public good', and consequently the inevitably elusive goal of optimal health care for all is receding (Saul, 1997). Nevertheless, the cost-effectiveness argument may act as a bridge to overcome this source of resistance. While we do not accept that in a civilized society this should be the sole or dominant criterion, it does make sense to be efficient with finite resources. Given the global prevalence and impact of mental disorders, choices do have to be made, and we believe that early psychosis will prove to be one of the 'best buys' (Murray & Lopez, 1996). Numerous groups of clinicians and researchers are rising to this challenge. In addition, the International Early Psychosis Association has now more than 2000 members from all around the world, and membership is growing. There appears to be a surprisingly widespread willingness to assist one another to forge ahead into new territory, making up for lost time using modern methods of communication. The early psychosis recipe is simple: develop a focus, explicate achievable goals, and attempt to actualize the plan. This 'strange new thing' is not really new, it is at last starting to be done in many places, and people, including consumers, carers, clinicians, managers and politicians, should now be seriously asking why it is not being attempted everywhere.

Acknowledgments

We are grateful to the Australian National Early Psychosis Project and members of the International Early Psychosis Association for making available information about their services. We wish to thank particularly Max Birchwood, Johan Cullberg, Jan Olav Johannesen, Don Linszen and Marco Merlo for their contributions.

References

AHMAC Mental Health Working Group. (1992). *National Mental Health Policy and Plan*. Canberra: Australian Government Publishing Service.

Alanen, Y. O., Ugelstad, E., Armelius, B., Lehtinen, K., Rosenbaum, B. & Sjostrom, R. (eds.) (1994). *Early Treatment for Schizophrenic Patients: Scandinavian Psychotherapeutic Approaches*. Oslo: Scandinavian University Press.

Alanen, Y. O. (1997). *Schizophrenia: Its Origins and Need-adapted Treatment*. London: Karnac Books.

Andreasen, N. C. (1983). *The Scale for the Assessment of Negative Symptoms (SANS)*. Iowa City: University of Iowa.

Andrews, G. (1997). Managing scarcity: a worked example using burden and efficacy. *Australasian Psychiatry*, **5**, 225–7.

Australian Bureau of Statistics (1991). *Census of Population and Housing Expanded Community Profile*. Canberra: Australian Bureau of Statistics.

Cameron, D. E. (1938). Early schizophrenia. *American Journal of Psychiatry*, **95**, 567–78.

Cuffel, B. J., Jeste, D. V., Halpain, M., Pratt, C., Tarke, H. & Patterson, T. L. (1996). Treatment costs and use of community mental health services for schizophrenia by age cohorts. *American Journal of Psychiatry*, **153**, 870–6.

Cullberg, J., Levander, S. & Claes-Göran, S. (1997). *The Parachute Project – Need-adapted Treatment for First Episode Psychosis. A Swedish Multicenter Care Development and Research Project*. Paper presented at the 12th International Symposium for the Psychotherapy of Schizophrenia, London, October 12–16, 1997.

Drury, V., Birchwood, M., Cochrane, R. & Macmillan, F. (1996). Cognitive therapy and recovery from acute psychosis: a controlled trial. I. Impact on psychotic symptoms. *British Journal of Psychiatry*, **159**, 593–601.

Edwards, J. & McGorry, P. D. (in press). Early intervention in psychotic disorders: a critical step in the prevention of psychological morbidity. In *Handbook of Psychotherapy with Psychotic and Personality Disorders*, ed. C. Perris & P. D. McGorry. Chichester, UK: Wiley.

Grimshaw, J. M. & Hutchinson, A. (1993). Clinical Practice Guidelines – do they enhance value for money in healthcare? *British Medical Bulletin*, **51**, 927–40.

Haines, S. A., Gleeson, J. F., Pennell, K. M. & McGorry, P. D. (1997). *Incorporating an Early Psychosis Focus in a Mainstream Psychiatric Setting: Early Psychosis Projects in Victoria*. Poster presented at the First UK International Conference on Early Intervention in Psychosis, Stratford-upon-Avon, England, June, 1997.

Hegarty, J. D., Baldessarini, R. J., Tohen, M., Waternaux, C. & Oepen, G. (1994). One hundred years of schizophrenia: a meta-analysis of the outcome literature. *American Journal of Psychiatry*, **151**, 1409–16.

Heinrichs, D. W., Hanlon, T. E. & Carpenter, W. T., Jr. (1984). The quality of life scale: an instrument for rating the schizophrenic deficit syndrome. *Schizophrenia Bulletin*, **10**, 388–98.

Jablensky, A., Sartorius, N., Ernberg, G., Anker, M., Korten, A., Cooper, J. E., Day, R. & Bertelsen, I. A. (1992). Schizophrenia: manifestations, incidence and course in different cultures. A World Health Organization ten-country study. *Psychological Medicine*, **20**. (Supplement).

Johannessen, J. O. (1996). *The Logic of Early Intervention in Psychosis*. Paper presented at 'Verging on Reality': The First International Early Psychosis Conference. Melbourne, June, 1996.

Kavanagh, D. (1992). Recent developments in expressed emotion and schizophrenia. *British Journal of Psychiatry*, **160**, 601–20.

Kuipers, E., Garety, P., Fowler, D., Dunn, G., Bebbington, P., Freeman, D. & Hadley, C. (1997). London–East Anglia randomised controlled trial of cognitive–behavioural therapy for psychosis. I: Effects of the treatment phase. *British Journal of Psychiatry*, **171**, 319–27.

Larsen, T. K., McGlashan, T. H. & Moe, L. C. (1996). First-episode schizophrenia: 1. Early course parameters. *Schizophrenia Bulletin*, **22**, 241–56.

McGlashan, T. H. (1996). Early detection and intervention in schizophrenia: research. *Schizophrenia Bulletin*, **22**, 327–45.

McGorry, P. D. (1996). The Centre for Young People's Mental Health: blending epidemiology and developmental psychiatry. *Australasian Psychiatry*, **4**, 243–6.

McGorry, P. D., Singh, B. S., Copolov, D. L, Kaplan, I., Dossetor, C. R. & van Riel, R. J. (1990). The Royal Park Multidiagnostic Instrument for Psychosis: Part II. Development, reliability, and validity. *Schizophrenia Bulletin*, **16**, 517–36.

McGorry, P. D., Edwards, J., Mihalopoulos, C., Harrigan, S. & Jackson, H. J. (1996). Early Psychosis Prevention and Intervention Centre: an evolving system for early detection and intervention. *Schizophrenia Bulletin*, **22**, 305–26.

McGorry, P. D., Copolov, D. L. & Singh, B. S. (1990). The Royal Park Multidiagnostic Instrument for Psychosis: Part I. Rationale and review. *Schizophrenia Bulletin*, **16**, 501–15.

McGorry, P. D. & Edwards, J. (1997). *Early Psychosis Training Pack*. Cheshire, UK: Gardiner–Caldwell Communications.

McGorry, P. D., Mihalopoulos, C. & Carter, R. C. (in press). *Is Early Intervention in First Episode Psychosis an Economically Viable Method of Improving Outcome?* Proceedings of the 1996 World Psychiatric Congress, Madrid, August, 1996.

Mental Health Branch, Commonwealth Department of Health and Family Services. (1997). *Youth Suicide in Australia: The National Youth Suicide Prevention Strategy*. Canberra: Australian Government Publishing Service.

Moncrieff, J. (1997). Lithium: evidence reconsidered. *British Journal of Psychiatry*, **171**, 113–9.

Moscarelli, M., Capri, S. & Neri, L. (1991). Cost evaluation of chronic schizophrenic patients during the first three years after the first contact. *Schizophrenia Bulletin*, **17**, 421–6.

Murray, C. J. L. & Lopez, A. D. (Eds.) (1996). *The Global Burden of Disease*. Cambridge, Mass.: Harvard School of Public Health.

National Early Psychosis Project (1998). *Clinical Practice Guidelines for Early Psychosis*. Melbourne, Australia: EPPIC Statewide Services.

Overall, J. E. & Gorham, D, R. (1962). The brief psychiatric rating scale. *Psychological Reports*, **10**, 799–812.

Parry-Jones, W. (1995). The future of adolescent psychiatry. *British Journal of Psychiatry*, **166**, 299–305.

Patton, G. (1996). An epidemiological case for a separate adolescent psychiatry? *Australian and New Zealand Journal of Psychiatry*, **30**, 453–66.

Pennell, K. M., McGorry, P. D., Haines, S. A., Urbanc, A., Pound, B., Dagg, B., Handley, P., Wigg, C. & Berry, H. (1997). *Australian National Early Psychosis Project: The Development and Promotion of a National Best Practice Model in Early Intervention in Psychosis – a Project Overview*. Paper presented at the Mental Health Services Conference, Sydney, Australia, 1997.

Rutter, M. (1995). *Psychosocial Disorders in Young People*. Chichester, UK: Wiley.

Saul, J. R. (1997). *The Unconscious Civilization*. Harmondsworth, UK: Penguin Books.

Thornicroft, G. & Tansella, M. (eds) (1996). *Mental Health Outcome Measures*. Berlin: Springer-Verlag.

Appendix 1. A consensus statement on strategies for prevention in early psychosis*

Goals, strategy and plan

There have been eight broad areas of some consensus.
1. There are potential benefits in terms of course and outcome in the early identification of first-episode psychosis.
2. There are potential benefits in terms of course and outcome in the provision of optimal treatment during and after this critical period of the first episode and thereafter.
   This includes:
   (a) a comprehensive biopsychosocial assessment during a neuroleptic-free phase
   (b) low dose 'antipsychosis' medication
   (c) comprehensive treatment involving integration of psychosocial and biological interventions
   (d) the development and refinement of specific psychological interventions.
3. There is value in the identification of high risk individuals, both asymptomatic and symptomatic (i.e. prodromal) with the aim of 'trialing' preventive strategies.
4. There is an advantage in the identification of early treatment resistance
   (a) Further investigation is required to examine risk factors for early treatment resistance
   (b) Evaluation of treatment strategies for early treatment resistance

* Formulated and agreed at the First International Conference on Early Psychosis: *Verging on Reality: Preventive Strategies in Early Psychosis*, Melbourne, June 1996. (McGorry, P. (ed.). 'Preventive Strategies in Early Psychosis. *British Journal of Psychiatry*, **172**, 1–136, Supplement 33, June 1998.)

needs to occur, including trials of new atypical antipsychotics and cognitive therapies.
5. Investigations need to be made into psychosocial and biological factors affecting the transition from: asymptomatic to prodromal to first-episode to recurrent episodes to treatment resistance, in order to examine the possibility of the prevention of the decompensation implicit in the evolution through these phases.
6. There is a need to better predict who can be taken off medication after remission, when this should occur, and how to do it.
7. It is important to establish a collaborative partnership with young people in assessment and treatment.
8. There is a need for early identification of and interventions for depression and drug abuse for example, and other treatable forms of comorbidity.

Strategies

1. Clinical

    (a) Need ongoing development of the critical elements of optimal models of care which are developed in partnership with consumers, families and carers, and take into account different psychiatric service systems, economic and sociocultural environments.

    (b) The clear enunciation and evaluation of models of practice and dissemination of these via material/literature. A number of manuals could be used for this purpose in the first instance.

    (c) The creation of networks of individuals and organizations (including consumer/carer groups) across different countries for collaboration.
    Need to explore the possibility of one centre taking responsibility for this. Maybe rotating across different international sites.
    Such a network could organize regular international meetings and could develop a newsletter to hold the network together.

Additional comments
1. Identify protective factors as well as risk factors.
2. Emphasize the prevention of disability.
3. Emphasize interventions for non-responders.
4. Emphasize the special needs of minority groups and indigenous peoples.

Plan
1. We should consider that this meeting (i.e. all attending) constitutes the first meeting of the network.
2. A bulletin of the consensus statements will be generated from this forum and sent to all founding members of the network.
3. The network agrees to meet at the time of future international forums.

Additional comments
1. How to include other interested parties in the network?
2. What name should the network use? The suggestion ultimately adopted was International Early Psychosis Association (IEPA).

2. Training

   (a) Training aspects could be focussed on at meetings of the network.
   (b) Workshops could be held at the same time as international meetings.
   (c) The development of other training, e.g. for short courses, diplomas could be considered.
   (d) Centre with established services could offer site visits/workshops.

Comments
1. Spell out who should receive training.
2. Should the model be better developed before being disseminated?
3. More controversial interventions should be negotiated at the regional level (e.g. prodrome interventions).

3. Research

   (a) Research activities in individual centres should be encouraged. In addition, multi-site studies should be facilitated, particularly in order to examine regional, national and cultural influences.
   (b) Research activities should include recommendations of consumers, be methodologically sound with adequate sample sizes and use 'core measures' that can translate across different centres.

4. Seeking a broader community/political endorsement

   (a) Systematic education of general public, consumer groups, governments in order to:

reduce stigma
increase community awareness
increase community endorsement/support of ongoing work in the field.
(b) Particular issues which could be included in the above are:
stigma
interventions including preventive, e.g. for those at high risk
cost effectiveness of interventions
youth suicide and violence.

Appendix 2. International Early Psychosis Association

1.   I am interested in becoming a member of the International Early Psychosis Association.

2.   Comments / Suggestions:

            ....
            ....
            ....
            ....
            ....
            ....

FROM: ....
            ....
            ....

TEL NO: ....

FAX NO: ....

EMAIL: ....

FAX TO: +61 3 9342 2941
            International Early Psychosis Association
            c/o EPPIC
            Locked Bag 10
            Parkville, Victoria, Australia 3052

Index

Note: page numbers in *italics* refer to figures and tables

absconding, risk assessment, 169
N-acetyl aspartate–creatine phosphocreatine ratio, 126
activities, return to normal, 315
activity level, EPPIC day programme, 420, 421
adaptation
　goals of therapy, 279–82
　issues, 277–8
　model, 276–7
　promotion, 279–82
adaptive tasks, 159–60
adolescents
　deviant behaviour, 55–6
　invulnerability perception, 81
　stresses, 410
Adult Community Treatment Team (ACTT), 219–21
affective psychoses, 28, 175
　cognitively oriented approaches, 266
　first-episode psychosis, 165
　insidious onset, 56
　prodromal symptoms, 33–4
　substance abuse comorbidity, 339
　suicide, 339
after-care models, 206
age at onset, 199–200, 277
　first-episode psychosis, 178, 184
　outcome predictors, 240
age barriers in early intervention, 453
aggression, preventive strategies, 167
agitation
　benzodiazepine therapy, 190
　management, 170
　neuroleptic therapy, 191
AIDS, psychosis risk, 171

alcohol, 200, 241
alcohol abuse xxiii, 188
　depression, 341
　prevention campaigns, 348
　schizophrenia, 363, 367
　suicide, 340–1
amphetamines
　persistent psychotic symptoms, 364
　precipitation of psychosis, 208
　schizophrenia, 363
Amsterdam Adolescent Psychiatry Unit, 466
antiprevention effect, 83
antipsychiatry paradigm, 449
antidepressants, 193
antipsychotic drugs, 115
　atypical, 191–2
　first-episode schizophrenia studies, 142–3
　home-based management, 216
　low dose, 186
antipsychotics
　novel xxi
　SSRI combination, 353
　TCA combination, 353
antisocial behaviour, suicide, 339
anxiety
　benzodiazepine therapy, 190, 370–1
　disorders
　　cognitively oriented approaches, 266
　　first-episode psychosis, 165
　late recovery phase, 322
　management, 170, 314
　medication, 195, *196–7*
　psychosis accompaniment, 330
　relapse, 313, 320

477

INDEX

anxiety (cont.)
  sedation, 215
  social, 284–5
apomorphine, 135–6
artistic activities, 424
assessment, neuroleptic-free phase, 169–70
at-risk mental state xviii, *41*
  transition to psychosis, 106–7
attachment, 312, 320
  theory, 267
attitudinal factors, 84
attributions, patient's sense, 273
Australian National Early Psychosis Project (NEPP), 458, 459–60
autoimmunity, 140

basal ganglia, 121
behaviour
  bizarre, 164
  changes, 37
  pathologizing, 320
  problems in mental retardation, 201
  self-destructive, 341
behavioural paradigm, 265
beliefs, core, 276
benzodiazepines
  anxiety treatment, 215, 370–1
  insomnia management, 170
  prescription, 190–1
  sleep pattern control, 188
Bern First Episode Programme, 466
biochemical evaluation of first-episode psychosis, 171, 172, *173*
biopsychosocial space, 272
biopsychosocial treatment, integrated, 327–9
bipolar disorder, 176
  prodrome duration, 38–9
  suicide, 339
Birmingham Early Psychosis Service, 465
body and soul group, 424
brain
  anatomical lateral symmetry, 132
  development, 119
  energy metabolism, 121–3
  morphology in schizophrenia, 118, 119
  size in schizophrenia, 118
brief limited intermittent psychotic symptoms (BLIPS) group, 101
Brief Psychiatric Rating Scale (BPRS), 105, 459
buddy system, 454

Camberwell Family Interview (CFI), 386
cannabis, 188, 200
  intoxication, 368–70

outcome predictor, 241
precipitation of psychosis, 208
psychotic symptoms, 365, 366, 368–70
relapse, 250, 368
schizophrenia, 363, 364
self-medication, 316
  hypothesis, 370
care
  access to xix, 51, 80
    delay, 52–3
    promotion, 85, 109
  continuing, 18–19
  continuity, 84
  interval before seeking, 53, 54
  models xix–xx
  paradigms, 226
  philosophy, 230–1
  see also pathways to care
career of patient, 185
carers
  families, 376
  neurotic disorders, 383
case conferences, 327, 330
case detection xix, 81–4
case management, 308–9
  acute phase, 313, 314–16
  brokerage model, 309
  cognitive–behavioural strategies, 323
  educational approach, 323
  EPPIC, 310–11
  intervention levels *324*
  NIPS project, 309
  phase-oriented approach, 323
  preventive, xxii–xxiii, 310
    integrated biopsychosocial treatment, 327–9
  recovery
    early, 316–18
    late phase, 318–23
    phase, 313
    prolonged, 323, *324*, 325–7
  refusal to accept treatment, 315
  service period, 320
  substance abuse, 311
  tasks, 313–23
  team, 330–1
  termination planning, 320
  therapist model, 309
  transition period, 320
case manager
  accessibility, 312
  awareness of relapse risk, 312–13
  case conferences, 330
  clinical dilemmas, 330
  debriefing, 330–1
  decision making, 313
  education, 327–8

INDEX

EPPIC day programme, 418, 420
flexibility, 312, 331
initial assessment, 312
knowledge, 327
objectives, 332
optimism maintenance, 312
outpatient (OCM), 394
recovery promotion, 312
skills, 327
specialist role, 330
staff conflict, 331
staff development, 327
supervision, 330
training, 331
see also clinician
caseness criteria in schizophrenia, 8
catatonia, 176
catering, 422–3
caudate nucleus, 120–1
causal attribution, 255
Central East Early Psychosis Project, 458–9
cerebral asymmetry development, 120
cerebral blood flow, 121
cerebral metabolic rate of oxygen, 121
cerebral tumours, psychosis risk, 171
cerebral ventricles, 116–18
child care, 200
chlorpromazine, 191, 216
choline–creatine-phosphocreatine ratio, 126
cholinergic pathways, 191–2
circling behaviour, 139
client needs assessment, 308
client–patient relationship, 311–13
clinical assessment, xx
first-episode psychosis, 162–70
clinical functioning, desynchrony with social functioning, 248
clinical history, 162–3
clinical outcome, 12
clinical practice guidelines, 456–8
clinical recovery, 232
clinicians
communication skills, 211–12
delay paradox, 65–6
home-based management, 210–13
illusion, 4
key, 449
mindset, 450–1
pathways to care, 65–6
treatment goals, 329
see also case manager
clozapine, 192, 327
STOPP combination, 294, 295
treatment resistance management, 256
comorbid syndromes, 282

cocaine
psychotic relapse, 368
psychotic symptoms, 364, 365
schizophrenia, 363
cognition, 343–4
cognitive behavioural therapy, 195, 198, 281, 454
case management, 323
first-episode psychosis, 186
individual intervention, 352
nurse training, 199
schizophrenia treatment, 290
suicide prevention, 350, 351–2
see also cognitive therapy
cognitive deficit, suicide ideation, 344
cognitive disputation technique, 285
cognitive distortions, 274
cognitive errors, 281
cognitive impairment, 130–1
cognitive interventions, 15
cognitive psychotherapy, 267–8
cognitive remediation, 266
cognitive strategies, 195, 197
coping, 268
cognitive therapy
depression, 248
early psychological adjustment, 254–5
principles, 267
programme, 257
relapse, 255
suicidal thinking, 248
treatment resistance management, 256, 257–8
see also cognitive behavioural therapy
cognitive work, adaptation, 280, 281
cognitively oriented psychotherapy for early psychosis *see* COPE
collaboration in therapy, 274, 472
Colombo technique, 162
communication
clinicians, 211–12
delay, 63
maximizing, 392
skills, 384
community
active rehabilitation, 230
education, 109
outreach models, 226
re-integration with home-based management, 217
community service, hospital service integration, 218
Community Treatment Order, 275
community-based treatment, 206
promotion, 82
comorbid disorders, 85
first-episode psychosis, 165, 177–8

479

competence paradigm, 389–90
compliance, medication adherence, 195
computed tomography (CT), 116–18, 172–3
concensus statement, 471–4
concentration loss, relapse, 320
confidentiality, 211
confrontation, limit setting, 167
congenital abnormalities, 172
constructivism, 267, 269
　developmental context, 269–70
　self, 269
consultation, 455
consumers
　compliance, 84
　delay paradox, 65
　empowerment, 73–4
　involvement, 455
　pathways to care, 65–6
　recall of events, 67
contagion prevention, suicide, 348
continuing care, 18–19
continuity of care, 84
convalescence period, 134
COPE xxii,, 273–88, 296, 412
　adaptation phase, 276–82
　appealing to self phase, 282
　assessment, 273–4
　research progress, 287–8
　therapeutic alliance, 274–6
coping
　cognitive strategies, 268
　families, 389–90
　help-seeking, 69
　skills, 426
　strategies, 317
　work, 280
cost-effectiveness of early intervention xxv, 442–3
counselling
　hospitalization, 171
　schizophrenia treatment, 290
counter-transference response, 313
creative expression, EPPIC day programme, 423–4
crisis, 155, 158
　acute care, 226
　intervention, 155, 309
　　model, 210
　phase, *214*, 215–16
critical period, 15, 226
　concept, 244–9
　prospective follow-up studies, 227
　reducing delay, 249
　relapse prevention, 249–51, *252*, 253
　schizophrenia, 311
　suicide risk, 239

therapeutic implications, 245
treatment, 55
cultural factors, 160–1
curbing techniques, 162
Cushing's syndrome, 171

D2 dopamine receptors
　antagonists, 190
　schizophrenia, 123–4, 126
daily living programme (DLP) model, 206–7
Davidson, Larry, 267–8
day programmes, 407–11
　COPE, 412
　definition, 408–9
　development, 407–8
　efficacy, 408–9
　evaluation, 410
　first-episode patients, 413
　function, 411–13
　goals, *418*
　milieu, 414–15
　patient role in recovery, 414
　severe mental illness, 410, 412
　structure, 411
　young people, 408, 409
　see also EPPIC day programme
death risk assessment, 166
decision making by case manager, 313
deficit functioning, 271
deficit syndrome, 326
deinstitutionalization, 5, 206, 308
delay, 52–3
　communication, 63
　concept xix
　first-episode psychosis, 53–5, 58–9
　gender, 54
　impact, 57–8
　negative consequences, 57
　paradox, 65–72
　reduction, 55, 65
　risk factors, 55–6
　secondary prevention, 73
　seeking care, 53, 54
　treatment experience, 72
delusional beliefs, 198, 256
delusional disorders, 175
delusions xxii
　bizarre, 341
　grandiose, 95, 96
　paranoid, 191
　STOPP, 292, 293–4
　treatment, 288–95
demoralization reduction, 411
denial, 64, 65, 66, 67, 69
　costs, 254
　engagement in treatment, 84

480

recovery style, 218
depression
  alcohol abuse, 341
  cognitive therapy, 248
  families, 390, 397
  from acute episode, 254
  outcome predictors, 240
  psychosis accompaniment, 330
  psychotic, 339
  recurrent, 241
  relapse, 320
    prediction, 241
  secondary morbidity, 207, 283
  treatment, 193
depressive delusions, 241
detection
  critical period xix
  early, 441–2
  psychosis in community, 44
determinants of outcome in severe mental disorder (DOSMD) study, 227, 236, 237, 249
detoxification, substance abuse, 370
development, 269, 270–1
  adult, 271
  first-episode psychosis, 160
  offtimedness, 384
  psychosis impact, 271–2
  reversal, 377
  stage, 275, 277
  stagnation, 376
  trajectory, 272
developmental needs of patient, 328–9
dexamethasone suppression test (DST), 133–4
diagnosis
  definitive, 28
  first-episode psychosis, 318
  health professionals, 70–1
diazepam, 216
disability, plateau effect, 233
discharge strategies, 320
discussion group, 426–7
disorganization symptoms of substance abuse, 366
distance learning, 454
distraction techniques, 317
distress management strategies, 314
disturbance, severe, 330
diurnal influences, 163–4
diversity of service, 444
dopamine agonists, 135–6
dopamine neural functioning, 134–5
dopaminergic neural dysfunction, 326
downstream effects, therapeutic input, 269
drug abuse
  outcome predictors, 241
  prevention campaigns, 348
  schizophrenia, 363
  suicide, 340–1
  see also substance abuse
drug treatment, 63, 64–5
  first-episode psychosis, 189–93, *194*, 195
  first-episode schizophrenia studies, 141–4
  self-medication, 69
  suicide behaviours, 353
  see also medication
drug-induced psychosis, 175, 176
  see also substance abuse
DSM-III and DSM-III-R, prodromal features, 34, 36–7
DSM-IV, 28, 37
duration of untreated psychosis (DUP), 6, 12
  brief psychosis, 13
  EE, 381, 382
  EPAT, 90–1, 93
  family impact, 377, 388
  outcome predictors, 242, 243–4
  reduction, 13
  relapse, 16
dyskinesia, spontaneous, 139–40
dysthymia, suicide, 339

Early Episode Psychosis Project, 461–2
early intervention, 12–17
  age band, 445–6
  age barriers, 453
  barriers, 467
  clinical practice guidelines, 456–8
  clinician mindset, 450–1
  concensus statement, 471–4
  consumer involvement, 455
  evaluation, 456
    techniques, 458–9
  focus, 452
    definition, 447–50
  goals, 447
  implementation obstacles, 450–3
  key clinicians, 449
  model of starting, 445–50
  morale, 451–2
  motivation, 445
  needs of group, 446
  pessimism, 450–1
  pilot phase, 450
  quality assurance, 456
  recognition of need, 52
  resources, 451
    allocation, 447, 448
  scoping, 444
  specific skills, 452

INDEX

early intervention, (cont.)
  sphere of action, 448
  strategies, 472–4
  see also EPPIC
Early Psychosis Assessment and Community Treatment Team (EPACT), 393–4
Early Psychosis Assessment Team (EPAT), 80, 85–97
  aims, 109
  cases, 91–7
  clinical service, 88–9
  community education, 87–8, 101–2
  DUP, 90–1, 93
  educational activities, 87–8
  engagement in treatment, 88
  family contact, 88–9
  GP referrals, 89–90
  home-based treatment, 89
  hours of operation, 86
  inclusion criteria, 87
  intake system, 86–7
  outcome, 90
  philosophy, 87
  police involvement, 90
  referral, 88, 89–90
    to PACE, 104
  response time, 90
  staffing, 86
Early Psychosis Prevention and Intervention Centre see EPPIC
Early Treatment and Identification of Psychosis (TIPS), 462–3
early warning signs, health professionals, 71
eating disorders, first-episode psychosis, 165
economic benefits of early intervention, 442
ecstasy, 365, 366
education
  about illness, 416
  case manager, 327–8
  consultation, 455
  families, 395
  home-based management, 220–1
  postgraduate, 454
  schizophrenia, 416
  suicide, 348
educational assessment, 174–5
educational attainment, 57
effectiveness of early intervention, xxv, 19
electroconvulsive therapy (ECT), 193
  suicide, 352, 354
electrodermal activity in schizophrenia, 129–30
electroencephalography (EEG)

first-episode psychosis, 174
  sleep, 127–8
emotions, pathologizing, 320
empowerment of consumers, 73–4
engagement, 314
  therapeutic process, 276
entrapment, 247, 248, 255
epidemiological catchment area (ECA) study, 38, 363
epidemiology, first-episode psychosis, 157
epilepsy, temporal lobe, 171
episode onset, 29, 30–1
EPPIC, 460–1
  case management xxiii, xxiv–xxv, 310–11
  catchment area, 446
  clinical guidelines 457
  entry point, 85
  evaluation techniques, 458
  family intervention, 399–400
  family services, 392–400
    assessment/engagement, 393–5
    philosophy, 392–5
    psychoeducation, 395–7
  family worker, 394
  home page, 88
  measurement indicators 457
  PACE association, 104
  project, 462
  service delivery model, 348
EPPIC day programme, 417
  assessment, 418, 420
  case manager, 418, 420
  content, 420–8
  creative expression stream, 423–4
  developments, 433
  evaluation, 428
  focus groups, 427–8
  follow-up study, 428–31, *432*
  goals, *418*
  health promotion stream, 424–6
  key worker, 418, *419*
  PAS, 429, 430, *431*
  personal skills development stream, 426–7
  progress monitoring, 428
  quality of life scale, 429
  referral, 418, 420
  SANS, 429, *430*, 431, *432*
  social recreational stream, 420–2
  structure, 417–18, *419*, 420
  vocational stream, 422–3
evaluation of early intervention, 456
  techniques, 458–9
evaluative model of individual response to psychosis, 247
event-related potentials (ERPs), 129

482

INDEX

evidence-based medicine, 444
evidence-based paradigm, 18
expectations, failed, 239
expressed emotion (EE), 379–83
  critical, 353
  DUP, 381, 382
  families,, 175, 246–7
  first-episode psychosis, 380–3
  predictive power, 380–1, 386
  reduction, 353
  relapse, 379–80, 380–1, 382
  staff, 187
extrapyramidal side-effects, 190, 191
extrapyramidal signs in schizophrenia, 137–9

false false positives, 11
family
  acute stress disorder, 388, 389, 390
  adaptive functioning, 389–90
  after detection, 388–9
  burden, 379
    development, 384
    first-episode psychosis, 383–4
  cognitive therapy programme, 257
  collateral information, 161, 163
  collusion with GP, 244
  competence, 389–90
  contacts, 239
  containment of individual, 209–10
  coping, 389–90
    ability, 220
    resources, 161
  crisis intervention
    access, 391
    model, 210
  critical caregivers, 376
  debriefing on hospitalization, 171
  denial, 244
  depression, 390, 397
  DUP, 377, 388
  dynamics, 175
  education, 99, 395
    psychoeducational, 265–6
  emotional support, 391
  EPAT, 88–9
  evaluation, 170
  expressed emotion, 175, 246–7
  first-episode psychosis, 379–87
  grief, 388–9, 390, 397
  group format, 397–9
  guilt, 397, 399
  help-seeking delay, 94, 95
  home-based management, 209–10, 220
  individual differences within, 389
  initial contact, 393–5
  interaction patterns, 209
  interactive sessions, 397–9
  intervention, xxiv, 199–200
    day programmes, 412
    EE predictive power, 386
    first-episode psychosis, 384–7
    preventive model, 376–9
    relapse prevention, 251, 253
    resources, 451
    service delivery model, 390–2
  limit setting for recovery phase, 199
  management plans, 210
  meeting needs, 387–90
  misapprehensions, 94–5
  multiple-family groups, 399
  non-compliance reinforcement, 85
  patient role, 208–9
  practical support, 391
  prodromal phase, 387–8
  prognosis information, 396
  psychoeducation, 391–2, 399
  psychosis course, 392
  rating scale, 209
  recovery phase, 389–90
  relapse effects, 246, 390
  services
    EPPIC, 392–400
    philosophy, 392–5
  substance abuse, 397
  support, 99, 170
    case management, 309
    first-episode psychosis, 161
    illness pattern, 379
    recovery environment, 378
    treatment plan involvement, 396
    treatment-resistant severe psychosis, 390
  unit, 377
  warning sign information, 388
  work, 454
  working with 400
fantasy world, 63–4, 65
fear of mental deterioration, 244, 254
financial problems, substance abuse, 366, 368
first-episode psychosis, 10, 13–14, *30*
  acute phase, 187
  age at onset, 178, 184, 199–200
  assessment, 186–7
  biochemical evaluation, 171, 172, *173*
  career of patient, 185
  clinical assessment, 162–70
  clinical problems, 156–7
  cognitive strategies, 195, 197
  cognitive–behavioural therapy, 186
  comorbid disorders, 165, 177–8
  confirmation, 175
  crisis, 155, 158

483

first-episode psychosis, (*cont.*)
  cultural factors, 160–1
  day programmes, 413
  delay, 53–4, 58–9
  diagnosis, 156–7, 175–8, 318
  diagnostic model, 177
  diagnostic problems, 176–7
  drug treatment, 189–93, *194*, 195
  EEG, 174
  engagement with patient, 159
  entry phase, 155–6
  epidemiology, 157
  expressed emotion (EE), 380–3
  family, xxiv, 14, 379–87
    burden, 383–4
    contact, 158
    intervention, 199–200, 384–7
    support, 161
  formulation, 175–8, 177
  home-based treatment, 206–8
  hospitalization, 170–1, 185
  illness phase, 187
  initial assessment, 155, 158–75
  initial treatment, 184–5
  insight, 164, 185–6
  interview technique, 161–2
  low dose medication, 186
  management misconceptions, 185–6
  medication administration, 193, 195
  mental state examination, 163–5
  needs, 269
  negative symptoms, 164–5
  neuroimaging studies, 172–3
  neuroleptic-free assessment phase, 169–70
  neuropsychological assessments, 174
  nursing interventions, 198–9
  onset, 156–7
  patient contact, 158
  patient needs, 14
  personal context, 159–61
  phase, 164
  physical examination, 172, *173*
  physical illness associations, 171
  prodromal features 33
  prognosis, 185, 318
  psychosocial interventions, 195, 198–200
  recognition, 61
  recovery phase, 187, 198
  remission, 13, 325–6
  risk assessment, 165–9
  seriousness, 156
  social support, 185
  sociocultural environment, 160–1
  speed of development, 160
  STOPP, 291–5

substance abuse, 176, 322–3
trauma, 158, 199
treatment
  location determination, 161
  phases, 214–15
  principles, 186–9
  resistance, 200
  understanding patient, 159–61
  vulnerability factors, 184
first-episode schizophrenia, xx–xxi
  electrodermal studies, 129–30
  event-related potentials, 129
  gender differences, 137
  immunological studies, 140–1
  movement disorders, 137–40
  neurobiology, 115–16
  neuroimaging studies, 116–27
  neurophysiology, 127–30
  neuropsychology, 130–3
  outcome of untreated illness, 143
  sleep EEG, 127–8
  treatment, 115–16
    studies, 141–4
flupenthixol, 142
fluphenazine, 142, 242
focus
  groups, 427–8
  specialist, 452
Friedreich's ataxia, 171
frontal lobe glucose metabolism, 122
fun and fitness group, 424–5
function predictors, 232

gardening, 423
gender, outcome predictors, 240
general practitioner (GP)
  awareness of psychotic disorders, 83
  high-risk individual identification, 98–9
  home-based management, 217
  illness detection, 71
  pathways to care, 73
  psychosis recognition, 59, 60, 244
  recognition of psychiatric disorders, 82
  referral to EPAT, 89–90
glucose metabolism in schizophrenia, 121–2
goal setting, recovery, 415, 416
Graves' disease, 140
grief, families, 388–9, 390, 397
group programmes for young people, 409
group-based interventions, 416
growth, adaptation, 280
growth hormone (GH), 134–5
growth model, 267, 272
guilt, families, 397, 399

hallucinations, xxii, 28

command, 341
STOPP, 292–3
treatment, 288–95
hallucinogens, 200, 365
haloperidol, 190, 191
harm minimization, 323
head injury, psychosis risk, 171
health belief framework, 247
health care costs, 57
health professionals
   community-based, 71
   diagnosis, 70–1
   early warning signs, 71
   pathways to care, 73
   support, 67–8
health promotion, 323, 424–6
help-seeking, xix, 68–70, 81–2, 102
   behaviour, 59–60
   coping, 69–70
   secondary prevention, 68
   symptoms, 69
heroin abuse, 367
herpes simplex encephalitis, 171
high-risk individual identification, 98–9
   community, 101
   interventions, 99
   strategies, 100
Hogarty, Gerard, 268
home visits, 84
home-based management, 206–8
   chlorpromazine, 216
   education, 220–1
   factors, 208–13
   family, 209–10, 220
   GPs, 217
   hospital support, 218
   individual, 208–9
   integrated programme, 207–8
   medication management, 215–16
   neuroleptics, 216
   outcome, 219–20
   package approach, 213–15
   physical investigations, 216–17
   pilot study, 218–21
   progress monitoring, 212
   psychoeducation, 217
   psychosocial issues, 217–18
   quality of life ratings, 219–20
   re-integration into community, 217
   recovery phase, 212
   strategies, 213–18
   structure for carers, 213
   treating team, 210–13
   treatment phases, 214–15
   vital signs monitoring, 217
   working timetable, 213
homelessness, 81, 82

risk assessment, 166
substance abuse, 366, 368
homovanillic acid (HVA), 134, 136–7
hopelessness
   relapse prediction, 241
   suicide, 352
      ideation, 343
      prediction, 240
hospital support, home-based
      management, 218
hospitalization, 61
   admission criteria, 170
   compulsory, 96, 97
   counselling, 171
   debriefing, 171
   first-episode psychosis, 170–1, 185
   non-traumatic, 218
   partial, 409–10
   police admissions, 170–1
   secondary morbidity, 207, 208
hospitals
   community service integration, 218
   risk of absconding, 169
   safety, 188
housing, 325
humiliation, 247, 255
Huntington's disease, 171
5-hydroxyindoleacetic acid (5–HIAA),
      134
hypodopaminergic activity, 138
hypofrontality, 122, 125

ICD-10, 28
identity
   concept, 254
   establishment, 317
   individual, 247
illness *see* mental illness
implementation of early intervention, 443
independence
   delay in young people, 376
   living skills, 412
index of awareness, 83
individuals
   experience, 412
   response to psychosis, 247
   view of world, 414
   see also high-risk individual
      identification
information-processing deficit, 266
initial treatment, 184–5
inpatients
   violence, 167–8, 187–8
   see also hospitalization
insight, 66–7
   first-episode psychosis, 164, 185–6
   lack, 330

insomnia, 170, 188
integrated mental health care model, 311–12
interactive learning, computer-assisted, 433
interleukin-2 (IL-2), 141
International Early Psychosis Network, 459, 475
interpersonal relationships, 255–6
interventions
　classification, 7
　cost effectiveness, 442–3
　foci, 391
　preventive, 329
　rationale, 272
　spectrum, 7
　strategies for relapse, 251
interview for retrospective assessment of the onset of schizophrenia (IRAOS), 37
interview techniques, 82, 161–2
intoxication, psychotic symptoms, 364
IQ, performance, 131, 132

key worker, EPPIC day programme, 418, *419*

language disturbance in schizophrenia, 119, 132
leadership roles, 452
least pathology assumption, 392
left temporal–hippocampal system, 133
lifestyle, return to normal, 208
Linehan model, 352
lithium, 192–3, 353
　first-episode schizophrenia studies, 142
　late recovery phase, 319
loss, 247, 255
lumbar puncture, 172
lymphokines, 141

magnetic resonance imaging (MRI), 118–21, 173
magnetic resonance spectroscopy, 126–7
management
　misconceptions, 185–6
　plans for families, 210
manic state, suicide protection, 344
manic symptoms, 96, 97
marijuana *see* cannabis
markers, xix
media control, 348
medication
　adherence, 195, 317
　anxiety, 195, *196–7*
　cessation *319*

decision tree, 193, *194*
depot, 328
duration, 319
long-term maintenance, 318
management strategies, 314
medicine, 249
minimally effective dose, 318
monitoring, 309
non-compliance, 328
perception by patient, 84
targeting, 99
see also drug treatment; self–medication
memory, 31, 32
mental deterioration
　critical period, 245–6
　fear, 239, 254
mental health service
　accessing, 83
　cultural appropriateness, 84
　delays, 83
　geographical access, 84
　GP knowledge, 83
　political agenda, 81–2
　treatment dissatisfaction, 83–4
mental illness
　chronic, 72
　client's awareness, 278
　concept, 63, 64
　day programmes, 410, 412
　diagnosis resistance, 66
　fear, 244
　label, 71–2
　lay stereotypes, 68
　model, 247
　negative stereotypes, 254
　onset, 29, 30
　pattern, 379
　phases, 187
　recognition, 66–8
　recovery, 413–17
　self-management, 329
　severe, 322
　stigma, 81–2, 244
　untreated, 242–4
　view of world, 414
mental retardation, 201
mental state
　at risk, 10
　examination, 163–5
mentor system, 454
mesiotemporal lobe, 120
methadone, 367–8
3,4–methylenedioxymethamphetamine (MDMA) *see* ecstasy
methylphenidate, 134–5, 136
misdiagnosis, 70
mood

disturbance, 176
psychoses, 28
stabilizers, 192–3
mood-related symptoms, 37
morbidity, plateau, 245–6
morbidity, secondary, 217, 272
   assessment, 284–5
   cognitive disputation technique, 285
   hospitalized patients, 207, 208
   psychopathology, 282–4
   treatment, 285–7
movement disorders, 137–40
multidisciplinary teams, 452
multiple sclerosis, 171
multiple-family groups,, 399

narrative reconstructions, 72
naturalistic studies, 456
needs
   assessment, 308
   first-episode psychosis, 269
neglect risk assessment, 166
negotiation approach, 314–15
neurochemistry/neuroendocrinology of schizophrenia, 133–7
neuroimaging, xx, 172–3
neuroleptic threshold, 190
neuroleptic-free assessment phase, 169–70
neuroleptics, xxi, 5
   choice, 190–1
   dosage, 191, 249–50
   early treatment, 231
   first-line treatment, 189–90
   frank psychotic features, 103
   home-based management, 216
   outcome, 231
      predictor, 241–2
   replacement of psychological interventions, 265
   response delay, 189–90
   side effects, 191
neurological conditions, 162
neurological soft signs, 139, 172
neurophysiology, xx
   first-episode schizophrenia, 127–30
neuropsychological function, 130–3
   assessment, 174
neuroreceptor studies, 123–4
neurotic symptoms, 32–3, 34
   non-specific, 37, 38
New Zealand National Intervention Interest Group, 462
non-compliance, 84–5, 318, 328
non-referral, 83–4
nursing
   interventions, 170, 198–9
   one-to-one, 198

obsessive compulsive disorder, 38, 165
occupational decline, 326
   post-morbid, 310
occupational functioning with substance abuse, 366
olanzapine, 191
onset, 27–8
   definition, 28–9
opiate abuse, 366, 367
optimism, 312, 451–2
outcome, 6
   clinical, 237–8
   EPAT referrals, 90
   evaluation, 444
   long-term, 237–8
   social, 237–8
   social isolation, 256
   socio-cultural influences, 249
outcome predictors, xxii, 239–44
   age at onset, 240
   depression, 240
   drug abuse, 241
   DUP, 242, 243–4
   early negative symptoms, 241
   family contacts, 239–40
   gender, 240
   neuroleptic medication, 241–2
   pathways to care, 244
   social contacts, 239–40
   time to presentation, 243
   untreated illness, 242–4
outpost syndromes, 36
outreach, assertive, 256
overlap model, 342

PACE, 87
package approach, 213–15
Parachute Project, 463–5
paranoid symptoms, 56, 191
parathyroid disorders, 171
parietal lobe, glucose metabolism, 122
paternalism, 65
pathways to care, xix, 51–2, 453
   clinician, 65–6
   consumer, 65–6
   experience, 66, 72
   help-seeking behaviour, 59–60
   initial treatment, 53–4
   outcome, 57
      predictors, 244
   personal experiences, 60–1, 62, 63–5
   referral, 70–2
   reluctance to use, 73–4
   risk factors for delay, 55–6
   topography, 58–60, 72–3
   treatment
      commencement, 60

487

pathways to care, (*cont.*)
  experience, 71–2
patients, warehousing, 5
peer support, 416
  substance abuse, 372
  supervision group, 454
performance IQ, 131, 132
Perris, Carlo, 267
Personal Assistance and Crisis Evaluation (PACE), 80
Personal Assistance and Crisis Evaluation (PACE) clinic, xx, 43, 99–108
  attenuated group, 100
  BLIPS group, 101
  BPRS scores, 105–6
  case detection, 101–2
  case management, 103
  clinical service, 103
  community development activities, 109
  disability level, 105–6
  drug education, 103
  ethical issues, 103
  false positives, 108
  help-seeking group, 102
  inclusion criteria, 100–1
  inclusive philosophy, 102
  monitoring for psychosis, 103
  primary care facilities, 101
  psychopathology, 105–6
  QLS, 105, 106
  referrals, 103–5, 108, 109
  SANS, 105, 106
  screening process, 109
  sequential screening, 101
  symptoms, 104–5
  transient psychotic episodes, 100–1
  transition to psychosis, 106–7
personal biography, 72
personal narratives, 72
personal skills development, 426–7
personal therapy, 268
personal vulnerability recognition, 314
personality
  deterioration in prodromal phase, 165
  developmental factors, 271–2
  difficulties in late recovery phase, 322
  inhibited traits, 339
  premorbid, 272
    disordered, 322
  psychosis interaction, 322
  schizotypal disorder, 28
  styles, 272
  traits, 272
pessimism, 450–1
phencyclidine, 364
phosphodiester, 126
phosphomonoester, 126

physical examination, 172, *173*
pimozide, 142
planum temporale, 119, 120
plateau
  effect, 233, 235–6
  morbidity, 246
police
  EPAT involvement, 90
  hospital admissions, 170–1
positron emission tomography (PET)
  first-episode schizophrenia studies, 121–4
  neuroceptor studies, 123–4
  neuroleptic therapy, 190
  radioligands, 123, 124
  regional brain energy metabolism, 121–3
post-modern approach, 269
post-traumatic stress disorder, 158, 254
  causes, 284
  secondary morbidity, 207
power to the people, psychoeducation, 426
precursor features, 10
precursor states, 40–2
prefrontal dysfunction, 174
premorbid adjustment
  scale (PAS), 429, 430, *431*
  schizophrenia, 129–30
premorbid functioning, 162, 232, 319
premorbid personality
  assessment, 174
  disorder, 322
  EPAT case, 94, 95
  first-episode psychosis, 160
premorbid phase, 29–30
  self idealization, 316
premorbid self, distortion, 316
preneuroleptic era, prospective follow-up studies, 227, 230–1
prepsychotic features, 9–10
prepsychotic individuals
  identification, 98–9
  see also high-risk individual identification
prevention
  foci, 391
  possibilities, 4
  psychotic disorder, 3–6
prevention, indicated, 27, 39–45
  false positives, 43–5
  PACE, 80
  prodrome, 39–42
prevention, secondary, 52
  delay, 73
  EPAT, 80
  help seeking, 68

INDEX

preventive intervention, 7–17
  cost-effectiveness, 12, 14, 18
  critical period, 15
  effectiveness, xxv, 19
  evidence-based, 18
  funding models, 18
  implementation, 17–19
  indicated, 7, 9–12
  phase-related, 14
  potential, 466
  relapse prevention, 16–17
  risk:benefit ratio, 11–12
  selective, 7
  spectrum, 8
  strategies, xviii
  subthreshold features, 7–8
  universal, 7
primary care
  facilities, 101
  system, 453
privacy, home-based management, 211
problem-solving skills, 99
  deficit in suicide ideation, 343
prodromal phase/prodrome xviii, 10, 29–31
  accessing patients, 97–108
  disability level, 37
  duration, 38–9, 244
  false positives, 98
  families, 387–8
  indicated prevention, 39–42
  individualized, 320
  interventions, 97–8
  length, 54
  personality deterioration, 165
  prospective application, 40–2
  relapse, 34–5, 251
  retrospective, 40
  transition to psychosis, 162
prodromal symptoms, 250
  affective psychoses, 33–4
  distress, 316
  diversity, 37
  DSM descriptions, 34–7
  false false positive 42
  false positive 42, 43–5
  negative, 38, 39
  outpost, 36
  positive, 38, 39, *41*
  prediction of psychosis, 33
  remission, 57
  retrospective descriptions, 31–2
  schizophrenia, 32–9
  self-medication, 316
prognosis
  first-episode psychosis, 185, 318
  information for families, 396

projects, 459–66
  see also EPPIC
prolactin, 137
prospective follow-up studies *228–9*
  acute symptoms, 232–3
  clinical outcome, 232
  early relapse, 236–7
  long-term outcome, 237–8
  outcome with neuroleptics, 231
  plateau effect, 233, 235–6
  pre-neuroleptic era, 227, 230–1
  residual symptoms, 232–3
  social outcome, 232
  suicide, 238–9
psychodynamic therapy, 267
psychoeducation, 85, 265–6, 268, 272, 317
  EPPIC family services, 395–7, 399
  families, 391–2
  home-based management, 217
  power to the people, 426
  self-management, 426
  substance abuse, 371
psychological interventions, 265–6
psychological techniques, 412
psychopathology, plateau effect, 233, 236
psychosis
  acute phase, 176
  critical period for intervention, xxii
  detection in community, 44
  distressing nature of experiences, 341
  duration of untreated, 58, 326
  duty to inform about risk, 103
  experience, 60–1, *62*, 63–5
  family interaction with illness course, 392
  forms, 175–6
  full-blown, xviii
  organic, 175
  phase-oriented classification, *178*
  revealed, 366
  risk factors, 43, 44
  spectrum disorders, 8
  symptom specificity, 81
  toxic, 366
  see also first-episode psychosis
psychosocial damage, extent, 442
psychosocial decline, 28
psychosocial development, 286
psychosocial functioning
  EPAT case, 94
  substance abuse, 368
psychosocial intervention xxi, 15, 195, 198–200
  formal, 232
  naturalistic, 232
  substance abuse, 371

489

INDEX

psychosocial issues, home-based management, 217–18
psychosocial recovery, capacity for, 12
psychostimulants, 200
psychotherapeutically-oriented treatment 309
psychotherapy, 5
　supportive, 199, 200
psychotic disorders
　early intervention, xvii
　fully-fledged, 11
　onset, xviii, 27–8
　prevention, xvii
　prodrome, 29–31
　recovery potential, 82
psychotic episode
　age at first, 81
　service access, 80–1
　transient, 100–1
psychotic states, transient, 319
psychotic symptoms
　attenuated, 37
　chronicity, 56, 57, 58
　positive, 28
　psychological techniques, 412

quality assurance, 456
quality of care evaluation, 444
quality of life
　case management, 310
　ratings for home-based management, 219–20
Quality of Life Scale (QLS), 105, 106, 458
　EPPIC day programme, 429

recognition, xix
　psychiatric disorders, 82–3
recovery
　chances for young people, 52
　environment, 414–15
　goal setting, 416
　group-based interventions, 416
　mental illness, 413–17
　patient role, 414
　personal strengths/attributes, 415
　phases, 415–16
　　first-episode psychosis, 198
　　home-based management, 212
　plus, 15
　potential, 82
　prolonged, 323, *324*, 325–7
　promotion, 312, 413
　relationships, 415
　social networks, 416
　theoretical models, 414
　time-tabling, 213

referral, xix, xx, 83–4
　EPAT, 88, 92, 93
　pathways, 70–2
　rapid, 53
rehabilitation, 226
relapse, xxii
　access to services, 251
　alert state, 251
　anxiety, 313
　awareness of risk, 312–13
　cannabis, 250
　cognitive interventions, 255
　duration, 250–2
　early signs, 251, 392
　expressed emotion (EE), 379–81, 382
　family impact, 246, 390
　family intervention, 251, 253
　frequent, 16–17
　identification of patient, 378
　intervention strategies, 251
　pattern recognition, 320–1
　potential, 317–18
　predictors, 240, 242
　prevention, 16–17, 99, 249–51, *252*, 253, 313
　prodrome, 251
　rate, 208, 318
　risk factors, 320
　severity, 250–1
　signature image, 251
　signs, 320
relationships, recovery, 415
relaxation techniques, 317
remission
　delayed, 14–15
　first-episode psychosis, 325–6
　prodromal symptoms, 57
resources
　early intervention, 451
　time limitation, 450
risperidone, 191, 192, 327
rhythm of life group, 423
risk assessment
　absconding from hospital, 169
　first-episode psychosis, 165–9
　non-adherence to treatment, 168
　suicide, 166
　victimization, 168
risk factors, xix
　potential, 98
　psychosis, 43, 44
routine, establishment, 415
Royal Park Multidiagnostic Instrument for Psychosis (RPMIP), 459

sarcoidosis, cerebral, 171
Schedule for the Assessment of Negative

490

INDEX

Symptoms (SANS), 105, 106, 429, 430, 431, 432, 458
schema, core, 276
Schilder's disease, psychosis risk, 171
schizophrenia
  alcohol abuse, 363
  amphetamines, 363
  brain
    development, 119
    morphology, 118, 119
    size, 118
  cannabis abuse, 363
  caseness criteria, 8
  caudate nucleus, 120–1
  cerebral asymmetry development, 120
  cerebral blood flow, 121
  cerebral ventricles, 116–18
  chronic course, 28
  cocaine, 363
  cognitive impairment, 130–1
  comorbid substance abuse, 365
  conceptual errors, 4
  critical period, 311
  D2 dopamine receptors, 123–4, 126
  delay, 53–5
  drug abuse, 363
  early diagnosis, 365
  early intervention, xvii
  early relapse, 236–7
  education, 416
  extrapyramidal signs, 137–9
  family history, 93–4
  glucose metabolism, 121–2
  health care costs, 57
  home-based treatment, xxi
  hypofrontality, 122, 125
  incipient, 27
  language disorder, 119, 132
  left temporal–hippocampal system 133
  mesiotemporal lobe, 120
  neurochemistry, 133–7
  neurodevelopmental model, 12
  neuroendocrinology, 133–7
  onset, 27–8
    assessment, 37–8
    insidious, 56
    phase, 8
  optimism, 5
  outcomes, 57, 233, 234
  performance IQ, 131, 132
  pre-psychotic features, 9–10
  prodrome, 29–31
    duration, 38–9
    symptoms, 32–9
  psychosocial decline, 57
  rapid access to treatment, 53
  septum pellucidum defects, 119
  spectrum disorders, 175
  substance abuse, 363
    symptoms independent of, 366
  suicide, 340
  temporolimbic dysfunction, 123
  threshold for treatment initiation, 8
  treatment seeking, 53–4
  ventricular size, 118, 119
  ventricular–brain ratio, 117
  vulnerability hypothesis, 364
  see also first-episode schizophrenia
schizophreniform psychosis, 176
schizotypal personality disorder, 28
scoping, 445–6
sealing over, 31, 275
  strategy, 249
sedative abuse, 367
selective serotonin reuptake inhibitors (SSRIs), 193, 353
self
  appealing to, 282
  cognitive appraisal, 255
  concept, 254
  constructivism, 269
  core concepts, 270
  discovery, 279
  enhanced sense, 414
  expected, 274
  focus in psychosis, 266–8
  future, 274
  ideal, 274
  implications of intervention, 272
  individual concept, 247
  objective stance, 275
  past, 274
  premorbid, 316
  present, 274
  psychosis impact, 271
  reintegration, 317, 415
  shoring up, 276–9
  social, 270
self-care skills, 384
self-construct, negative, 198
self-destructive behaviour, 341
self-efficacy, 270
  concept, 276
  psychosis impact, 271
  recovery, 268
self-esteem, 198
  building, 294
  fragility, 256
  physical fitness, 425
self-evaluation, 255
self-evaluative beliefs, 255
self-instructional training, 267
self-management, illness, 329
self-medication, 69

491

INDEX

self-medication, (cont.)
  cannabis, 316
  substance abuse, 366–7
  hypothesis, 364
self-regard, lowering, 247
self-regulation, 270
self-stigmatization, 198, 282
  social phobia, 284
septum pellucidum defects, 119
serotonergic depletion, 341
serotonin, 191
serotonin–dopamine antagonist drugs, 191
sertindole, 191
service, 459–66
  access, 80–5
  assessment, 309
  monitoring, 309
  period for case management, 320
  plan development, 308
  utilization, 368
  see also EPPIC
service delivery, 308–9
  models, 155
    family intervention, 390–2
    suicide, 347–8
sex chromosome abnormalities, 171
sexual abuse, 322
Simpson Angus extrapyramidal sign scale (SAEPS), 138
single photon emission computed tomography (SPECT), 124–6
site visits, 454–5
skills
  development, 377
  training, 218
sleep
  deprivation, 188
  EEG findings, 127–8
  rapid eye movement (REM), 127–8
  slow-wave, 128
social activity, 281–2
  EPPIC day programme, 420, 421
social assessment, 174–5
social contacts, 239–40
social deterioration, 326
  critical period, 245–6
social functioning
  desynchrony with clinical functioning, 248
  schizophrenia, 130
  substance abuse, 366
social isolation, 256
  EPPIC day programme, 420–1
social network, 352–3
  erosion, 377
  recovery, 416

social phobia, 38, 164
  secondary morbidity, 283
  self-stigmatization, 284
  subsequent to psychosis, 283–4
social position, individual concept, 247
social recovery, 232
  early, 255–6
social rehabilitation, 309
social relationships, 415
social self, 270
social services, 348
social skills training, 99, 266, 427
  day programmes, 412
social support, 185
sociocultural environment, 160–1
sociocultural influences, outcome, 249
solipsism, 269
somatic complaints, 82
speakers, expert, 454–5
specialling, 198
speed of psychotic relapse, 368
spontaneous dyskinesia, 139–40
staff, expressed emotion, 187
stereotypes, detoxifying, 279
stigma, 276
  mental illness, 244
Strauss, John, 267–8
stress
  families, 388, 389, 390
  management, 99, 207, 416
    EPPIC day programme, 424
  minimization, 325
stress–vulnerability framework, 378
stress–vulnerability model, 177, 317, 318
stress–diathesis model, 279
stressors
  external, 255
  psychosocial, 188
Study of Cognitive Re-alignment Therapy for Early Schizophrenia (SOCRATES), 290
subarachnoid haemorrhage, psychosis, 171
substance abuse, 81, 82, 188, 363–4
  benzodiazepines for anxiety alleviation, 370–1
  case management, 311
  comorbidity with affective disorder, 339
  complicating disorders, 200
  detoxification, 370
  disorders, xxiii
  distinction from schizophrenia symptoms, 365
  drug availability, 368
  families, 397
  financial problems, 366, 368
  first-episode psychosis, 165, 176, 322–3

492

homelessness, 366, 368
late recovery phase, 322
occupational functioning, 366
onset, 364–6
outcome, 323
peer-based support, 372
psychoeducation, 371
psychosocial functioning, 368
psychosocial intervention, 371
risk assessment, 166
schizophrenia, 363
   consequence alleviation, 367
   course, 366–70
   response to treatment, 370
   treatment with, 370
self-medication, 366–7
   hypothesis, 364
service utilization, 368
social functioning, 366
structured treatment programmes, 371
subjective relief, 368
symptoms independent of schizophrenia, 366
vulnerability hypothesis, 364
see also drug abuse; drug-induced psychosis
suicidal thinking, cognitive therapy, 248
suicidality
   dynamic state, 341, 342
   model, 341–7
   predictive indicators, 349
   and suicide behaviour model, 341–4
      clinical application, 345–7
   transient, 350
suicide xxii, xxiii
   access to methods, 349
   affective disorder, 339
   alcohol abuse, 340–1
   antisocial behaviour, 339
   assessment schedules, 349–50
   attempt outcome, 342
   behaviours, 341–7
   bipolar disorder, 339
   clinical management, *354–5*
   cognitive styles, 343
   contagion prevention, 348
   critical period of risk, 239
   drug abuse, 340–1
   dysthymia, 339
   ECT, 352, 354
   education, 348
   EPPIC service model, 348
   gender, 340
   government social services, 348
   hopelessness, 352
   incidence, 338
   lethal method removal, 349
   media control, 348
   pharmacological treatment, 353
   physical treatments, 353, 355
   prediction, 240, 344
   prevention, 349
      interventions, 351
      primary, 347
   previous attempts, 339, 340
   prospective follow-up studies, 238–9
   protective factors, 344–5
   psychological interventions, 350–1
   rate, 347
   risk, 192, 320
      assessment, 166, 349–50
      detection, 349–50
      factors, 239, 342–4, 346
      prevention/management, 347–53, *354*, 355
   schizophrenia, 340
   serious mental illness, 338–55
   service models, 347–8
   training programmes, 348
suicide ideation
   early recovery phase, 345
   hopelessness, 343
   intensity, 341
   monitoring, 350
   post-discharge from hospital, 345–6
   problem-solving deficits, 343
   state/trait dependent features, 343–4
   transition from prodrome to psychosis, 345
   vulnerability, 342
support
   network, 376–7
   peer-run group, 416
supporting relationships, 325
symptoms
   acute, 232–3, *234*
   alleviation, 364
   checklist, 162
   clinical history, 162
   disclosure, 69
   groups, 235–6
   influence over, 293
   monitoring, 99
   physical, 82
   positive, 288–95
   prodromal, 250
   reduction with day programmes, 411
   refractory, 192
   residual, 232–3, *234*
syndrome
   full-blown, 42
   prodrome in retrospect, 40

syphilis, cerebral, 171
Systematic Treatment for Persistent Positive Symptoms (STOPP), 289, 291–5, 296
systemic lupus erythematosus, 140, 171
targeting age groups, 449
teams, multidisciplinary, 210–11
temazepam, 215
temporohippocampal dysfunction, 174
temporolimbic dysfunction, 123
termination of treatment, planning, 320
therapeutic alliance, 268
  breakdown, 167
  COPE, 274–6
  development, 159
  home-based management, 211
therapeutic input, downstream effects, 269
therapeutic process, engaging in, 276
therapeutic window for neuroleptics, 190
therapist
  characteristics, 274
  model, 309
therapist–case managers, 311
thinking, distortions, 281
thioridazine, 191
  STOPP combination, 294
thiothixene, glucose metabolism, 121–2
thyroid disorders, 171
thyrotropin releasing hormone (TRH) stimulation test, 133
time
  structure in use, 415
  to presentation as outcome predictor, 243
training
  programmes, 348
  staff, 453–4
transition period, 106–7, 471–2
  case management, 320
trauma
  first-episode psychosis, 158, 199, 254
  hospitalization, 170
  model of individual response to psychosis, 247
treatment
  commencement, 60
  critical period, 55
  delay, 3–4, 12
  engagement, 84–5
  experience, 71–2
  flexible, 409
  harmful effects, 189
  illness phase, 187
  initiation
    critical period, xix
    delays, 6
    threshold, 8
  integrated interventions, 188–9
  involuntary, 275
  location, 187–8
    determination, 161
  methods
    acute phase, 314
    coping strategies, 317
    early recovery, 316–18
    negotiation approach, 314–15
  non-adherence risk, 168
  plan
    family involvement, 396
    formulation, 310
  principles, 186–9
  programmes, 371, 372
  public perception, 68
  rapid access, 53
  refusal to accept, 315
  resistance, xxiii, 14–15, 200, 323, 325, 471
    identification, 378
    illness recognition, 66, 67–8
    managing, 256–7
  seeking, 73
  see also delay; drug treatment
tricyclic antidepressants, 193, 353

ventricular size, 118, 119
ventricular–brain ratio, 117
verbal memory function deficit, 174
victimization risk, 168
violence, inpatients, 167–8, 187–8
vital signs monitoring in home-based management, 217
vitamin B$_{12}$ deficiency, 171
vocational attainment, 57
vocational path, EPPIC day programme, 422–3
vocational relationships, 255–6
voices, 61, 63, 69
vulnerability
  factors, 184
  hypothesis, xxiii, 364
  late recovery phase, 320
  personal, 320
  prediction, 318–19
  psychotic disorder, 11
  risk assessment, 168

warning signs, information for families, 388
Wechsler Adult Intelligence Scale–revised (WAIS–R), 132

wellness maintenance, 416
WHO Disability Assessment Schedule, 232, 237
Wilson's disease, 171
Wisconsin Card Sorting Test (WCST), 125, 132
withdrawal, psychotic symptoms, 364
work experience opportunities, 433

Printed in the United Kingdom
by Lightning Source UK Ltd.
101732UKS00001B/81